2nd Edition

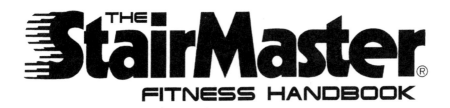

THE StairMaster® FITNESS HANDBOOK

A User's Guide

To Exercise Testing

And Prescription

• • •

Foreword by:
Bruno Balke, M.D., Ph.D.

James A. Peterson, Ph.D., FACSM
Cedric X. Bryant, Ph.D., FACSM

Book design: Laura Griswold
Cover design: Craig Johnson
Typing: Roseanne Kiesz

Library of Congress Catalog Card Number: 95-070429
ISBN: 1-5716-024-6

StairMaster , StairMaster, Crossrobics, 4000 PT, 4000 CT, Stepmill, Gravitron, and 6000 are registered trademarks and 1650 LE, CardioSquat, 2650 UE, Kayak, 7000 PT, 2000 AT, Spinnaker, 3000 CE, 3600 RC, and 5000 are trademarks of StairMaster Sports/Medical Products, Inc. All non-StairMaster product brands used in the text are trademarks of their respective manufacturers.

Published by   Sagamore Publishing, Inc.
               P.O. Box 673
               Champaign, IL 61824-0673
               (217) 359-5940
               Fax: (217) 359-5975

FOREWORD

Life is action—movement affects and forms total life! Insufficient physical challenges in our civilization have been shown to result in functional degeneration, as evidenced by the enormous number of heart and vascular diseases in countries with the highest standards of living.

Shortly after the end of the last great war, it was not unusual for any pursuit of voluntary physical exercise to be ridiculed. As a consequence, "physical fitness" in American children and adults was at an undesirably low level, as shown by several pertinent studies.

With the founding of the American College of Sports Medicine in 1954, a significant change in the lethargic behavior and attitudes of the general population was initiated. Medical doctors and exercise physiologists undertook numerous scientific investigations into the effects of inactivity, as well as of physical training on a regular basis, on health and fitness. The leadership provided by the spoken words, the writings and the personal examples of these individuals served as a major stimulus for the growing number of exercise enthusiasts in this country.

Since "fads" come and go, many individuals were concerned that this new level of active participation in sports and recreational activities might be a termporary phenomenon. Such an undesirable consequence, however, seems most unlikely to occur since too many men and women have experienced the many benefits that accrue in their own lives as a consequence of individual adherence to any of the many positive forms of physical activity.

Forty years ago, the author of this foreword was engaged in teaching a theoretical, as well as practical, course concerned with the physiological reactions and functional adaptations to regularly performed "aerobic" exercise. The "students" were medical officers at the United States Air Force School of Aerospace Medicine in San Antonio, Texas. One of the officers who participated in the training program experienced personal changes in his own body attendant to a more healthy lifestyle. Subsequently, he declared his intention to stir up the mood of the American population to become more active. And indeed, he did just that by coining the term "AEROBICS," as a replacement for the somewhat dreadful words "physical education" and "calisthenics." This new term caught on quickly. As a result, many aerobic types of physical activity became not only more popular, but even "fashionable."

iii
• • •

Since that time, millions of people have joined the fitness "band wagon." The enthusiasm and efforts of these individuals have contributed to the awareness concerning the innumerable benefits that await those who engage in a sound exercise program. For those of you who are already exercise "converts," *The StairMaster® Fitness Handbook* was written to help preserve your discipline and desire to maintain a level of optimal performance capacity into "old age." For those of you who have been advised to change to a healthier lifestyle or have decided on your own for whatever reasons to become more physically active, this book was designed to provide the basic understanding regarding the "why" and "how" you can exercise reasonably and regularly.

The reader should keep in mind that not all of the chapters are written for everyone. Some of the chapters may only have a unique appeal to health professionals who want to reinforce their knowledge or understanding of the scientific basis of matters about which they are going to "preach." Other chapters, or parts of them, may be more important initially to those individuals who are just on the verge of embarking on a new adventure of initiating a sound exercise program.

In a book with contributions by several authors with similar interests, many repetitions were unavoidable. Such repetitions, however, can only serve to reinforce certain important issues.

StairMaster Sports/Medical Products, Inc. should be commended for making *The StairMaster Fitness Handbook* available, not only to its customers, but also to anyone who is interested in the health benefits of a sound exercise program— regardless of the type of equipment used.

Bruno Balke, M.D., Ph.D.

• •

"We doctors can now state from our experience with people, both sick and well, and from a growing series of scientific researches that 'keeping fit' does pay richly in dividends of health and longevity."

Paul Dudley White, M.D.

CONTRIBUTORS

Rosemary Agostini, M.D.
Sports Medicine & Family Practice
Virginia Mason Sports Medicine Center
Clinical Assistant Professor of Orthopedics
University of Washington School of Medicine
Seattle, Washington

Donald B. Bergey, M.A.
Exercise Coordinator
Cardiac Rehabilitation Program
Dept. of Medicine, Health
and Sport Science
Wake Forest University
Winston-Salem, North Carolina

Walter M. Bortz, II, M.D.
Clinical Associate Professor of Medicine
Stanford University School of Medicine
Palo Alto, California

Cedric X. Bryant, Ph.D.
Associate Director of Sports Medicine
StairMaster Sports/Medical Products, Inc.
Kirkland, Washington

Dennis L. Colacino, Ph.D.
Professor
New York Medical College
Valhalla, New York

William J. Considine, P.E.D.
Undergraduate Chairman
Physical Education, Health & Health/Fitness
Springfield College
Springfield, Massachusetts

Debra J. Crews, Ph.D.
Assistant Professor
Dept. of Exercise and Sport Science
University of North Carolina at Greensboro
Greensboro, North Carolina

Karol J. Fink, M.S.
Nutritional Sciences Program
University of Washington
Seattle, Washington

B. Don Franks, Ph.D.
Professor and Chair
Dept. of Kinesiology
Louisiana State University
Baton Rouge, Louisiana

Barry A. Franklin, Ph.D.
Director
Cardiac Rehabilitation & Exercise Lab
Division of Cardiology
William Beaumont Hospital
Royal Oak, Michigan

Larry W. Gibbons, M.D.
Medical Director
The Cooper Clinic
Dallas, Texas

James E. Graves, Ph.D.
Associate Professor and Chair
Dept. of Health & Physical Education
Syracuse University
Syracuse, New York

Gary Gray, P.T.
Director
Gary Gray Physical Therapy
Adrian, Michigan

Sue Haapaniemi, M.S.
Division of Cardiology
Cardiac Rehabilitation & Exercise Lab
William Beaumont Hospital
Royal Oak, Michigan

Ronald J. Hagen, M.S.
Director
Human Performance Lab
StairMaster Sports/Medical Products, Inc.
Kirkland, Washington

Elizabeth Hart M.A.
Dept. of Exercise & Sport Science
University of North Carolina
at Greensboro
Greensboro, North Carolina

George Havenith, Drs.
Senior Scientist
TNO Institute for Perception
Soesterburg, The Netherlands

Kirk Hendrickson, B.S.
Division of Cardiology
Cardiac Rehabilitation & Exercise Lab
William Beaumont Hospital
Royal Oak, Michigan

David L. Herbert, Esq.
Senior Partner
Herbert, Benson & Scott,
Attorneys at Law
Canton, Ohio

William G. Herbert, Ph.D.
Professor and Director
Laboratory for Exercise, Sport & Work
Physiology
Virginia Polytechnic Institute
Blacksburg, Virginia

George J. Holland, Ph.D.
Professor and Co-Director
Exercise Physiology Laboratory
California State University at Northridge
Northridge, California

Reed H. Humphrey, Ph.D., P.T.
Assistant Professor of Physical Therapy
Medical College of Virginia
Virginia Commonwealth University
Richmond, Virginia

W. Larry Kenney, Ph.D.
Associate Professor of Applied Physiology
Noll Human Performance Laboratory
Pennsylvania State University
University Park, Pennsylvania

Steven F. Loy, Ph.D.
Associate Professor and Co-director
Exercise Physiology Laboratory
California State University
Northridge, California

Julie E. Mullen, M.S.
Manager
Grand Ohio Athletic Club
Chicago, Illinois

Ralph A. Paffenbarger, M.D., DPH
Professor of Epidemiology, Emeritus (Active)
Stanford University School of Medicine
Palo Alto, California

James A. Peterson, Ph.D.
Director of Sports Medicine
StairMaster Sports/Medical Products, Inc.
Kirkland, Washington

Michael L. Pollock, Ph.D.
Director
Center for Exercise Science
University of Florida
Gainesville, Florida

Lee Rawls, M.S.
Director
Product Development
StairMaster Sports/Medical Products, Inc.
Kirkland, Washington

Paul M. Ribisl, Ph.D.
Director
Cardiac Rehabilitation Program
Dept. of Medicine, Health, & Sport Science
Wake Forest University
Winston-Salem, North Carolina

Steven J. Riddle, M.S.
Director of Fitness Services
University Hospitals of Cleveland
Cleveland, Ohio

Thomas P. Sattler, Ed.D.
Professor of Kinesiology
University of Illinois at Chicago
Chicago, Illinois

James S. Skinner, Ph.D.
Professor
Dept. of Exercise Science and
Physical Education
Arizona State University
Tempe, Arizona

Karl G. Stoedefalke, Ph.D.
Professor
Dept. of Exercise & Sport Science
Pennsylvania State University
University Park, Pennsylvania

Robyn M. Stuhr, M.A.
Exercise Physiologist
Health Education Center
Virginia Mason Medical Center
Seattle, Washington

Linda Terrien, R.N., B.S.N.
Division of Cardiology
Cardiac Rehabilitation & Exercise
Laboratories
William Beaumont Hospital
Royal Oak, Michigan

Gerald D. Thompson, M.S.
Dept. of Kinesiology
Louisiana State University
Baton Rouge, Louisiana

Paul M. Vanderburgh, Ed.D.
Assistant Professor of Health Fitness
Springfield College Health Fitness
Springfield College
Springfield, Massachusetts

Susan Wentz, M.D.
Assistant Professor
Dept. of Family Medicine
School of Medicine
Case Western Reserve University
Cleveland, Ohio

Bonnie Worthington-Roberts, Ph.D.
Professor and Director
Nutritional Sciences Program
University of Washington
Seattle, Washington

CONTENTS

If you should have any questions pertaining to the information presented in this book, please contact:

StairMaster® Sports/Medical Products, Inc.
Attn.: Department of Sports Medicine
12421 Willows Road NE, Suite 100
Kirkland, WA 98034

PROLOGUE:

ABOUT THIS BOOK

*T*he *StairMaster® Fitness Handbook* is an extension of the corporate philosophy of StairMaster® Sports/Medical Products, Inc. to lend support to projects that are designed to enable individuals to become more knowledgeable about what constitutes "sensible exercise." Previous endeavors that reflect this corporate commitment to disseminate information relating to the benefits and parameters of sensible exercise include the sponsorship of several educational symposia, colloquia, clinics (e.g., the StairMaster International Conference on Aging, the Fifty Plus-StairMaster Project, the national series of Gary Gray Chain Reaction Physical Therapy Seminars; several cooperative projects with the American College of Sports Medicine; an AACVPR symposium on the application of contemporary exercise equipment in cardiac rehabilitation, the national series of "Shaping the Future of Exercise" seminars; etc.), and the development of one of the most extensive programs of independently conducted, applied research in the therapeutic and fitness equipment industry.

Collectively, the *StairMaster Fitness Handbook* features the writings of 40 individuals whose contributions enabled this book to become a reality. The contributors' thorough mastery of their subject matter served as the basis for providing a comprehensive overview of several critical issues relating to exercise, including *why* you should exercise, *what* physiological responses occur as the result of exercising, and *what* type of exercise prescriptions produce optimal results. Every attempt was made to make the information included in this book as user-friendly as possible.

As you read the *StairMaster Fitness Handbook*, you should keep in mind that becoming knowledgeable about exercise is only one of many essential ingredients in your personal recipe for sensible exercise. If you want to make your "exercise experience" as productive and enjoyable as possible, you need to take several steps. Undoubtedly, the most critical step is that you make an unwavering commitment to exercise on a regular basis. For most individuals, that commitment will be based—at least in part—on an understanding of the fact that regular exercise participation makes sense for almost everyone and that exercise truly has medicinal properties. Hopefully, *The StairMaster Fitness Handbook* will serve to facilitate that understanding and, as a result, strengthen your resolve to exercise in a safe and appropriate manner.

CHAPTER 1

• •

PHYSICAL ACTIVITY, PHYSICAL FITNESS, AND HEALTH: AN OVERVIEW *

by

Ralph S. Paffenbarger, Jr., M.D., DPH

• • •

*A*ddressing the basic parameters of physical activity—how much, how often, and what type—in order to identify how to best reduce the risk of disease, increase longevity, and improve the quality of an individual's life is a substantive undertaking? Precise answers to these questions may provide the best motivation to become and remain active, especially as a person tries to fit exercise into an otherwise busy schedule of conflicting commitments. Likewise, knowing at what point further effort becomes fruitless, or perhaps even harmful, will help prevent discouragement, injury, "burnout," or perhaps worse catastrophes.

Though a great deal is known about the relation between activity and health, the message unfortunately still hasn't gotten through to the masses. Only 22% of adults in the United States are active at the level recommended for health benefits in Objective 1.3 of Health People 2000 (US Dept. of Health & Human Service). Twenty-four percent are completely sedentary, while the remaining 54% are inadequately active. Unfortunately, such sedentary lifestyles could have dire consequences in the years to come. Statistics confirm that the United States is a greying nation. It seems inevitable that as Americans grow older, their sedentary habits will begin to catch up with them, creating a huge population of frail, older men and women, at enormous cost to themselves in suffering and to society in lost productivity and resources.

---

* Note: The material contained in this chapter is adapted from *LifeFit, a complete guide to exercise, health, and longevity for men and women over 40*, by R.S. Paffenbarger and E. Olsen, Human Kinetics Publishers, Champaign, Illinois (in press).

It may be that the ongoing failure of Americans to become and remain more physically active, despite all that is known about the benefits of an active lifestyle, results, at least in part, from the somewhat confusing messages they've been getting over the years—messages that have ranged from the "marathon-or-else" school of thought of 15 years ago to the more recent "less is more" approach. Thus, a book like *The StairMaster Fitness Handbook*, which brings together much of the best information about activity and health available today, is a valuable resource for those individuals who want to become active and stay active.

THE BEGINNING

The idea that physical activity and fitness lead to good health, general well-being, and longevity is hardly new. For over 4000 years in Asia, from the time of Huang Ti (the so-called mythical Yellow Emperor) to the present day, there has been a virtually unbroken tradition that assigns to appropriate physical exercise an essential role in the maintenance of physical, mental, and even spiritual well-being. Not surprisingly, the parks in China today are filled with men and women practicing Tai Chi Ch'uan and other disciplines that probably are not that much different from those exercises advocated for health and longevity by Huang Ti around 2500 B.C.

Here in the West, however, such tradition has been less coherent. The European Ancients all recognized that a vigorous, physically active life was a life well lived. Of course, in both the East and the West, the Ancients' notion that physical activity and physical vigor were central to the good life was as much a matter of common sense and survival in rough-and-tumble times, as it was a result of sound scientific observation or philosophical inclination.

Thus, it was left to the Greek physician, Galen, (129-200 A.D.), enjoying the relative peace and quiet of the Roman Empire, to suggest that sometimes exercise could be over done. The Greco-Roman ideal of a sound mind in a sound body was weakened further with the collapse of the Roman Empire, followed by the Dark Ages, the rise of the Church, and finally the Enlightenment, all of which tended in various ways to drive a wedge between mind and body, or body and soul. A rather unsympathetic view of vigorous exercise persisted through the centuries that followed, so that by the late 19th century, when the European medical community began to look seriously once again at the question of exercise and health, it was not to establish the value of exercise, but rather to test the prevailing *fear* that vigorous exercise might kill some of the best and brightest of the British elite—the young rowers at Oxford and Cambridge.

During these early periods in history, some individuals were examining the health benefits of physical activity. In 1713, for example, Bernardini Ramazinni described the poor health of sedentary tailors in Italy, as contrasted with the general well-being of fleet-footed messengers. Dr. Edward Smith, in 1863, found London tailors to be no more healthy than Ramazinni had described their Italian counterparts 150 years earlier. Smith's tables of age-specific mortality rates showed tailors had 50-75% greater mortality in mid-life than physically active farmers. Some three-quarters of a century later, considerable attention was being directed at coronary heart disease (CHD). In 1939, O.H. Hedley published an analysis of 5000 cardiovascular deaths in Philadelphia during the period of 1933-1937 in which he found death rates higher among professional and managerial men than among laborers.

PHYSICAL ACTIVITY, CHD, AND ALL-CAUSE MORTALITY

It was not until the 1940s when Jeremy N. Morris and his colleagues in England initiated efforts to look at the association between occupational physical activity and CHD that the medical community first began to understand that both vocational and leisure-time physical activity relate to good health and increased longevity. In their astute observations, Morris et al. found that highly active conductors on London's double-decked buses were at lower risk of heart disease than bus drivers, who sat all day at the steering wheel. What disease conductors did develop was less severe, and they were more likely to survive the acute effects. Morris and his colleagues also found that postmen delivering mail on foot had lower rates of CHD than sedentary clerks and telephonists. Furthermore, the findings of Morris et al. also suggested that a gradient existed for positions of intermediate physical activity.

Epidemiologists have continued to collect and analyze quantitative evidence that habitual physical activity, high levels of physical fitness, not smoking, low-fat diets, and certain other lifestyle habits and personal characteristics lessen the risks of CHD and other chronic diseases. These studies, involving college alumni, British civil servants, Seventh Day Adventist men, Alameda County (California) residents, U.S. railroad workers, individuals of Finnish descent, men of the British Regional Heart Study, and others, have all lent support to the observation that life is extended by physical activity, largely by protecting individuals against cardiovascular disease.

Observations of the nearly 15,000 individuals aged 45-84 who participated in the Harvard Alumni Health Study, for example, revealed lower risks of death with higher levels of each activity pattern in gradient or step-wise fashion. Energy expenditure by the alumni was measured through questionnaires, on which they reported how much they walked, how many stairs they climbed, and any leisure-time sports they played. From these self-reports, a physical activity index (PAI) was calculated. Compared to the least active alumni (less than 1000 kcals per week), risk of early mortality was one-quarter lower among the intermediate group (1000-2499 kcals), and one-third lower among the most active men (2500 kcals or more). Of particular interest was the fact that a prompt and persistent advantage existed for those individuals who were involved in sustained activities requiring 4.5 METs or more of intensity (i.e., moderately vigorous recreational activities likely to increase the heart rate, deepen breathing, and bring sweat to the brow). Any increase in survival for less vigorous recreational activities (i.e., sports play of a relatively undemanding nature) seemed to occur only at age 75 and beyond.

The concepts of activity and fitness have become more inclusive in the past 40 years, extending beyond the narrow "aerobic" and cardiovascular parameters which formerly "defined" them to now include considerations of muscular fitness and flexibility. At the least, this more expansive view of activity and fitness has critical implications for exercise prescription.

PHYSIOLOGICAL FITNESS AND ALL-CAUSE MORTALITY

In parallel with observations on physical activity and longevity, a number of studies have revealed important relationships of physiological fitness (a condition) to health. The results of these investigations point in the same direction as the physical activity (a behavior) findings which were reviewed in the previous section. Populations in Finland, Belgium, Sweden, Canada, and the United States (perhaps most notably, groups at the Cooper Institute for Aerobic Research in Dallas, Texas) have had their aerobic fitness levels assessed in a laboratory in an effort to determine what correlation these subsequent measurements had to longevity.

In the Cooper Institute study, for example, death rates were found to be lowest (18.6 per 10,000 person-years) among the most fit and highest (64.0) among the least fit men, tracking closely the results from studies of physical activity levels and mortality just cited. Corresponding rates for women were 8.5 and 39.5 per 10,000 person-years. Trends remained after standardizing for differences among fitness quintiles in cigarette smoking habit, blood cholesterol, blood pressure, and blood glucose levels, and parental history of CHD. Since physical activity habits and fitness levels often are linked, these findings may imply that the beneficial effects of physical activity on health and longevity are mediated by physiological fitness status.

These concepts were united rather effectively in the Multiple Risk Factor Intervention Trial (MRFIT) studies where baseline levels of physical fitness which had been determined from exercise treadmill tests were compared to tertiles of leisure-time physical activity. Both treadmill time and the proportion of subjects achieving a target heart rate were significantly higher with increasing levels of leisure-time physical activity, whereas resting and intermediate exercise heart rates were lower. The upper one-third of the subjects, in terms of physical activity status, had a normal or average estimated mean functional capacity, whereas the bottom one-third was below average in fitness. Thus, the relative risks of CHD in the MRFIT men corresponded both to their levels of physical activity and physical fitness.

Since the early 1980s, further studies of disease rates and physiological fitness have shown that it is physical activity, rather than aerobic fitness, that is essential for protecting against cardiovascular disease and other diseases. The Copenhagen Male Study, for example, found that physically active men who were nonetheless measured as having a low level of physical fitness had the same low risk for CHD as their equally active, but more fit colleagues. The key point to remember is that it is the relative level of *physical activity*, more than any other factor, which determined the subjects' risk for premature mortality.

CURRENT ACTIVITY, NOT HISTORICAL

Physical activity should also be contemporary, not historical, to be "beneficial." Among studies involving college alumni, for instance, participation in intercollegiate athletics had no relation to mortality later in life. Only *contemporary* physical activity was related to morbidity and mortality. Morris et al. found that rates of CHD were similarly high among men who had not played vigorous sports previously and those who had stopped playing athletics less than five to more than 40 years previously. More interestingly, men who reported being vigorously active at the time of their entry into the study had the same low incidence, whether or not they had been physically active at a previous time in their lives.

WHAT IS KNOWN

Thus, with the accumulation of such evidence, it can now be concluded with considerable confidence that:

- Physical activity extends longevity, *protects* against the development of CHD, stroke, hypertension (HTN), obesity, non-insulin-dependent diabetes mellitus (NIDDM), osteoporosis, colon cancer, and depression.
- Physical activity improves quality of life.
- Of particular importance as the population ages, physical activity helps maintain full functioning and independence among the elderly.
- Relationships between physical activity and improved health are not merely expressions of hypotheses or selection bias, but are likely cause-and-effect relations through alternations in definable mechanisms.
- Some of these mechanisms include: a reduced oxygen demand at any given level of physical activity, lowered heart rate and blood pressure, a reduced tendency for blood to form clots where arteries have narrowed, an increased elasticity in the arteries, formation of collateral arteries, and so on, all of which reduce the risk of infections and certain types of cancer; an increased insulin sensitivity that reduces the risk of NIDDM and the host of health problems associated with it; and changes in the brain and brain chemistry that may improve cognitive functioning and mood.
- Finally, an exercise prescription can be developed for individuals which offers the amount and type of physical activity necessary to provide optimal health, longevity, and quality of life.

TOWARD AN EXERCISE PRESCRIPTION

Any activity is better than none, of course, and, to a point, more is better than less. The available evidence indicates that the least amount of activity for optimal health is a total of 1500-2000 kcals a week expended using the large muscles of the legs, arms, and trunk, preferably in a sustained, rhythmic fashion. Such an approach to being physically active has been shown to provide most of the possible protection against nonfatal and fatal CHD and other hypertensive-metabolic-atherosclerotic disease. This total weekly physical activity can include both intermittent light activities (i.e., 1-4.4 METs) of daily living such as gardening, chasing after the kids, raking the leaves, and leisurely walking—"puttering around"—for a total of about an hour a day. However, it should also include regular, moderately intense, sustained activity of at least 30 minutes three times a week that elevates the heart rate, causes you to perspire, and increases your rate of breathing (i.e., most typically in the form of recreational activities).

INTENSITY OF EFFORT

Some uncertainty remains as to whether quantity alone or intensity of physical activity is of *primary* importance in protecting against premature mortality. It appears, however, from the Harvard Alumni Study data and data from other studies as well (e.g., Morris et al.), that some sustained, moderately vigorous physical activity is necessary for optimal health and longevity. For the purposes of analysis, the Harvard alumni were separated into those activities which required less than 4.5 METs of effort and those who included some weekly activities requiring 4.5 METs or more. With increasing levels of energy expenditure, up to about 3500 kcal per week, both light and moderately vigorous activities are associated with a reduced risk of all-cause mortality. Higher weekly outputs confer little further benefit, but throughout, the risk is significantly lower with moderately vigorous than with less vigorous activities. This substantial parallel is evident even if those men who had a relatively low energy output (less than 1000 kcal per week) were to be omitted for premonitory inferences.

STRENGTH AND FLEXIBILITY

Limited data exists that shows that resistance training offers the same health benefits provided by aerobic activities. The most likely explanation for the absence of such findings is that this is an area that simply hasn't been studied extensively. Those studies which have been conducted on the topic have clearly shown that resistance training does provide significant health benefits. Somewhat surprisingly, contrary to what seems to be intuition and common sense, it also appears that as individuals age, strength training becomes *increasingly* important.

For decades, the basic "fitness message" has focused on the value of aerobic exercise training. Sound aerobic training is, of course, particularly beneficial in helping individuals get through "middle-age" free of heart disease and all the other afflictions associated with a generally sedentary society. As individuals reach their 60s, 70s, 80s, and beyond, however, they begin to face other risks and challenges, including an increased level of frailty.

The very old probably aren't "destined" genetically to die of such things as heart disease, otherwise they wouldn't have made it to become "very old."

Rather, they too often die of the effects of an inadequate level of muscular fitness, which can lead to increasing difficulty getting through the day without help from others, trouble negotiating stairs or getting out of chairs without help, and most seriously, an increasing risk of falls. About 40% of individuals 65 and over fall at least once a year. For most, these falls are relatively minor, but for many they result in possible life-threatening bone fractures. Even the *fear* of falling can begin to severely restrict an individual's lifestyle, leading to social isolation and lack of activity that create a downward spiral to increasing disability and dependence on others for the tasks of daily living.

Whether or not individuals are "old" is a matter not just of chronology, but of their ability to function effectively and independently. Much of what conventional wisdom calls "aging" is instead the complications of disease and *disuse*, something over which individuals have a high degree of control. In truth, individuals probably do *tend* to lose some strength as a normal consequence of growing older. It must, however, be asked whether what is "typical" in a largely sedentary society is truly "normal." Though some *normal* loss of strength may be likely with aging (even training athletes seem to lose muscle strength after the age of 60 or 65, for reasons that aren't fully understood), most older adults almost certainly lose much more strength than they need to, even when they are completely "healthy" (or at least free of overt disease), because they tend to reduce their activity levels.

Numerous studies have shown that older men and women who strength train improve not only their muscular strength level, but also their ability to live more independent and productive lives. When they incorporate strength training activities into their exercise routines, older adults, even those who have been sedentary for a number of years, can achieve significant gains in strength, reversing the trend toward extreme, even disabling weakness, and slowing the decline in strength typically associated with age.

Like strength training, proper stretching becomes even more important as individuals grow older, to help prevent or delay the musculoskeletal stiffening that contributes to increased frailty and interferes with independent living. Stretching regularly also helps prevent injury, since a flexible muscle or tendon is less prone to pulls or tears than a tight one. Accordingly, while stretching is not a substitute for either aerobic or anaerobic activities, it should be an integral part of a sound exercise program.

A LAW OF DIMINISHING RETURNS

Beyond the aforementioned 2000 kcal level, it appears that additional *physical* health benefits come only with increasing effort, and eventually level off at about 3500 kcals per week. However, while exercising beyond this level may not provide additional benefits in terms of *physical* health, additional effort may well continue to provide significant psychological and philosophical effects, as well as continued opportunities for engagement with others and improvements in quality of life.

The Future

In the future, we will be better able to further refine what constitutes a sound exercise prescription and to more clearly understand what specific types of activity provide the most benefits in terms of avoiding various specific diseases.

We will increase our understanding of the role of strength and flexibility training in health and longevity and the proper use of exercise equipment for effective conditioning, motivation, and injury prevention.

We will come to understand more thoroughly why men and women drop out of exercise programs, and what strategies are most effective in motivating people to engage in and stick with an active lifestyle.

We will take into account the observations of Dr. Claude Bouchard and his colleagues that genetic variation may account for a substantial portion of individual differences in response to regular physical activity, in particular its effect on physiological fitness and health. This genetic inheritance involves four major components of physiological fitness: cardiorespiratory, morphological, muscular, and metabolic. Accordingly, future epidemiological observations will closely study the familial patterns of these attributes.

In the next five to 10 years, we will learn more about the effect of physical activity and physiological fitness on the risk of developing progressive diseases, especially site-specific cancers, chronic obstructive pulmonary disease, arthritis, and certainly the myriad of neurologic-psychiatric conditions. In particular, increasing attention will be given to the specific effects of exercise and fitness on women's health.

We will begin study of the kinds, the amounts, and the intensities of physical activity to be advised for the *old* and the *oldest old* (an almost entirely unexplored area). We will also begin to consider the *social* effects of increased physical activity, total-body fitness, and lengthened life in both sexes. Will this increase or decrease the burden on health care and other support systems? What new services or social structures will be necessary to meet the needs or expectations of a growing population of vigorous older adults?

Finally, we will learn more about the effects of *change* in exercise and fitness patterns, combined with changes in other lifestyle factors, and what role these effects have on the prevention or the delay of recurrent or extended disease. The interaction and integration of exercise and fitness with *diet*, a prominent adjunctive area of concern, will help with the design of appropriate recommendations for prudent living. We will learn more about the extension of longevity to its optimum, and how to promote the enhancement of a high quality of living. In other words, we will learn more about how to better preserve God's greatest gift to each of us—life. ❏

AN OVERVIEW

• • •

BIBLIOGRAPHY •

1. Åstrand, P.O., Rodahl, K. *Textbook of Work Physiology*, 3rd ed. New York, NY: McGraw-Hill, 1986.
2. Blair, S.N., et al. "Physical fitness and all-cause mortality: A prospective study of healthy men and women." *JAMA* 262:2395-2401, 1989.
3. Bouchard, C., Shephard, R.J., Stephens, T., Sutton, J.R., McPherson, B.D. (Eds). *Exercise, Fitness, and Health*. Champaign, IL: Human Kinetics, 1990.
4. Bouchard, C., et al. (Eds.) *Physical Activity, Fitness, and Health*. Champaign, IL: Human Kinetics Publishers, 1994.
5. Cooper, K.H. *Aerobics*. New York, NY: M. Evans and Company, 1968.
6. Ekelund, L.G., et al. "Physical fitness as a predictor of cardiovascular mortality in asymptomatic North American men: The Lipid Research Clinics Mortality Follow-up Study." *N Engl J Med* 319:1379-1384, 1988.
7. Fiatarone, M.A., et al. "High-intensity strength training in nonagenarians." *JAMA* 263:3029-3034, 1990.
8. Foreman, J. "Longer life, the next frontier." *Boston Globe*, Sept. 28, 1992.
9. Frontera, W.R., et al. "Strength conditioning in older man: Skeletal muscle hypertrophy and improved function." *J Appl Physiol* 64:1038-1044, 1988.
10. Haskell, W.L., Leon, S.A., Caspersen, C.J., Froelicher, V.F., Hagberg, J.M., Harlan, W., et al. "Cardiovascular benefits and assessment of physical activity and physical fitness in adults." *Med Sci Sports Exerc* 24(6 Suppl):S201-S220, 1992.
11. Hein, H.O., et al. "Physical fitness or physical activity as a predictor of ischaemic heart disease? A 17-year follow-up in the Copenhagen Male Study." *J Int Med* 232:471-479, 1992.
12. Helmrich, S.P., Ragland, D.R., Leung, R.W., Paffenbarger, R.S. "Chronic disease in former college students: XLII, Physical activity and reduced occurrence of non-insulin-dependent diabetes mellitus." *N Engl J Med* 325:147-152, 1991.
13. Kaplan, G.A., et al. "Mortality among the elderly in the Alameda County Study: Behavioral and demographic risk factors." *Am J Public Health* 77:307-312, 1987.
14. Lakka, T., et al. "Relation of leisure-time physical activity and cardiorespiratory fitness to the risk of acute myocardial infarction in men." *N Engl J Med* 330:1549-1554, 1994.
15. Lee, I.M., Paffenbarger, R.S. "Chronic disease in former college students: XLIX, Physical activity and its relation to cancer risk: A prospective study of college alumni. *Med Sci Sports Exerc* (in press).
16. Mittleman, M.A., Maclure, M., Tofler, G.H., et al. "Triggering of acute MI by heavy physical exertion." *N Engl J Med* 329:1677-1731, 1993.
17. Morgan, W.P. "Physical activity, fitness and depression." In: *Physical Activity, Fitness and Health*. Bouchard, C., Shephard, R.J., Stevens, T. (Eds.). Champaign, IL: Human Kinetics, 1994.
18. Morris, J.N., et al. *Lancet* 2:1053-1057, 1111-1120, 1953.
19. Paffenbarger, R.S., et al. "Physical activity, all-cause mortality, and longevity of college alumni." *N Engl J Med* 314:605-613, 1986.
20. Paffenbarger, R.S., et al. "The association of changes in physical-activity level and other lifestyle characteristics with mortality among men." *N Engl J Med* 328:538-545, 1993.
21. Paffenbarger, R.S., et al. "Changes in physical activity and other lifeway patterns influencing longevity." (Submitted for publication)
22. Pekkanen, J.B., et al. "Reduction of premature mortality by high physical activity: A 20-year follow-up of middle-aged Finnish men." *Lancet* 1:1473-1477, 1987.
23. Saltin, B. "Sedentary lifestyle: A underestimated health risk." *J Int Med* 232:467-469, 1992.
24. Work, J. "Strength training: A bridge to independence for the elderly." *Phys Sportsmed* 17:134-140, 1989.

CHAPTER 2

• •

EXERCISE IS MEDICINE

by

Larry W. Gibbons, M.D.
and
Karl G. Stoedefalke, Ph.D.

• • •

C. Everett Koop, during his tenure as the Surgeon General of the United States, had one of his researchers add up all of the people known to be suffering from the various major diseases reported by the National Center for Health Statistics. Somewhat astonishingly, the researcher found that the total exceeded the entire population of the United States. The major point to be inferred from this fact is that health—specifically the lack of health—is perhaps the most critical issue currently facing the American society.

Attempts to identify the factors which have been major contributors to this virtual epidemic of medical problems have produced a litany of probable reasons why such a large number of individuals are so apparently unhealthy: poor eating habits, a sedentary lifestyle, stress, poor health habits (i.e., smoking), ad infinitum. At the same time, a number of studies have been undertaken to identify what—if anything—can be done to diminish either the number or the severity of medical problems affecting the public. These studies have provided considerable evidence that exercise has substantial medicinal benefits for individuals of all ages.

Two of the most widely publicized efforts to investigate the possible relationship between exercise and disease were longitudinal studies, each of which involved more than 10,000 subjects. Several years ago, in a renowned study of 17,000 Harvard graduates, Ralph Paffenbarger, M.D., found that men who expended approximately 300 calories a day—the equivalent of walking briskly for 45 minutes—reduced their death rates from all causes by an extraordinary 28% and lived an average of more than two years longer than their sedentary former classmates. A more recent study conducted by Steven Blair, P.E.D., of the Institute of Aerobics Research in Dallas documented the fact that a relatively modest amount of exercise has a significant effect on the mortality rate of both men and women. The higher the fitness level, the lower the death rate (after the data was adjusted for age differences between subjects in this eight-year investigation of 13,344 individuals). An analysis of the extensive data yielded by both studies suggests one inescapable conclusion—*EXERCISE IS MEDICINE.*

REDUCING YOUR RISK FOR CAD

The number one cause of death of men and women in the United States is coronary artery disease (CAD). In 1991 alone more than 800,000 deaths could be directly attributed to CAD. Unfortunately, even though CAD has been found to begin relatively early in life (sometimes as early as the teenage years for males), the symptoms of this horrific condition do not occur until the disease is far advanced in an individual. Almost twenty-five percent of the individuals with CAD suffer a fatal heart attack as their initial symptom of this disease. Given the nature of CAD, "prevention" is, without question, the most appropriate approach to this pandemic medical problem.

Of all the major interventive steps that an individual can take to help prevent the onset of CAD—change of lifestyle, cessation of cigarette smoking, weight control, and eating a nutritionally balanced diet,—exercise has generally been found to be the cornerstone of an effort that combines several interventions. Exercise has been shown to have a substantial effect on the most critical (and modifiable) risk factors for CAD.

Exercise helps to prevent CAD by affecting an individual's blood lipid level in a positive way. For example, regular exercise has been found to raise high density lipoprotein (HDL—the "good" type) cholesterol levels. HDL cholesterol is more important than low density lipoprotein (LDL—the "bad" type) cholesterol, apparently because of its ability to help protect against CAD by its efforts to collect cholesterol in the body's blood system and help dispose of it safely in the liver. By transferring cholesterol to the liver, HDL helps prevent the accumulation of lipids on walls of the arteries (a process commonly referred to as atherosclerosis). By facilitating the formation of HDL and helping to slow the eventual breakdown of HDL, exercise enables individuals to have higher levels of this cardioprotective lipoprotein.

Exercise also helps to prevent CAD by enabling individuals to keep their blood pressure level under control. High blood pressure (a condition commonly referred to as hypertension) is a state in which the blood pressure is chronically elevated above optimal levels. Regular exercise has been found to lower both systolic and diastolic blood pressure. The average lowering of blood pressure with exercise has been shown to be approximately 10 mm Hg and 8 mm Hg for systolic and diastolic blood pressure, respectively. Recent studies show that a 7 mm Hg reduction in diastolic blood pressure, for example, will reduce the incidence of CAD by approximately 29% and the incidence of stroke by 46%. Not surprisingly, individuals who already suffer from high blood pressure can significantly lower their mortality risk by exercising on a regular basis.

Exercise has also been shown to help prevent CAD by aiding some people (not all) in their attempts to quit smoking. Some evidence exists to suggest that an individual's craving for cigarettes is reduced with exercise participation. Other studies have found that many individuals who had previously smoked voluntarily gave up this habit once they became involved in a program of regular physical activity. Unfortunately, the addictive qualities of nicotine (nicotine is a drug which is six to eight times more addictive than alcohol) override, in many instances, a smoker's capacity to adequately consider the beneficial consequences of exercise. At the present time, statistics indicate that more than 50 million Americans still smoke.

Exercise has also been found to play a major role in lowering body fat. Obesity is a significant risk factor for CAD. Individuals who are "over-fat" have a substantially higher risk of heart disease—particularly when the body fat is accumulated around their waists. Regular exercise helps to improve body composition in primarily two ways. One way is by increasing caloric expenditure, and thereby creating a caloric deficit. If a previously sedentary individual walks two miles a day at a speed of 4 mph, five days a week, that person can expect to lose about 9.5 to 11.0 pounds over a one-year period of time—provided caloric intake remains stable.* The other way in which exercise helps to improve body composition is by ensuring that the majority of weight loss is from fat rather than lean body tissue. In addition to its positive effects on body composition, exercise also helps to counteract several of the negative consequences of being over-fat, such as high blood pressure, glucose intolerance, a low level of HDL cholesterol in the blood, and low self-esteem.

MORE EXERCISE, LESS DRUGS

In recent years, many health experts have concluded that medical science has achieved (for many chronic health problems) about as much as can be expected in the battle against sickness and death. Furthermore, based upon an increasing amount of evidence, many experts have surmised that additional expenditures for health care cannot and will not produce the financial benefits that could be achieved if every American adopted better health practices—particularly a physically active lifestyle. In the past three decades, several major epidemiological studies have demonstrated that regular physical activity is associated with an improved quality of life and longevity. And yet, several chronic health problems and conditions exist that are still treated solely with conventional medical therapy. For whatever reason, many members of the medical community are unaware of the therapeutic—as opposed to preventative—role that exercise can have in health care.

In numerous instances, exercise can be an extremely effective adjunct treatment modality for individuals suffering from a diverse array of chronic

---

* Authors' note: These calculations are based on individuals of average size —women (60 kg) and men (70 kg).

medical problems. As a result, properly prescribed exercise programs can lower health care costs, not only by reducing the incidence or severity of health problems in many cases, but also, when illness does occur, by diminishing an individual's reliance on drugs and limited medical resources.

Any listing of the medical problems and health-related conditions that can be at least partially treated and controlled by exercise would be extensive. Among the most significant of these health concerns are the following:

1. **Hypertension** is a condition, as previously stated, in which an individual's resting blood pressure is chronically above optimal levels. An estimated 60 million American adults have high blood pressure. Hypertension adds to the workload of the heart and arteries and contributes to heart failure and arteriosclerosis. Research has shown that low-intensity (50-70% of $\dot{V}O_{2\,max}$) aerobic exercise can lower systolic blood pressure by 5 to 25 mm Hg and diastolic blood pressure by 3 to 15 mm Hg in mild-to-moderate hypertensives. Of the several possible mechanisms by which training could lower resting blood pressure, a decrease in sympathetic nervous system activity has received the most experimental support. A reduction in sympathetic nerve activity could lower one or both of the two principal determinants of blood pressure (mean arterial blood pressure equals the product of cardiac output and total peripheral resistance).

2. **Anxiety and depression** are the two most prevalent of all mental disorders in the United States. During any given six-month period, up to twenty percent of the U.S. population is affected by either or both of these common symptoms of an individual's failure to properly cope with mental or emotional stress. Exercise can have a positive effect on reducing the $22 billion that is expended in direct costs on mental health care in the United States every year. Exercise has been shown to increase the brain's emission of alpha waves—the brain waves associated with a relaxed meditation-like state of mind. Researchers have also speculated that exercise decreases depression by altering the levels of certain neurotransmitters (norepinephrine, dopamine, and serotonin) in the brain. The majority of studies have involved subjects engaging in aerobic forms of exercise. The ability of resistance exercise to relieve anxiety and depression remains to be seen.

3. **Hypercholesterolemia** is a condition in which the amount of cholesterol in your blood is above an optimal level. Approximately one-fourth of all American adults have blood cholesterol levels above 240 mg/dl (mortality rates for coronary heart disease climb steadily when serum cholesterol levels rise above 180 mg/dl). Numerous studies have documented the fact that physically active people have cholesterol profiles consistent with a lower risk of coronary heart disease. Exercise training produces two very positive plasma lipid and lipoprotein changes in the individual suffering from hypercholesterolemia: it lowers the plasma triglyceride

level and raises the high density lipoprotein (HDL—the so-called "good" lipoprotein particle in your blood) level. To date, this training effect has been more consistently demonstrated in males than in females.

4. **Low back pain** is the most costly medical problem in American society for the 30-60 age group. Across all age groups, it has been estimated that more than 30 million Americans are afflicted with this painful malady. Despite its seriousness, a fail-safe treatment for low back pain has yet to be identified. In a number of instances, however, exercise has been found to be an effective means for both preventing and treating low back pain by enabling an individual to restore proper muscular balance (between abdominal and low back muscles) and to achieve proper flexibility (primarily in the iliopsoas, erector spinae, and hamstring muscle groups).

5. **Peripheral vascular occlusive disease (PVOD)** is a major health problem in the United States that affects over 14 million individuals at any given time. Resulting from restricted (reduced) blood flow to (most commonly) the lower extremities due to arterial obstruction, PVOD can be very painful and may lead, in some instances, to the development of gangrene and eventual amputation. Exercise training has been shown to be effective in controlling PVOD and in improving the physical capabilities of PVOD sufferers. While the exact mechanisms for these positive responses are not precisely known, researchers advance several plausible explanations. The following mechanisms have been most often suggested: an increase in collateral circulation whereby previously "dormant" blood vessels are used to reroute blood around the site of obstruction; reduced blood viscosity allowing for an easier passage of blood through the narrowed vessel; selective redistribution of blood away from inactive muscles in order that exercising muscles receive a greater supply of blood; biomechanical alteration of gait in which walking patterns are changed such that the metabolic demands placed upon the muscles affected by the disease are reduced; greater extraction of oxygen from the blood by the exercising muscles; and improved pain tolerance resulting from repeated pain exposures during training. Whatever the responsible mechanism(s), a leading authority has stated that exercise training is the most successful and cost effective treatment for PVOD.

6. **Osteoporosis** is an age-related disorder that is characterized by a decreased bone mineral content and has been estimated to be responsible for 1.3 million bone fractures per year. Some evidence exists that exercise retards bone mineral loss. Studies have shown that appropriate exercise can even increase bone density. When gravity stress or muscle movement stress is applied to the bone, the pressure produces a desirable adaptive response within the bone. Training-induced improvements in muscle strength and balance may provide an added benefit by preventing the falls that cause a great number of the fractures occurring among the elderly.

7. **Diabetes mellitus** is the name given to a group of disorders (collectively called diabetes) characterized by metabolic abnormalities, of which the most prominent is an improper handling of glucose (sugar) by the body's cells, resulting in elevated blood glucose levels (the hallmark sign of diabetes). Diabetes is a very serious health problem in the United States. It is the cause of approximately 36,000 deaths annually and is a contributing factor in an additional 95,000 deaths. It is also costly. More than $18 billion is spent in the U.S. to treat diabetes each year. The majority of diabetics are classified as either Type I/insulin-dependent (the pancreas doesn't produce sufficient amounts of insulin), or Type II/non-insulin dependent (the body's cells don't respond appropriately to the insulin produced by the pancreas). Exercise has been shown to be a beneficial adjunct therapy for both types (particularly Type II). A clearly demonstrated effect of aerobic forms of exercise is improved glucose uptake by exercising muscle, which can last up to 72 hours following the exercise bout. By exercising on a regular basis, some individuals with Type II diabetes who require medication to control their blood sugar levels are able to reduce or eliminate their need for drugs. Finally, exercise improves a diabetic's blood lipid profile and helps control their blood pressure. By raising HDL-C levels, lowering triglyceride levels and blood pressure, exercise helps protect the diabetic's blood vessels from atherosclerosis (fatty deposits in the arteries). It should also be noted that evidence is accumulating which shows that strength training exercise may also enhance the ability of the body's cells to utilize glucose.

One of the most overriding insights that can be acquired from the aforementioned information concerning the documented relationship between regular exercise and the major health concerns is that exercise can provide a terrific R_X for effective health care. "More exercise, less drugs" should be the standard prescription—not the exception—for those individuals interested in achieving and maintaining a healthy lifestyle.

SLOWING DOWN THE AGING CLOCK

A critical question regarding the aging process centers around whether exercise can slow down the irreversible physiologic changes that occur over the course of an individual's lifetime. The answer is unequivocally "yes," although no one can be certain of the precise extent to which exercise can influence the manner in which an individual's bodily systems respond to aging.

Several of the major changes that occur as an individual ages are of substantial importance. Of particular interest is the fact that many of the changes that accompany aging are similar to those associated with a sedentary lifestyle. At the very least, a physically active lifestyle should have a positive impact on the amount of deterioration experienced by the various physiologic systems of the body since physical activity should help to preserve or maintain higher levels of physiologic function.

One of the primary means by which exercise can exert a positive effect on the aging process involves the cardiorespiratory system. Numerous investigative efforts have shown that elderly individuals who exercise maintain a higher proportion of their cardiorespiratory fitness level than those who don't. As evidence of this, even though $\dot{V}O_{2\ max}$ declines in everyone as we get older, physically active individuals are able to slow their average rate of decline in $\dot{V}O_{2\ max}$ to a level approximately half that of their sedentary counterparts. Other positive physiological responses include an increase in plasma volume, hemoglobin, muscle glycogen, mitochondrial and oxidative enzyme activity, oxygen pulse (the amount of oxygen delivered to the working muscles per contraction of the heart), and a reduction in both blood lactate concentrations and heart rate at submaximal work rates.

The other major way that exercise impacts the rate and degree of aging is through its effects on the musculoskeletal system. Several recent studies have supported the contention that strength training can have positive effects on the rate of deterioration of the musculoskeletal system typically observed in older persons. The results of these studies indicated that strength did not decrease substantially with age as it often does (for example, individuals typically suffer a 20-30 percent loss in strength by age 65). In fact, many individuals exhibited dramatic increases in strength. Some subjects in these studies also experienced muscle hypertrophy (an increase in muscle size), in contrast to the usual decrease that occurs. These increases in muscle strength and size tend to translate into improved gait, balance, mobility, and, consequently, better functional capabilities and a lower susceptibility for falling. Also, strength training and low-impact weight-bearing aerobic exercises have been shown to produce increases in bone mineral content in elderly adults.

The American Medical Association's Council on Scientific Affairs states unequivocally that exercise can improve the quality of life for the elderly. Limited functional capabilities and "slowing down" are not, and should not, be viewed as inevitable consequences of attaining a certain age. The available scientific data indicate that much of the decline in function of a physiologic system is dependent upon the degree to which that system is used. In other words, many changes associated with old age are influenced more by lifestyle than by simply the passage of time. Regardless of how old you are, if you eat right and exercise more, you'll live better. A strong argument could be made that an individual's dignity and sense of independence are inexorably intertwined. The cornerstone of both factors is the ability to be able to do things for yourself. Exercise enhances the likelihood that you will have that ability.

FIT TO LIVE

The old adage, "add life to your years, as well as years to your life," has considerable merit. A sound exercise program can contribute to the quality of your life in countless ways. Are the positive consequences which result from exercising worth the effort involved? Without question. Put another way, is the squirt worth the squeeze? Without a doubt. Should you make exercise an integral part of your daily routine? Of course, you should. In many ways, your life depends on it. ❑

BIBLIOGRAPHY ••

1. American College of Sports Medicine. *Guidelines for Exercise Testing and Exercise Prescription.* Philadelphia, PA: Lea & Febiger, 1991.
2. American College of Sports Medicine. *Resource Manual for Exercise Testing and Exercise Prescription.* Philadelphia, PA: Lea and Febiger, 1988.
3. Bouchard, C., Shephard, R.J., Stephens, T., et al. (Eds). *Exercise, Fitness, and Health.* Champaign, IL: Human Kinetics Publishers, 1990.
4. Duncan, J.J., Farr, J.E., Upton, S.J., et al. "The effects of aerobic exercise on plasma catecholamines and blood pressure in patients with mild essential hypertension." *JAMA* 254:2609-2613, 1985.
5. Eckert, H.M., Montoye, H.J. (Eds). *Exercise and Health.* Champaign, IL: Human Kinetics Publishers, 1984.
6. Ernst, E. "Physical exercise for peripheral vascular disease—a review." *Vasa* 16:227-231, 1987.
7. Franklin, B.A., Gordon, S., Timmis, G.C., et al. (Eds). *Exercise in Modern Medicine.* Baltimore, MD: Williams & Wilkins, 1989.
8. Gordon, N.F., Scott, C.B., Wilkinson, W.J., et al. "Exercise and mild essential hypertension: Recommendations for adults." *Sports Med* 10(6):390-404, 1990.
9. Hiatt, W.R., Regensteiner, J.G., Hargarten, M.E., et al. "Benefit of exercise conditioning for patients with peripheral arterial disease." *Circulation* 81:602-609, 1990.
10. Horton, E.S. "Role and management of exercise in diabetes mellitus." *Diabetes Care* 11:201-211, 1988.
11. Morgan, W.P., O'Connor, P.J. "Exercise and mental health." In *Exercise Adherence.* Dishman, R.K. (Ed). Champaign, IL: Human Kinetics Publishers, 1988.
12. Peterson, J.A., Wheeler, J. *The Goodbye Back Pain Handbook.* Grand Rapids, MI: Masters Press, 1988.
13. Sinaki, M. "Exercise and osteoporosis." *Arch Phys Med Rehabil* 70:220-229, 1989.
14. Tipton, C.M. "Exercise, training and hypertension: An update." *Exerc Sport Sci Rev* 19:447-505, 1991.

CHAPTER 3

• •

GUIDELINES FOR PRE-EXERCISE HEALTH SCREENING

by

Steven J. Riddle, M.S.
and
Susan Wentz, M.D.

• • •

*P*rior to beginning a new exercise program, it is important to evaluate your health status to identify any existing medical conditions or risk factors that you may have. This is even more pertinent for those who have previously been sedentary and are unaccustomed to strenuous physical activity. This chapter focuses on screening and evaluation procedures which, when followed, will allow you to enter into an exercise program with very little risk of medical or physical complications. Our primary purpose here is not to make any medical diagnoses, but to determine if you are at high risk for, or experiencing symptoms of, cardiopulmonary or metabolic disease.

For the vast majority of people, exercise is safe and promotes improved health. Noted Swedish exercise physiologist P. O. Åstrand probably summed it up best with the following quote: "All men and women should submit to a thorough physical exam before deciding not to exercise regularly." Many people have one or more known health problems that have been diagnosed and/or treated by a physician. If you are in this group, then you must rely on guidance from a knowledgeable health-fitness instructor or your physician for appropriate fitness programs. If, however, your health status has been recently analyzed by a physician and/or a health professional and no existing health problems or major risk factors were found, you are ready to begin (or continue) a fitness program. Most people lie somewhere within this continuum. They do not have any known major health problems or obvious symptoms, but have never had their health status thoroughly checked or their health risk properly assessed.

THE HEALTH RISK APPRAISAL

The vast majority of medical conditions, symptoms, and risk factors that are predictive of future cardiovascular disease or additional medical problems can be identified by a well-designed health assessment or medical history questionnaire. This tool, often referred to as a "health risk appraisal" or HRA, has a more specific function related to exercise in that it can identify existing medical conditions that have the potential to be significantly exacerbated by physical activity.

An HRA must be simple, easily understood, and require minimal time to complete to be practical and effective. A health risk appraisal can be self-administered, provided you have access to an acceptable instrument and possess an appropriate level of understanding regarding how to interpret the information obtained by the process. In most instances, the evaluation of your health status is most accurately done by a medical or health/fitness professional.

OVERVIEW

This chapter is designed to take you through the proper steps to determine your need for medical evaluation prior to initiating a new exercise routine. Depending on the expected intensity of your exercise activities, you will use one of two health risk appraisals. If the intensity of your exercise activities will be low or "light," a simple screening questionnaire will be sufficient to assess your need for additional screening. If, however, your intensity will be moderate to high, you will need to use a more intensive HRA to determine your current "health risk category."

The American College of Sports Medicine (ACSM) defines **three primary health risk categories** for individuals who wish to participate in an exercise program.

- *Apparently Healthy* - Individuals with no diagnosed cardiopulmonary disease, no signs or symptoms of disease, and no more than one major coronary risk factor.
- *Higher Risk* - Individuals who have two or more major coronary risk factors and/or demonstrate signs or symptoms that are suggestive of active cardiopulmonary or metabolic disease.
- *With Disease* - Individuals who have been diagnosed with cardiac, pulmonary, or metabolic disease at any time in the past.

The ACSM has also established recommendations for obtaining medical clearance based on the risk category into which you fall. These guidelines are clearly defined later in this chapter and will be the basis of your decision to seek additional medical screening prior to beginning any exercise activities at a moderate or vigorous intensity.

PRE-EXERCISE HEALTH SCREENING
• • •

The following sections of this chapter will briefly describe the initial considerations, health risk appraisals, and other tools used to guide you in your self-administered risk assessment. A step-by-step summary will take you through the actual procedures required to identify your health risk category and readiness for exercise.

AGE CRITERIA

The first consideration in your decision to seek medical evaluation before beginning to exercise is your age. The ACSM has established age guidelines (below) that should be followed closely. Note that the intensity of your exercise is an important factor as well.

- It is recommended that all men over 40 and women over 50 undergo medical evaluation and/or diagnostic exercise testing prior to beginning or participating in **moderate** (50% - 70% of maximal heart rate) or **vigorous** (> 70% of maximal heart rate) intensity exercise activities.
- Men under 40 and women under 50, who are free of known symptoms of disease, and plan to participate in **moderate** or **vigorous** intensity exercise activities should first complete an appropriate medical/health questionnaire to identify any significant health risk.
- Individuals of any age who are free of known symptoms or disease (screened by simple HRA) can begin an exercise regimen as long as the exercise begins at a low intensity (i.e., < 50% of maximal heart rate) and proceeds gradually, and the individual is alert for any unusual signs or symptoms.

EXERCISE INTENSITY

Once age criteria are considered, the specific HRA questionnaire you use is dependent upon the intensity at which you plan to exercise or the nature of the intended activities.

LOW INTENSITY EXERCISE

If your exercise activities are non-competitive and will be at a low intensity, a simple health risk appraisal called a **Physical Activity Readiness Questionnaire** (PAR-Q) is sufficient to identify any need for additional medical screening (refer to Figure 3-1). It has been shown to be effective in appropriately referring those who need medical screening, while not excluding the majority of people who will benefit from participation in regular low-intensity activity.

MODERATE-TO-HIGH INTENSITY EXERCISE

If your exercise program will include competitive, or moderate-to-high intensity (vigorous) activities, then a more comprehensive health risk appraisal called a **Health Status Questionnaire** (HS-Q) will be necessary so that your health risk category can be appropriately determined. Since some moderate or vigorous exercise will usually be included in a fitness program, the HS-Q will be used by most people.

The Health Status Questionnaire

The following are brief explanations of each of the sections on the HS-Q. It is also a descriptive version of the HS-Q algorithm which determines your health risk category based on your HS-Q responses. In order to best understand the sections that follow, refer to the actual HS-Q and HS-Q algorithm (pp. 26-30) as you proceed. The step-by-step instructions provided in Table 3-1 will guide you through your health risk assessment. Sections 1-4 are designed to help you determine your health risk category and, therefore, make a knowledgeable decision as to whether to seek medical evaluation and/or diagnostic exercise testing prior to beginning your new exercise program. Sections 5-6 are designed to be used by a health/fitness professional to make informed and realistic recommendations in developing your fitness plan.

HS-Q Section 1: Cardiopulmonary/Metabolic Disease

This section will identify the presence of documented cardiac, pulmonary, or metabolic disease such as diabetes mellitus. Any "yes" answer here places you in the "with disease" category. Medical clearance is certainly necessary before initiating any exercise program. Your physician should identify any limitations or restrictions that are necessary, and your exercise should be supervised by qualified exercise professionals.

HS-Q Section 2: Medical History

This section is designed to identify the presence of any diseases, serious medical conditions, or orthopedic problems that could be worsened by physical activity. Medical evaluation is required if you have a positive history for any of the items addressed in the first three questions. The presence of orthopedic or joint injuries or other physical problems may mean that certain activities should be avoided so that these problems are not aggravated to the point where they prevent you from exercising safely. It is recommended that you seek medical consultation if any of these problems exist.

HS-Q Section 3: Cardiopulmonary/Metabolic Symptoms

This section will identify any signs or symptoms you may be experiencing that are suggestive of cardiac, pulmonary, or other metabolic disease. Any "yes" answer here places you in the "higher risk with symptoms" category. If this is the case, medical evaluation and/or diagnostic exercise testing is recommended prior to initiating exercise activities **at any level of intensity.**

HS-Q Section 4: Coronary Risk Factor Profile

This section is designed to identify the presence of major risk factors which are known to contribute to the development of heart attacks and other manifestations of cardiovascular disease. Reducing these risk factors is an important focus of any health enhancement effort. A "yes" answer indicates the probable presence of a major risk factor.

- If you have two or more of these risk factors, you are placed in the "higher risk" category. It is recommended that you seek medical evaluation and/or diagnostic exercise testing before undertaking **vigorous physical activity.**
- If you have two or more of the major risk factors but none of the symptoms outlined in section 3, medical evaluation and exercise testing may not be necessary if you limit your activity to **light** or **moderate intensities**, progress gradually, and do not participate in competitive activities.

HS-Q Section 5: Fitness

This section is helpful to a health/fitness professional who is assessing your current level of fitness and will be developing recommendations as to the type, intensity, frequency, and duration of exercise activities that will best serve your current needs.

HS-Q Section 6: Lifestyle and Behavioral

This section is also very helpful to the health/fitness professional (and yourself) in evaluating the behavioral and lifestyle issues that will affect the type of exercise plan that best fits your lifestyle. Too often exercise is begun with unrealistic goals, inappropriate expectations and no consideration for "real-life" constraints that may limit participation and subsequent results. Planning for obstacles, evaluating your daily schedule, and basing your exercise plan on activities you have enjoyed in the past should enhance long-term adherence to your exercise program.

Table 3-1. Step-by Step Summary
Six Easy Steps to Assess Your Health Risk Prior to Exercise

Follow the step-by-step instructions below to complete your thorough health risk assessment.

1.   Review the age criteria on page 24:

     •   If you exceed the age criteria and plan to participate in moderate-to-vigorous intensity activities, discontinue this step-by-step sequence. Simply complete the HS-Q and seek medical evaluation first. The HS-Q may be helpful to your doctor and/or health professional in their evaluation.

2.   Determine the approximate intensity you intend to maintain during exercise using the Intensity Worksheet on page 25.

3.   Fill out the appropriate HRA questionnaire:

     •   If your exercise workouts will consist of low-intensity activity and you are free of any known cardiovascular or pulmonary disease, complete the Physical Activity Readiness Questionnaire (PAR-Q) on page 25.
     •   If your exercise workouts will include any moderate intensity or vigorous activities, complete the Health Status Questionnaire (HS-Q) on pages 26-29.

4.   After completing your HRA, use the appropriate algorithm:

     •   If you completed the PAR-Q, follow the instructions on the PAR-Q. Consult your physician if you answered "yes" to any of the seven questions. If all of your responses were no, you may begin low-intensity exercise activities.
     •   If you completed the HS-Q, use the HS-Q Algorithm on page 29 to determine your health risk category based on your answers in sections 1-4.

5.   Use the Health Risk Category Table on page 30 to determine what action to take based on your risk category and symptoms.

6.   After obtaining medical clearance (if necessary), seek out a qualified health/fitness instructor who can advise you on a safe and effective exercise routine based on sections 5 and 6 of your HS-Q.

AGE CRITERIA

The ACSM has established age guidelines (below) that should be followed closely. Note that the intensity of your exercise workouts is an important factor as well. The exercise intensity worksheet is also provided below.

*It is recommended that **all males over 40** and **females over 50** undergo medical evaluation and/or diagnostic exercise testing prior to beginning or participating in **moderate** or **vigorous** intensity exercise activities.*

PRE-EXERCISE HEALTH SCREENING

• • •

If the criteria above describes you, follow the instructions in step 1 of the Step-by-Step Summary (refer to Table 3-1). If you are not affected by the above criteria, proceed to step 2.

EXERCISE INTENSITY WORKSHEET

The intensity of your exercise activities is an important factor in assessing your need for additional medical screening prior to beginning your exercise program. The ACSM defines two categories of exercise intensity which are described below. Define your expected intensity of exercise based on the descriptions below and proceed with step 3 which is to complete the appropriate health-risk appraisal.

1. **Low-Intensity Activity** is defined by the ACSM as being well within the individual's current capacity and can be sustained comfortably for a prolonged period (i.e., 60 minutes). Steady walking, easy cycling, light stair climbing, stretch-and-tone classes, and steady lap swimming are good examples of "low intensity" activity.

2. **Moderate-to-High Intensity or "Vigorous" Activity** is defined by the ACSM as exercise that causes significant increases in breathing and heart rate and usually cannot be sustained for more than 15-20 minutes by untrained individuals. Power walking, jogging, aerobic dance, step aerobics, stair climbing, active sports and games, and any type of weight lifting are good examples of "moderate-to-high intensity" activity.

My exercise intensity is best represented by (circle one):   #1   or   #2

PAR-Q & YOU

Par-Q is designed to help you help yourself. Many health benefits are associated with regular exercise, and the completion of PAR-Q is a sensible first step to take, if you are planning to increase the amount of physical activity in your life.

For most people, physical activity should not pose any problem or hazard. PAR-Q has been designed to identify the small number of adults for whom physical activity might be inappropriate or those who should have medical advice concerning the type of activity most suitable for them.

Common sense is your best guide in answering these few questions. Please read them carefully and check the "YES" or "NO" box opposite each question if it applies to you.

YES NO

____ ____   1.   Has your doctor ever said you have heart trouble?

____ ____   2.   Do you frequently have pains in your heart and chest?

____ ____   3.   Do you often feel faint or have spells of severe dizziness?

___ ___	4.	Has a doctor ever said your blood pressure was too high?

___ ___   4.   Has a doctor ever said your blood pressure was too high?

___ ___   5.   Has your doctor ever told you that you have a bone or joint problem, such as arthritis, that has been aggravated by exercise or might be made worse with exercise?

___ ___   6.   Is there a good physical reason not mentioned here why you should not follow an activity program even if you wanted to?

___ ___   7.   Are you over age 65 and not accustomed to vigorous exercise?

IF YOU ANSWERED:

YES to one or more questions:

If you have not recently done so, consult with your physician by telephone or in person BEFORE increasing your physical activity and/or taking a fitness appraisal. Tell your physician what questions you answered YES to on PAR-Q or present your PAR-Q copy.

After medical evaluation, seek advice from your physician as to your suitability for:
• Unrestricted physical activity, starting off easily and progressing gradually.
• Restricted or supervised activity to meet your specific needs, at least on an inital basis. Check in your community for special programs or services.

NO to all questions:

If you answered PAR-Q accurately, you have reasonable assurance of your present suitability for:
• A graduated exercise program—a gradual increase in proper exercise promotes good fitness development while minimizing or eliminating discomfort.
• An exercise test—simple tests of fitness (such as the Canadian Home Fitness Test) or more complex types may be undertaken if you so desire.
Remember to postpone physical activity if you have a temporary minor illness, such as a common cold.

* *Developed by the British Columbia Ministry of Health. Conceptualized and critiqued by the Multidisciplinary Advisory Board on Exercise (MABE). Translation, reproduction, and use in its entirety is encouraged.*

HEALTH STATUS QUESTIONNAIRE

Name				Phone (H)
Address				Emergency Contact
				Emergency Contact
City		Zip		Emergency Contact
DOB:	Age	Sex M F		Emergency Contact

PRE-EXERCISE HEALTH SCREENING

• • •

SECTION 1) CARDIOPULMONARY/METABOLIC DISEASE

Y   N   Have you ever had a **heart attack, bypass surgery, angioplasty,** or been diagnosed with **coronary artery disease** or other heart disease? If yes, describe:

Y   N   Do you have **emphysema, asthma,** or any other chronic lung condition or disease?

Y   N   Are you an **insulin dependent diabetic?**

SECTION 2) MEDICAL HISTORY

1.   Mark any of the following for which you have been diagnosed or treated:
     ___Kidney problem   ___Heart problem   ___Phlebitis   ___Concussion
     ___Mononucleosis   ___Cirrhosis, liver   ___Stroke   ___Asthma

2.   Mark any medications taken in the last six months:
     ___Blood thinner   ___Epilepsy medicine   ___Nitroglycerin
     ___Diabetes medicine   ___Heart rhythm medicine   ___Insulin
     ___Blood pressure med.   ___Diuretic (water pill)   ___Digitalis
     ___Cholesterol medicine
     ___Other:_ _____

3.   List any surgeries you have had in the past (e.g., knee, heart, back, etc.):

Y   N   Have you ever had **back problems,** any problems with **joints** (e.g., back, knee, hip, shoulder, elbow, neck), or been diagnosed with **arthritis?**
        If yes, describe:_____

Y   N   Do you have **any other medical conditions** or health problems which may affect your exercise plan or safety in any way?
        If yes, describe:_____

SECTION 3) CARDIOPULMONARY AND METABOLIC SYMPTOMS

Y   N   Do you ever get unusually **short of breath** with very light exertion?
Y   N   Do you ever have **pain, pressure, heaviness,** or **tightness** in the chest area?
Y   N   Do you regularly have **unexplained pain** in the abdomen, shoulder, or arm?
Y   N   Do you ever have severe **dizzy spells** or episodes of fainting?
Y   N   Do you ever feel **"skips," palpitations,** or runs of fast heart beats in your chest?
Y   N   Has a physician ever told you that you have a **heart murmur?**
Y   N   Do you **regularly** get lower leg pain during walking that is relieved at rest?
Y   N   Do you have any joints that **often** become swollen and painful?
        Where: _____

SECTION 4) CORONARY RISK FACTOR PROFILE

Y N Have you had **high blood pressure** (>160 or >95) on more than one occasion? Please list any **medications** you take for high blood pressure:

Y N Have you ever been told that your blood **cholesterol** was high (240 or higher)? Cholesterol level _____

Y N Do you currently **smoke** 10 or more cigarettes per day?
_____ **cigarettes/day**   _____ **years smoked**

Y N Have you ever been told that you have **high blood sugar** or **diabetes**?

Y N Has anyone in your **immediate family** (parents, siblings) had any heart problems or coronary disease before **age 55**? Describe:

Y N Do you feel you are more than 30 lbs. **overweight**? What do you feel is your realistic **ideal weight**? _____ lbs

SECTION 5) FITNESS

0 1
2 3   Circle the average number of times per week you participate in planned
4 5   moderate-to-strenuous exercise of at least 20 minutes in duration (brisk
6 7   walking, jogging, cycling, swimming, stair climbing, weight lifting,
       active sports such as tennis, aerobic classes, etc.):

Y N Can you briskly walk one mile without fatigue?

Y N Can you jog two miles continuously at moderate pace without discomfort?

Y N Can you do 20 push-ups?
Please list your body weight:
Now: _____ lbs   1 year ago: _____ lbs   Age 21:_____lbs

SECTION 6) LIFESTYLE AND BEHAVIORAL

1. Describe any **cardiovascular exercise** you have done in the past (what, when, how often, for how long):

2. Describe any **muscular strength/weight training** you have done in the past (same as above):

3. List any **major obstacles** that you feel you will have to overcome to stick with your exercise plan long-term (or what has stopped you in the past):

PRE-EXERCISE HEALTH SCREENING
• • •

4. Have you ever participated in **aerobic** or **aerobic step** classes? Yes   No

5. Please list any **recreational physical activities** (e.g., tennis, golf, etc.) in which you regularly participate and how often:

6. List any **favorite** activities you would like to include in your exercise plan:

7. List any activities that you definitely **do not like** and do not want to include:

8. Which do you prefer? ___group exercise ___exercising on your own

9. List your two most important goals or reasons why you want to exercise regularly:
    #1._____ #2._____

10. Your occupation:_____

11. Do you spend more than 25% of work time at the following:
    (mark all that apply):
    ___Sitting at desk ___Lifting/carrying loads ___Standing
    ___Driving   ___Walking

12. Number of **hours** worked per week: ___hours   Any flexible hours? Y N

13. Write in the best exercise times for you during a **typical week**:

	M	T	W	TH	F	S	S
AM							
PM							

14. Where do you plan to exercise? ___Club ___Home ___Outside
    Other_____

15. If at home, list available equipment:_____

HS-Q ALGORITHM

Refer to Health Status Questionnaire as you follow this algorithm to determine health risk category

> ### Age Criteria
> The ACSM recommends that all men over 40 and women over 50, regardless of their risk category, obtain medical clearance and, more specifically, undergo a maximal graded exercise test prior to beginning a vigorous or high-intensity exercise program.

Table 3-2. Health Risk Category Table

The following table is set up to provide clear recommendations after you have determined your risk category from the HS-Q. The recommendations are based on the guidelines set forth by the ACSM.

Please remember that these guidelines are well-established and represent the current standards of the health and fitness industry. Exceptions and special cases will, however, always exist. If you have any doubt about your medical status, please seek medical consultation before beginning your exercise activities. It is always better to be conservative and to make sure that a situation does not develop where you are not able to exercise at all due to medical or physical complications.

	Risk Category	Recommendations
1	Apparently Healthy	You can begin with low-intensity exercise and gradually increase to moderate or vigorous intensity without medical evaluation or testing.
2A	Higher Risk - asymptomatic	You can begin low-intensity exercise without medical evaluation. Qualified supervision is recommended. Medical evaluation/testing should be sought prior to moderate- or vigorous-intensity exercise or competitive activities.
2B	Higher Risk - with symptoms	Medical examination and or diagnostic testing should be completed to evaluate symptoms prior to beginning any type of exercise regimen. Qualified supervision is recommended during exercise.
3	With Disease	Appropriate medical clearance and/or diagnostic testing must precede exercise. Limitations or restrictions should be set by a physician or qualified health professional. Exercise should be supervised by qualified fitness personnel.

PRE-EXERCISE HEALTH SCREENING
• • •

SAFETY FIRST

For years, many professionals in the medical community have ascribed to three basic rules for rehabilitating their patients—rules which also have direct application for individuals who want to engage in a sound exercise program:

Rule #1. Create an environment for optimal healing (results).
Rule #2. Above all else, Do No Harm.
Rule #3. Be as aggressive as you can, without breaking Rule #2.

Obviously, all of the positive benefits of exercise will be inconsequential to you if your safety is compromised by the activity. In order to minimize the possibility that such an event might occur, an appropriate HRA should be administered prior to engaging in any type of exercise test or physical activity program for the first time.

An HRA is a tool whose primary purpose is to help protect you from experiencing any serious adverse events during your participation in exercise. The basic objective of pre-activity screening is not diagnostic, but rather to determine risk, whether it be cardiovascular, orthopaedic, metabolic, etc. An HRA, if properly used, should be able to:

- determine if you have a medical condition or risk factor that could be exacerbated by exercise,
- be used to develop appropriate exercise tests and prescriptions, and
- be used to educate and motivate you to initiate and sustain necessary lifestyle behavioral changes.

Given the many desirable consequences of sound exercise, it is sometimes too easy and too tempting to jump right into an exercise program without spending a few moments to ensure that your safety will not be compromised. Accordingly, you should view an HRA as a user-friendly form of "safety insurance" . . . insurance that you need and deserve. ❑

BIBLIOGRAPHY •••••••••••••••••••••••••••••••••••••••

1. American College of Sports Medicine. *ACSM's Health/Fitness Facility Standards and Guidelines.* Champaign, IL: Human Kinetics Publishers, 1992.
2. American College of Sports Medicine. *Guidelines for Exercise Testing and Prescription,* 4th Ed. Philadelphia, PA: Lea & Febiger, 1991.
3. American Heart Association. *1988 Heart Facts.* Dallas, TX: American Heart Association, 1988.
4. Chisholm, D.M., collis, M.L., Kulak, L.L., et al. "Physical activity readiness." *Brit Col Med J* 17:375-378, 1975.
5. Fardy, P.S., Yanowitz F.G., Wilson, P.K. *Cardiac Rehabilitation, Adult Fitness, and Exercise Testing,* 2nd Ed. Philadelphia, PA: Lea & Febiger, 1988.
6. Howley, E.T., Franks, B.D. *Health Fitness Instructor's Handbook,* 2nd Ed. Champaign, IL: Human Kinetics Publishers, 1992.
7. Koeberle, B.E. *Legal Aspects of Sports Medicine.* Canton, OH: Professional Reports Corporation, 1990.
8. Nieman, D.C. *Fitness and Sports Medicine: An Introduction.* Palo Alto, CA: Bull Publishing Company, 1990.
9. Shephard, R.J. "PAR-Q, Canadian home fitness test and exercise screening alternatives." *Sports Med* 5:185-195, 1988.

CHAPTER 4

••

ASSESSING AND ADDRESSING HEALTH RISK FACTORS

by

Reed H. Humphrey, Ph.D., P.T.

• • •

*I*t is no secret that the major causes of death and disability in the United States today result largely from preventable diseases, such as chronic diseases involving the heart and lungs. Clear evidence indicates that a healthy lifestyle that includes exercise is important in both the primary prevention of heart and lung disease, as well as in reducing the risk of further problems in individuals suffering from these diseases. Physical activity may also play an important role in reducing the risk of certain types of cancer.

Despite a consistent and gradual decline in mortality, heart disease remains the leading cause of death and disability in the United States. The focus of this chapter, then, will be the identification of the recognized risk factors associated with premature heart disease and the effects of a regular exercise program in reducing those risks. However, because most chronic diseases are associated with the same group of health factors, the management of heart disease risk factors transfers to the reduction in risk for the wide assortment of other chronic diseases. Recent studies have exquisitely demonstrated the effects of exercise on both reductions in heart disease as well as all-cause mortality. So, by effectively managing the risks associated with heart disease, you will really be reducing the risk of many premature diseases, and improving the quality—and probably the quantity—of your life.

CHRONIC DISEASE, RISK FACTORS, AND YOUR RISK

Risk factors may be thought of as those factors present in your lifestyle that are associated with an increased likelihood of a premature health problem.

For example, a heart attack, or myocardial infarction, may occur as a result of coronary artery disease. This is a progressive form of heart disease wherein the coronary arteries—those arteries that supply the heart—become occluded, and the heart tissue is damaged from lack of oxygen. Unfortunately, too often the first sign of the disease is sudden death. In those that survive, recovery can be complicated, disabling and expensive. It has been estimated that greater than 90% of premature heart disease is preventable.

The occlusion of the coronary arteries, like most chronic diseases, occurs in an accelerated fashion because of the presence of certain risk factors. Exercise, when combined with a healthy lifestyle, can be thought of as a way to slow down, perhaps even reverse, the progression of the disease.

One question that immediately comes to mind is: How do we know which lifestyle habits are truly risk factors for a disease? While various ways of approaching this question exist, probably the most powerful method is to start with a large community of individuals and carefully study them, and the generations that follow, to evaluate their lifestyles in relation to how frequently various diseases occur. For heart disease, the most famous community study in the United States has been taking place in Framingham, Massachusetts. Some factors that are not controllable, like age, gender and family history of heart problems were identified as risk factors for heart disease. Over the many years of this study, certain *controllable* factors began to emerge that were independently associated with premature heart problems: cigarette smoking, high blood pressure, and high total cholesterol levels. More recently, a sedentary lifestyle has been shown to exhibit similar risk characteristics. This is a very important addition to this group of independent risk factors, when you consider the prevalence of inactivity in the United States. Table 4-1, adapted from the *Journal of the American Medical Association*, provides an excellent resource to assess your heart disease risk factor profile.

As you determine the presence or absence of risk factors, it is important to keep in mind that the presence of risk factors does not mean you will get the disease prematurely, nor does the absence of risk factors mean you are immune from premature disease. Rather, the presence of risk factors simply places you in a group of individuals with a similar risk factor profile. Within this group, some will have a premature onset of heart disease, others will never develop the disease. But, as the number of risk factors present increases, the proportion of those prematurely suffering from the disease likewise increases. Hopefully, this brief explanation helps to explain why some individuals who have many apparent risk factors don't get sick, while others who are seemingly very healthy can become ill. It should, however, also be apparent that the *risk* of getting sick prematurely is increased with the presence and number of risk factors. Fortunately, it is a risk you have a reasonable degree of control over.

Essentially, while you are able to assess your risk factor profile, you can't determine your specific individual risk of premature chronic illness. You *can*, however, identify those aspects within your lifestyle that you can exert control over, so as to move yourself to a group with a better risk factor profile—and a lower probability of premature disease.

Table 4-1. Coronary Artery Disease Risk Factors
Positive Risk FactorsComments.

Positive Risk Factors	Comments
1. Age	Men > 45 years, women > 55 or premature menopause without estrogen replacement therapy.
2. Family History	Myocardial infarction or sudden death before 55 years of age in father or male first-degree relative, or before 65 years of age in mother or other first-degree relative.
3. Current cigarette smoking	
4. Hypertension	Blood pressure ≥ 140/90 mm Hg, confirmed by meaurements on at least two separate occasions or on antihypertensive medication.
5. Hyperlipidemia	Total serum cholesterol > 200 mg/dl (if lipoprotein profile is unavailable) or HDL < 35 mg/dl.
6. Diabetes mellitus	Persons with insulin dependent diabetes mellitus (IDDM) who are > 30 years of age or have had IDDM for > 15 years, and persons with non-insulin dependent diabetes mellitus (NIDDM) who are > 35 years of age should be classified as patients with disease.
7. Sedentary lifestyle	

Negative Risk Factor	Comments
1. High HDL cholesterol	> 60 mg/dl; if HDL is high, subtract on risk factor from sum of risk factors, since high HDL decreases CAD risk.

Note: Obesity is not listed as an independent positive risk factor because its effects are exerted through other risk factors (e.g., hypertension, hyperlipidemia, diabetes). Obesity should be considered as an independent target for intervention. Sedentary lifestyle/physical inactivity is not listed as a positive risk factor in the referenced paper. However, the American Heart Association, in a recent position paper, states that physical inactivity should be treated as an independent target for behavioral intervention.

RISK FACTORS YOU CAN'T CONTROL BUT NEED TO KNOW

Age, family history, and gender are three risk factors that you simply can't control, but need to know about. Age is important since it should alert those over the thresholds identified in Table 4-1 to take special notice of other risk factors that may be present. Obviously, waiting until one is at the age threshold to begin a program of risk reduction is unwise, since chronic diseases develop over a lifetime. The sooner one starts, the better the outlook. On the other hand, it is never too late to get started. Significant improvements in health and fitness can be attained even in the very elderly.

The presence of premature illness, as outlined in Table 4-1, within the family suggests a genetic tendency which cannot be altered. While unfortunate, this should only serve to emphasize the importance of managing controllable risk factors that may be present. Having a positive family history does *not* guarantee premature illness, it only suggests that the predisposition exists. That is, given the same risk factor profile as someone else who has a negative family history, the *probability* of greater risk lies with the person who has a positive family history, but that is all that it means. Since you can't do anything about that, you must focus your energy on those factors you can change.

Regarding gender, males have a higher incidence of heart disease than females. Many believe this is largely due to the hormone estrogen, since after menopause the risk of heart disease increases significantly in women. However, although we don't know the precise reason, the incidence of heart disease in women between 1980-1988 (the most recent period for which data is available) virtually doubled, suggesting that women in today's society appear to be at a higher risk than previously thought.

CONTROLLABLE RISK FACTORS

Cigarette smoking is a powerful risk factor for all chronic diseases. It is a pervasive risk factor that increases risk in proportion to the quantity of cigarettes smoked. Aside from impairing the delivery of oxygen into the bloodstream, increasing cardiac stress, and the rate of atherosclerosis, smoking causes a chronic inflammation of the lungs that is associated with various diseases of the lungs, eventually causing irreparable damage to lung tissue. Remarkably, with regard to heart disease, quitting smoking reduces risk significantly.

Because smoking and exercise are virtually incompatible behaviors, little is known about the two behaviors in combination. However, the powerful effects of smoking relative to the progression of chronic disease suggests that exercise cannot be used to offset the negative effects of smoking. For the few exercisers that continue to smoke, the benefits afforded by exercise are likely suppressed by smoking.

Frequently, individuals state they can't quit smoking due to the inevitable weight gain that follows. While evidence does exist to support this contention, the substitution of exercise to increase energy expenditure can virtually eliminate the tendency for weight gain due to smoking cessation. More importantly, gaining a few pounds versus the reduction in risk from quitting smoking is no contest relative to overall long-term health. It is *always* better to stop smoking.

High blood pressure, defined in Table 4-1 as a resting systolic blood pressure of 140 mm Hg and higher, or a diastolic blood pressure of 90 mm Hg or higher, remains an important independent risk factor for chronic diseases. The contraction of the heart reflects the systolic pressure, while the pressure between beats (diastole) reflects the diastolic pressure. *Both* are important and should be viewed as two separate measures. Both should be normalized as quickly as is feasible. An important consideration is that *any* reduction in blood pressure is associated with a reduced risk. That is, while a reduction from 150 to 144 mm Hg isn't below the 140 threshold, it still is a significant reduction. Traditional approaches to lowering blood pressure include: reduced sodium consumption, decreasing excess body fat, stress management, exercise, and, when prescribed by a physician, medication. In many cases, a combination of many of these strategies is necessary to effectively lower blood pressure. If medication is prescribed, it is critical that it not be discontinued without first consulting your physician. Because high blood pressure frequently does not produce symptoms, it is important to comply with the regimen of treatment as prescribed and have your blood pressure checked regularly.

Although the exact mechanism of exercise in helping to normalize blood pressure is not known, it is likely through a variety of mechanisms. The normalization of body fat and weight, associated reduction in psychological stress, improved physiological fitness of the cardiovascular system, and accompanying adoption of positive health behaviors such as better nutrition probably all combine to bring about a lower blood pressure.

Hyperlipidemia, a total serum cholesterol of over 200 mg/dl or an HDL cholesterol of less than 35 mg/dl, is an important risk factor. Often a source of controversy and confusion over the years, it is clear that an elevated total cholesterol or a low HDL level are *both* independent and important risk factors. While it is fashionable to look at the ratio between total cholesterol and the HDL (having a ratio of less than four to five is optimal), it is important to have normal total and HDL levels. The higher the level of total cholesterol, the higher the risk of premature disease. As with blood pressure, incremental decreases in total cholesterol result in a decrease in risk; for every one percent decrease in serum cholesterol mortality from coronary heart disease declines approximately two percent.

Genetic predisposition, as with most risk factors, plays an important role in hyperlipidemias. Beyond the genetic influence, decreases in total cholesterol are associated with changes in nutritional habits, as outlined in chapter 16 of this book. Exercise is likely to positively influence total cholesterol levels when it is associated with weight loss. Probably the more important effect of exercise is in raising the HDL levels of cholesterol in the blood. HDL, more commonly referred to as the "good" cholesterol in contrast to LDL cholesterol, which is more atherogenic, has been demonstrated to increase with exercise training and is typically at high levels in endurance trained individuals. Thus, independent of weight loss, regular exercise will tend to raise HDL cholesterol without significant effects on the total cholesterol, with a net lowering of the cholesterol:HDL ratio. This general effect should serve to emphasize the importance of engaging in a complete program of good health behaviors to lower disease risk.

The presence of diabetes mellitus as outlined in Table 4-1 constitutes an important risk factor. The prevalence of this disease increases with age, and by the age group 65-74, at least ten percent of all race and gender groups report having diabetes. Type I diabetes (insulin dependent or juvenile-onset) and Type II (non-insulin dependent or adult onset) result in an elevated blood sugar level (hyperglycemia), either from a pancreatic dysfunction (Type I) or decreased peripheral tissue insensitivity to insulin (Type II). Exercise has been shown to be beneficial in many respects for diabetic patients, particularly Type II. Managing body weight is a critical consideration for the diabetic, and exercise provides an excellent means to attain this goal. The American College of Sports Medicine provides specific guidelines for exercise and diabetes, and these should be carefully adhered to in order to enhance the safety and effectiveness of exercise.

The negative effects of a sedentary lifestyle, relative to premature heart disease, are virtually as powerful as those risk factors previously outlined. Earlier in this chapter, it was noted that recent epidemiological studies have clearly demonstrated the importance of physical activity in the reduction of both heart disease and all-cause mortality. Obviously, exercise directly counters the health risk of a sedentary lifestyle, while indirectly influencing nearly all the other risk factors for chronic disease. The methodologies for exercise programming are well outlined in this book, and, when followed, provide the physiological adaptation necessary to achieve important risk reduction. It is important, however, to keep the concept of *comprehensive* risk reduction in mind. Reducing negative health risk behaviors from a combined program of nutrition, behavior, and exercise intervention is the best insurance against premature chronic disease. The benefits of regular physical activity are illustrated in Table 4-2.

Not listed in Table 4-1 as independent risk factors, but important to consider as negative health risks that contribute significantly to chronic disease are obesity and psychosocial distress. In Table 4-1, it is the position of the American Medical Association that obesity's effects are exerted through other risk factors such as elevated blood pressure, hyperlipidemias, and diabetes. However, obesity should be targeted for intervention, since excess body fat is associated with the myriad of risk factors previously discussed. Research clearly shows that the only effective long-term solution to weight management is a combination of diet and exercise. Chapter 17 addresses the specific topic of exercise and weight control, but the optimal balance between body fat and lean body mass is best brought about by a comprehensive program of sound nutrition and regular exercise that focuses not only on aerobic exercise, but muscular fitness as well.

Table 4-2. Benefits of Regular Physical Activity

1. Improvement in Cardiorespiratory Efficiency

   a. Increased maximal oxygen consumption due to both central and peripheral adaptations.
   b. Lower oxygen cost for a given absolute submaximal workload.
   c. More efficient submaximal cardiovascular responses (lower heart rate and blood pressure).
   d. Increased work threshold for the accumulation of lactate.
   e. Increased work threshold for the onset of disease symptoms (e.g., angina pectoris).

2. Reduction in Coronary Artery Disease Risk Factors

   a. (Modestly) reduced systolic and diastolic pressures.
   b. Increased HDL cholesterol, decreased triglycerides.
   c. Reduced body fatness.
   d. Reduced insulin needs, improved glucose tolerance.

3. Decreased Mortality and Mobidity

   a. Primary Prevention   Lower activity and/or fitness levels are associated with higher death rates from CAD.
   b. Secondary Prevention   No single randomized exercise study has had a sufficient number of patients and duration to demonstrate the protective effects of exercise; however, most randomized trials report a positive effect of exercise on longevity. Meta-analyses (pooled data across studies) involving post myocardial infarction patients provide supportive evidence that a comprehensive cardiac rehabilitation program can reduce premature mortality from cardiovascular events, but probably not non-fatal reactions.

4. Other Postulated Benefits

   a. Decreased anxiety and depression.
   b. Enhanced feelings of well-being.
   c. Enhanced performance of work, recreational, and sports activities.

Adapted from Huhn, R.P. *Cardiopul Phys Ther J* 4(3):4-8, 1993.

Psychosocial distress, as manifested by depression, anger, hostility, and social maladjustments, contributes significantly to chronic disease. As quality research continues to emerge, the importance of this grouping of risk factors increases. While the results of exercise studies are mixed in their effectiveness, it is believed that, in general, exercise provides a mechanism to relieve negative psychological stress and improve many of the markers of psychosocial distress (refer to chapter 10). Clearly, while exercise may play a role in managing this grouping of risk factors, direct intervention as part of a comprehensive health program is needed.

In summary, this chapter has addressed the assessment of health risk factors in chronic disease, specifically heart disease, and the role of exercise in helping to manage these behaviors (refer to Table 4-3). It is important to remember that the nature of risk factors is continually changing, as we gain more information from the scientific literature. The risk factors and their values in 1994 are different than those identified in 1954, and will continue to change. As you assess your risk factor profile, it is critical that you prioritize those controllable factors that may be present, and set about a plan to change them, one at a time. Starting an exercise program lays a great foundation from which to begin a systematic plan of improving your health and reducing disease risk. ❏

Table 4-3. Summary of Results of Studies Investigating the Relationship Between Physical Activity or Physical Fitness and Incidences of Selected Chronic Diseases.

Disease or condition	Number of studies	Trends across activity or fitness categories and strength of evidence
All-cause mortality	***	▼▼▼
Coronary artery disease	***	▼▼▼
Hypertension	**	▼▼
Obesity	***	▼▼
Stroke	**	▼
Peripheral vascular disease	*	►
Cancer		
Colon	***	▼▼
Rectal	***	►
Stomach	*	►
Breast	*	▼
Prostate	**	▼
Lung	*	▼
Pancreatic	*	►
Non-insulin dependent diabetes	*	▼▼
Osteoarthritis	*	►
Osteoporosis	**	▼▼
Functional capability	**	▼▼

*   Few studies, probably less than five; ** several studies, approximately 5-10; *** many (>10) studies.

\#   No apparent difference in disease rates across activity or fitness categories; ▼ some evidence of reduced disease rates across activity or fitness categories; ▼▼ good evidence of reduced disease rates across activity or fitness categories, control of potential confounders, good methods, some evidence of biological mechanisms; ▼▼▼ excellent evidence of reduced disease rates across activity or fitness categories, good control of potential confounders, excellent methods, extensive evidence of biological mechanisms, relationship is considered causal.

BIBLIOGRAPHY •••••••••••••••••••••••••••••••••••••••

1. American College of Sports Medicine. *Guidelines for Exercise Testing and Prescription*, 4th Ed. Philadelphia, PA: Lea & Febiger, 1991.
2. American Heart Association. *1991 Heart and Stroke Facts*. Dallas, TX, 1991.
3. Blair, S.N., Kohl, H.W., Gordon, N.F., Paffenbarger, R.S. "How much physical activity is good for health?" *Annu Rev Publ Health* 13:99-126, 1992.
4. Centers for Disease Control and Prevention. *Cardiovascular Disease Surveillance: Ischemic Heart Disease*, 1980-1989. Issued 1993.
5. Hadden, W.C., Harris, M.I. Prevalence of diagnosed diabetes, undiagnosed diabetes and impaired glucose intolerance in adults 20-74 years of age, United States, 1976-1980. Vital and Health Statistics, Series II. No. 237 DHHS Publ. No. (PHS) 87-1687. DHHS, Washington, DC, 1987.
6. Huhn, R.P. "Cardiac rehabilitation in the cost containment environment." *Cardiopul Phys Ther J* 4(3):4-8,1993.
7. Lipid Research Clinics Program: The Lipid Research Coronary Primary Prevention Trial Results, II. "The relationship of reduction in incidence of coronary heart disease to cholesterol lowering." *JAMA* 251:365, 1984.
8. Ornish, D., Brown, SE, Scherwitz, L.W., Billings, J.H., et al. "Can lifestyle changes reverse coronary heart disease?" *Lancet* 336:129-133, 1990.
9. Powell, K.E., Thompson, P.D., Casperson, C.J., Kendrick, J.S. "Physical activity and the incidence of coronary heart disease." *Annu Rev Publ Health* 8:253-287, 1987.
10. Shaper, A.G., Wannamethec, G. "Physical activity and ischaemic heart disease in middle-aged British men." *Br Heart J* 66:384-394, 1991.
11. Steinfeld, B. "Cancer and the protective effect of physical activity: The epidemiological evidence." *Med Sci Sports Exerc* 24(11):1195-1209, 1992.
12. Summary of the second report of the NCEP expert panel on detection, evaluation, and treatment of high blood cholesterol in adults. *JAMA* 269:3015-3023, 1993.
13. Williams, M. *Exercise Testing and Training in the Elderly Cardiac Patient*. Champaign, IL: Human Kinetics, 1994.

CHAPTER 5

UNDERSTANDING GRADED EXERCISE TESTING

by

George J. Holland, Ph.D.
and
Steven F. Loy, Ph.D.

• • •

*O*nce you reach a decision to start exercising, your physician may recommend that you undergo a graded exercise test (GXT) before you begin your exercise regimen, a procedure which is commonly referred to as an exercise stress test. Such a recommendation from your physician may raise a number of questions in your mind regarding a GXT: What does a GXT involve? Why should you undergo a GXT? Is it safe? What information does it provide? Etc. This chapter addresses the aforementioned questions and other relevant issues concerning graded exercise testing in an attempt to remove much of the confusion and mystery that sometimes surrounds this increasingly utilized evaluative procedure.*

WHAT A GXT INVOLVES

A GXT can be administered in a variety of locations, including a physician's office, at a hospital, or at a professionally supervised health and fitness facility. Regardless of where a GXT is administered, special equipment to handle any medical emergency that may arise and a sufficient number of appropriately trained professionals must be present. According to the guidelines established by the American Heart Association (AHA), all individuals who administer GXTs should be trained in cardiopulmonary resuscitation (CPR), and at least one of the technicians in the testing area should also be trained and certified in advanced cardiac life support. Also, in accordance with AHA guidelines, a physician should be on the premises (i.e., in the building) at all times.

---

* Individuals interested in obtaining information concerning the administration of a GXT should refer to the bibliography for this chapter.

To prepare for a GXT, you should abstain from food, tobacco, alcohol and caffeine for a minimum of three hours before your test—since all of these substances affect your physiological responses to exercise. In addition, you should wear comfortable shoes (e.g., sneakers, walking shoes, etc.) and loose-fitting clothes (e.g., a t-shirt and gym shorts). If you are a woman, it is advisable that you wear a loose-fitting blouse that (preferably) buttons down the front—this permits easier attachment of the ECG electrodes. Women, undergoing a GXT, should not wear nylon bras (since nylon material tends to interfere with the ECG tracings).

Prior to the start of a GXT, a resting electrocardiogram (ECG) is performed to check for cardiac abnormalities that exist in the absence of "stress" and to provide a basis for comparison with your physiological responses during the exercise session. Both resting blood pressure and heart rate are assessed and monitored throughout a GXT. Electrodes (sensors) are placed on your chest during a resting ECG. These sensors remain in place during a GXT, so that the rhythm and electrical activity of your heart can be monitored continuously. At rest, an ECG may indicate that your heart is receiving adequate amounts of blood and oxygen, but when you're stressed (i.e., during exercise), an ECG may reveal signs that your heart is receiving insufficient amounts of blood and oxygen.

A variety of modalities (e.g., a treadmill, a stationary cycle, a stair climbing machine, etc.) can be used to provide the exercise stress. The motor-driven treadmill is the device most commonly used in the United States for graded exercise testing. In general, a GXT initially involves placing a relatively low level of exercise-induced stress on your cardiovascular system. Subsequent increases in work demand are then gradually incorporated into the exercise protocol that you are required to perform by raising either the speed or grade (incline) of the treadmill. Because the goal of a GXT is simply to determine the capability limits of your cardiovascular system, you need not worry about the treadmill reaching "warp" speed or being raised to a grade that simulates Mount Everest.

Two different types of GXTs can be administered. One is referred to as a symptom-limited maximal GXT and the other as a submaximal GXT. The symptom-limited maximal GXT is the more common of the two types of GXTs and involves the progressive increase of the exercise intensity until you display signs or symptoms of exertional intolerance. The submaximal GXT, on the other hand, progressively increases the level of exercise intensity until you reach some predetermined end point (e.g., 85% of your maximum heart rate) or until a sign or symptom of exertional intolerance occurs before the end point has been reached.

WHO SHOULD HAVE A STRESS TEST?

The current guidelines of AHA indicate that if you are under age 40 (male and female) and undergo a normal physical examination, which indicates no symptoms of cardiovascular disease, no major coronary risk factors, no physical findings (including murmurs and hypertension), you can be considered free of disease and do not require GXT before undertaking a new exercise regimen. If you are 40 years of age or older, have had an abnormal physical examination (murmurs, etc.) or possess two or more coronary risk factors, you should have a GXT before embarking on a vigorous exercise program (refer to Table 4-1 for a listing of the coronary risk factors).

In guidelines recently revised by the American College of Sports Medicine (ACSM), a GXT is not recommended prior to initiation of an exercise program if you are an asymptomatic male 40 years or younger, or female 50 years or younger. If you are an older asymptomatic adult (males 40 plus, females 50 plus), you may initiate a moderate exercise regimen (intensity 40-60% $\dot{V}O_{2\,max}$) without a GXT. A GXT is recommended for all older adults planning a vigorous exercise program (intensity greater than 60% $\dot{V}O_{2\,max}$).

The ACSM uses the same criteria of two or more major coronary risk factors as the basis for recommending a GXT prior to an individual's beginning an exercise program. Gradual moderate exercise is, however, permitted without a GXT for individuals without coronary artery disease (CAD) symptoms, but with two or more CAD risk factors. Individuals with two or more risk factors, but without symptoms, should undergo a GXT before vigorous exercise. The ACSM recommendations regarding who should be required to take a GXT and the attendant level of requisite supervision are outlined in chapter 3.

How Safe Is A GXT?

Like most medical procedures, a GXT is not without some risk. The risk can be minimized by proper screening and by having the test administered by properly trained personnel. As stated previously, personnel involved in conducting a GXT should be thoroughly familiar with the equipment and trained to handle emergency situations should they arise. Although untoward events (e.g., heart attacks) are well publicized, they are extremely rare (less than one per every 500 symptom-limited GXTs). The risk of a fatal clinical complication is much lower (less than 1 in 10,000).

What Information Does A GXT Provide?

In the early stages of CAD, individuals usually do not exhibit symptoms of coronary insufficiency, while either at rest or during nonstrenuous activity. During exercise, however, signs or symptoms of CAD often become manifest, as the demands for oxygen increase beyond what the diseased arteries can supply. If the oxygen demand and supply imbalance is relatively large, it can cause anginal chest pain—a hallmark sign of CAD. Smaller oxygen imbalances can cause changes in heart rate, blood pressure, and heart rhythm and may elicit changes on the ECG. An abnormal ECG during a GXT is only suggestive that a cardiac problem is present since the results of such tests are not always accurate. Approximately 16% of GXTs result in false positives (i.e., the test erroneously indicates that an individual has heart disease). Unfortunately, a higher proportion (34%) of false negative (i.e., the test incorrectly indicates that an individual is free of heart disease) GXT results occur. Accordingly, when evaluating your test results, your physician will consider all of the following: how long and through what stage you exercised, what your heart rate and blood pressure responses were, whether any rhythm disturbances of heart occurred and when they occurred, whether any ECG abnormalities appeared, and how you looked and felt.

AFTER THE GXT

Once you have taken a GXT, you should discuss the results with your doctor. If no problems are discovered, the information obtained from the GXT should be used to help design an appropriate exercise program for your specific goals, needs, interests, and fitness level. Should your physician feel that your stress test was not accurate, or was inconclusive, he or she may recommend a thallium exercise stress test* in order to improve diagnostic accuracy.

Remember, it is impossible to "flunk" a GXT. If a problem is detected, it is much better to identify it in the controlled setting of your physician's office, a hospital, an exercise science laboratory, or a medically supervised health and fitness club than in your own home. Finally, no matter who you are, you can benefit from participating in an exercise program based on the information obtained from a properly conducted GXT. ❏

BIBLIOGRAPHY •

1. American College of Cardiology/American Heart Association. "Guidelines for exercise testing." *Am J Cardiol* 8:725-738, 1986.
2. American College of Sports Medicine. *Guidelines for Graded Exercise Testing and Prescription*, 4th Ed. Philadelphia, PA: Lea & Febiger, 1991.
3. American College of Sports Medicine. *Resource Manual for Graded Exercise Testing and Prescription*, 2nd Ed. Philadelphia, PA: Lea & Febiger, 1988.
4. American Heart Association. "Exercise standards." *Circulation* 82:2286-2322, 1990.
5. Ellestad, M.H. *Stress Testing: Principles and Practice*, 3rd Ed. Philadelphia, PA: F. A. Davis Company, 1986.
6. Foster, C. "Stress testing: Directions for the future." *Sports Med* 6:11-22, 1988.
7. Franklin, B.A., Gordon, S., Timmis, G.C. (Eds). *Exercise in Modern Medicine*. Baltimore, MD: Williams & Wilkins, 1989.
8. Froelicher, V.F. *Exercise and the Heart: Clinical Concepts*. Chicago, IL: Year Book Publishers, 1987.

---

* A radioactive dye (thallium-201) is injected into your arm, and its passage is traced through your heart during a graded exercise test to more definitively determine if CAD is present, and if so, to what degree of severity. For more information on thallium exercise stress testing, refer to items 3, 6, 13, and 15 in the bibliography.

9.   Froelicher, V.F. *Exercise Testing and Training*. Chicago, IL: Year Book Publishers, Inc., 1983.

10.   Gibbons, L., Blair, S.N., Kohl, H.W., et al. "The safety of maximal exercise testing." *Circulation* 80:846-854, 1989.

11.   Holland, G.J., Heng, M.K., Weber, F. "Exercise testing for asymptomatic adults." *Cardiovasc Rev Reports* 9(6):38-40, 1988.

12.   Holland, G.J., Hoffman, J.J., Vincent, W., et al. "Treadmill vs. Steptreadmill ergometry." *Phys Sportsmed* 18:79-85, 1990.

13.   Holland, G.J., Weber, F., Weng, M.K., et al. "Maximal steptreadmill exercise and treadmill exercise by patients with coronary heart disease: A comparison." *J Cardiopul Rehabil* 8:58-68, 1988.

14.   Iskandrian, A.S., Wasserman, L.A., Anderson, G.S., et al. "Merits of stress thallium-201 myocardial perfusion imaging in patients with inconclusive exercise electrocardiograms: Correlation with coronary arteriograms." *Am J Cardiol* 46:553-558, 1980.

15.   Pollock, M.L., Wilmore, J.H. *Exercise in Health and Disease: Evaluation and Prescription for Prevention and Rehabilitation,* 2nd Ed. Philadelphia, PA: W. B. Saunders Company, 1990.

16.   Ritchie, J.L., Trobaugh, G.B., Hamilton, G.W., et al. "Myocardial imaging with thallium-201 at rest and during exercise: Comparison with coronary arteriography and resting and stress electrocardiography." *Circulation* 56:66-71, 1977.

17.   Skinner, J.S. (Ed). *Exercise Testing and Exercise Prescription for Special Cases*. Philadelphia, PA: Lea & Febiger, 1987.

CHAPTER 6

•••••••••••••••••••••••••••••••••

LEGAL CONSIDERATIONS FOR GRADED EXERCISE TESTING AND EXERCISE PRESCRIPTION[*]

by
David L. Herbert, Esq.
and
William G. Herbert, Ph.D.

• • •

As was discussed in chapter 5, graded exercise (stress) testing (GXTs) procedures are assessment techniques which are widely used for a variety of purposes. In general, the two main uses of GXTs involve exercise testing and exercise prescription. Medical professionals, for example, have traditionally employed GXTs to diagnose the status of individuals with known or suspected coronary heart disease. In fact, the use of exercise stress testing procedures within the medical provider section has grown dramatically in the past few years. The rise in the popularity of GXTs within the medical community is reinforced by recent statistics which indicate that GXTs are currently used by medical personnel as a prognostic indicator for almost half of all acute heart patients.[1]

The use of GXTs to provide much of the basis for exercise prescription has also grown in popularity in recent years. Prescribing exercise based on a thorough analysis of baseline GXT results is frequently employed for relatively healthy individuals with a primary interest in fitness, as well as for individuals with a medically related condition.

The sharp increase in the use of GXTs has also given rise to a number of rather significant legal issues associated with such evaluative practices. These issues

---

[*] Note: This chapter is focused specifically for those professionals involved in conducting graded exercise testing or prescribing exercise. Individuals with a general interest in fitness, however, may find this information enlightening.

[1] " *TRENDS*, "Dramatic Increase in Diagnostic Testing for MI Patients Reported," *THE EXERCISE STANDARDS & MALPRACTICE REPORTED* 2(2):28, 1988.

center upon: (1) the relative safety of stress testing procedures; (2) the propriety of non-physician personnel carrying out such procedures; and (3) the legal risks associated with the performance of these tests.

SAFETY CONCERNS ASSOCIATED WITH TESTING

In 1971, the results of a large-scale study of exercise stress testing procedures were reported by P. Rochmis and H. Blackburn.[2] An analysis of the results of this study, as well as other studies that have been conducted since, indicate a rather low incidence of serious risk associated with GXT procedures (approximately one-half to one in 10,000 tests).

Most individuals within the medical community consider GXTs to be relatively safe, especially when supervised by a physician. Many individuals also believe that these tests may be carried out by appropriately trained/certified non-physicians.[3] Some professionals, however, feel that GXTs should only be conducted or supervised under the direction of a physician.[4] The preliminary results of a recently completed analysis of a twelve-year study of more than 41,000 GXTs indicates that specifically trained non-physicians may safely perform GXTs, at least in a hospital setting.[5]

Prescribing exercise on the basis of GXT results can involve a myriad of safety concerns. Each of the concerns is inextricably related, in many instances, to how well the GXT is administered and how accurately the GXT results are interpreted. Improper exercise prescription or exercise prescription without the development of adequate baseline information can result in participant injury and even death. Unfortunately, the diverse settings within which exercise prescriptions are developed are not (as a rule) offered the opportunity for uniform statistics to be compiled regarding the safety of specific prescriptions for particular patient populations. Medico-legal fact patterns have arisen, however, which should provide an appropriate basis for examining and better understanding the GXT safety issues involving exercise prescription, as well as testing procedures.

---

[2] "Exercise Tests: A Survey of Procedures, Safety and Litigation Experience in Approximately 170,000 Tests," *JAMA* 217:1061-1066, 1971.

[3] *BLESSEY*, "Exercise Testing By Non-Physician Health Care Professionals: Complication Rates, Clinical Competencies and Future Trends," *THE EXERCISE STANDARDS AND MALPRACTICE REPORTER.*

[4] *GIBBONS M.D.*, "Editorial - The Safety of Maximal Exercise Testing," *J. CARDIOPUL REHABIL* 7:277, 1987.

[5] *NEWS & REPORTS*, "New Study: Specially Trained Non-Physicians Can Safely Supervise GXTs," *THE EXERCISE STANDARDS AND MALPRACTICE REPORTER* 5(1):10, 1991.

LEGAL CONSIDERATIONS

• • •

The Practice And Unauthorized Practice of Medicine

The practice of medicine is universally regulated by state licensing laws defining the practice, specifying who may conduct the activities and under what circumstances.[6] Those individuals who engage in such activities without proper licensure run the risk of being charged with the crime of the unauthorized practice of medicine (generally a misdemeanor), as well as having their conduct, in the event of some untoward event and suit, judged in accordance with the standard of care for those practicing medicine, Id. Non-physicians cannot escape such a comparison without having liability attached to their conduct.

In the exercise field, many potential concerns arise that are related to the unauthorized practice of medicine. This situation is particularly true for testing procedures and exercise prescriptions. Generally, if GXTs are carried out within a medical setting and for medically related purposes, or if a prescription of exercise is provided for the treatment of a disease, condition, or infirmity, then nearly universal agreement exists that those carrying out such procedures are engaged in the practice of medicine. In the event that such procedures are carried out for non-medical purposes in a non-health care setting (e.g., for fitness assessment evaluations and/or by non-medical personnel), then in all likelihood, such procedures are not medical in nature. It is in those areas, between these two extremes, that questions and potential legal concerns arise. These concerns are complicated by the diversity of state laws and administrative regulations impacting the practice of medicine and other allied health care professions.

The State of North Carolina Medical Examiners, for example, issued a statement in June 1987 declaring: "When a non-physician administers a graded exercise test, the standard of care in North Carolina is that a physician is to be in the room or the immediate area.[7]" Obviously, expressions of concern similar to this one can raise significant legal issues as to who can properly conduct GXTs, and under what circumstances.

Little doubt exists that the debate regarding the propriety of a non-physician performing GXTs and/or prescribing physical activity is certain to continue for the foreseeable future. Concurrently, it is also reasonably certain that this debate will continue to be impacted by a variety of statements from a myriad of prominent professional associations. These statements concerning the applicable standards of practice will impact the provision of service and may affect court interpretation of state legislative practice statutes and regulations. The interrelationship of these laws and professional practice standards are brought into sharp focus in various court proceedings dealing with issues related to informed consent, negligence and malpractice. A comprehensive examination of these issues points out the potential

---

6 *HERBERT & HERBERT, LEGAL ASPECTS OF PREVENTIVE AND REHABILITATIVE EXERCISE PROGRAMS*, 2nd Ed., 113-144 (Professional Reports Corporation, Canton, Ohio, 1989).

7 *TRENDS*, "Physician Must be Present For Administration of Graded Exercise Tests," *THE EXERCISE STANDARDS & MALPRACTICE REPORTER* 1(5):75, 1987.

legal factors that should be considered, either when administering GXTs or when prescribing exercise.

INFORMED CONSENT

The law of informed consent requires—among other things—that every patient be informed of the material and relevant risks associated with any contemplated medical procedure, before the procedure is commenced. In quasi-medical or non-medical settings, the medical doctrine of informed consent may or may not apply. Some form of consent, however, will always be required for any procedure involving human clients.

In both the settings involving either the testing of exercise subjects or the provision of exercise prescriptions, the law has impacted the informed consent process. For example, in the 1985 case of Hedgecorth v. United States,[8] an elderly patient underwent a physician-supervised GXT at a VA hospital. He had a significant adverse medical history and had recently undergone another GXT procedure at another facility, the results of which were not obtained by the VA hospital. While he underwent a pre-test informed consent process, no disclosures as to either risk of stroke or blindness due to stroke were disclosed to him by his physicians. During the test, he suffered a stroke and later blindness due to the stroke. He and his wife subsequently brought suit contending that the physicians were negligent in their provision of information to him and that the consent process was thus void, rendering the physicians liable for all adverse consequences which occurred related to the procedure. A jury returned a verdict of nearly one million dollars to the patient and his wife. While the risk of stroke and the resultant risk of blindness due to stroke associated with GXT procedures must be considered minute, the case has resulted in a "rethinking" of the informed consent process for such procedures. In fact, it may have provided the impetus for the recent decision of the American College of Sports Medicine (ACSM) to revise its recommended informed consent disclosure form to include the risk of stroke.[9]

In another GXT-related informed consent case, a plaintiff's estate brought suit contending that the physician did not disclose the risk of death to the decedent and, as a consequence, the consent was void, rendering the physician liable for the untoward event which occurred after the test.[10] Despite these contentions, a jury returned a defense verdict upon the estate's lawsuit. A subsequent appeal

---

[8] Hedgecorth v. United States, 618 F. Suppl. 627 (E. D. Mo. 1985), analyzed in *HERBERT*, "Informed Consent Documents For Stress Testing To Comport With Hedgecorth v. United States," *THE EXERCISE STANDARDS AND MALPRACTICE REPORTER* 1(6):81-88, 1987.

[9] HERBERT, "Sample Informed Consent Forms From the AHA, AACVPR and the ACSM," *THE EXERCISE STANDARDS AND MALPRACTICE REPORTER* 5(1):7-8, 1991.

[10] Smogor v. Enke, 874 F. 2d 295 (5th Cir. 1989), analyzed in *HERBERT*, "Exercise Stress Testing Lawsuit Results in Defense Verdict," *THE EXERCISE STANDARDS AND MALPRACTICE REPORTER* 4(2):23-24, 1990.

resulted in a finding that a written informed consent form had been signed by the decedent which specifically "informed him of the risk of death."[11] Consequently, the defense verdict was upheld. Quite a different result could have occurred had no such statement been contained within the informed consent document. Sample informed consent forms for GXT procedures which do not utilize full disclosures including the risk of stroke and death in addition to other more traditional risks, should be viewed with cautious circumspection.[12]

The informed consent doctrine also impacts the prescription process. Risks associated with prescribed activities should be reviewed and discussed with patients prior to providing advice as to particular exercise. Shortcomings in this area can lead to significant litigation. For example, in the Utah case of Mikkelsen v. Haslam,[13] the plaintiff, who was affected with a congenitally dislocated right hip, sought physician advice and recommendation as to her condition. She subsequently underwent a total hip replacement and a period of rehabilitation. She contended that her physician eventually endorsed her participation in snow skiing. Later, during her participation in the activity, she fractured her femur and fell. Evidence indicated that the injury was due to a deteriorating condition of the bone. She subsequently brought suit contending that the physician was negligent in his provision of advice. The issues raised in the case will ultimately be decided by a jury trial.[14]

In another case, Contino v. Lucille Roberts Health Spa,[15] a chiropractor prescribed aerobic dance exercise for a back patient. She subsequently sought spa membership to engage in the recommended activity. She fell while doing the activity and later brought suit against the facility contending she was injured due to overcrowding, improper supervision, and negligent leadership. The facility joined the chiropractor who prescribed the activity in the litigation. In considering the chiropractor's potential liability, the court determined that the pleadings in the case set forth an "ample basis" for prescriber liability based upon the allegation that the chiropractor's advice was negligent.[16]

A number of other cases involving GXT procedures and the prescription of exercise, but not entailing factors specifically related to informed consent, should

---

[11] Smoger v. Enke, p. 297.

[12] HERBERT, "Sample Informed Consent Forms From the AHA, AACVPR and the ACSM," supra.

[13] Mikkelsen v. Haslam, 764 p. 2d 1384, 1988.

[14] "Provider's Alleged Advice To Ski May Result In Liability," THE EXERCISE STANDARDS AND MALPRACTICE REPORTER 4(1):13-14, 1990.

[15] Contino v. Lucille Roberts Health Spa, 509 NYS 2d 369 (A.D. 2 Dept. 1986).

[16] LITIGATION AND COURT RULINGS, "Chiropractor's Advice To Patient To Take Aerobic Dance Class May Be Negligent," THE EXERCISE STANDARDS AND MALPRACTICE REPORTER 1(3):45-47, 1987.

also be considered. These cases, while not subject to common classification, deal with issues of negligence and malpractice.

Negligence And Malpractice

Negligence is generally regarded as a failure to govern one's conduct to a generally accepted standard or duty. A cause of action upon the basis of negligence is established upon proof of DUTY, BREACH OF DUTY, PROXIMATELY CAUSING HARM/DAMAGE TO ANOTHER. Such a cause of action may be based upon a substandard act or an omission to act. Malpractice is simply negligence committed in the course and scope of a professional, patient/client relationship.

For GXT and exercise prescription procedures, a number of issues and cases dealing with negligence/malpractice have arisen. Examining these issues and cases can lead to a better understanding of the legal factors associated with same. In the "classic" exercise testing case of Tart v. McGann,[17] the patient/plaintiff underwent a physician-supervised GXT procedure as part of his regular physical process to maintain his commercial airline pilot's license. During the fourth stage of the test, the plaintiff pilot testified that he began to feel tired and fatigued, but in light of the physician's encouragement, continued on with the test. After completing the test, he suffered a heart attack and brought suit contending that the physician should have terminated the test due to his outward but nonverbalized manifestations of fatigue.

Of particular importance during the jury trial was the question of the duty of the physician to stop the test in light of the pilot's facial expressions of fatigue. While expert testimony differed on the physician's duty to terminate the test under such circumstances, the standards of the American Heart Association (AHA) were used to "judge" provider conduct in the case. Although a defense verdict was eventually rendered, the plaintiff received a substantial settlement. Thereafter, the provider population began to grapple with the issue of physician obligation to stop such procedures based upon evaluations of the patient's level of fatigue and distress.[18]

In other GXT-related cases, negligence/malpractice claims have been put forth dealing with a variety of issues, including improper placement of electrocardiographic leads, allegedly resulting in missed ST-segment changes,[19] falls from

---

[17] Tart v. McGann, 697 F. 2d 75 (2d Cir. 1982).

[18] EDELMAN, "The Case of Tart vs. McCann: Legal Implications Associated With Exercise Stress Testing," THE EXERCISE STANDARDS AND MALPRACTICE REPORTER 1(2):21-26, 1987.

[19] Kolodney v. U.S., U.S. Dist. Ct., Maryland, 1975, CIVIL CASE NO. M-74-108.

treadmills, or inappropriate supervision or instruction as to their use. [20],[21],[22]

One of the most significant cases of alleged negligence dealing with the prescription of physical activity involves a California malpractice arbitration case focusing upon the death of a patient, Ricardo Camerena. Mr. Camerena was a 40-year-old patient who sought a physical examination and clearance prior to starting an exercise program. While he was given a physical, a resting electrocardiogram and blood tests, no GXT was performed. Following completion of this examination no restrictions were placed upon his activities. He died shortly thereafter while jogging, due to a heart attack.

His estate subsequently brought a claim against the physician contending that the physician was negligent in not conducting a GXT to screen him for silent ischemia prior to the decedent's commencement of activity. The arbitration panel ruled in favor of the estate and awarded the family $500,000.00. The plaintiff's lawyer subsequently claimed that the case stood for the proposition that **all** men 40 years of age or older required a GXT prior to beginning such activities. Some practitioners have contended that such testing is now a necessary defensive medicare tactic.[23] While such contentions have been strongly contested by some individual practitioners in the medical profession[24] and questioned by some subsequent statements of professional societies,[25] the substantial possibility always exists for such claims to be brought upon the prescription of activity which is not preceded and based upon the results and interpretation of a properly conducted and performed GXT.[26]

Negligence/malpractice cases are greatly affected by statements of professional associations. These statements, oftentimes referred to as standards, parameters of practice, or guidelines, can impact the provision of service, as well as the

---

[20] Figure World v. Farley, 680 S.W. 2d 33 (Tex. App. 3 Dist. 1986), analyzed in *LITIGATION AND COURT RULINGS:* "Participant Injuries Suffered While On Jogging Treadmill Can Be Facility's Responsibility," *THE EXERCISE STANDARDS AND MALPRACTICE REPORTER* 1(4) 161, 1987.

[21] Malkiewicz v. Overlia, No. 470493 (1987), *LITIGATION AND COURT RULINGS*, "Treadmill Fall Results In Defense Verdict," *THE EXERCISE STANDARDS AND MALPRACTICE REPORTER* 2(2):30, 1988.

[22] Tucker v. Trotter Treadmills, Inc., 779 P. 2d 524 (Mont. 1989), *LITIGATION AND COURT RULINGS*, "Suit Against Treadmill Manufacturer Dismissed," *THE EXERCISE STANDARDS AND MALPRACTICE REPORTER* 4(1):11-12, 1990.

[23] *KEIFETZ AND WATKINS*, "Routine Stress Tests Now Defensive Tactic," *MEDICAL TRENDS* 30(14):1, 8 (1989).

[24] *ASSEY*, "Screening for Silent Myocardial Ischemia," *AFB* 38(6):13-146, 1988.

[25] *AHA/ACC/ACP*, "Clinical Competence In Exercise Testing," *CIRCULATION* 82(5):1884-1888, 1990.

[26] *LITIGATION AND COURT RULES*: "Are GXTs Required For Screening Of All Men Over 40?," *THE EXERCISE STANDARDS AND MALPRACTICE REPORTER* 2(2):30, 1988.

outcome of negligence/malpractice suits. As a result, they must be considered within the scope of any review of this subject.

STANDARDS OF PRACTICE

The provision of services through GXT procedures or by way of exercise prescription is greatly affected by the written expression of the standard of care for these services. Standards of practice for these services have been developed and promulgated by the ACSM and the AHA, as well as the American Association for Cardiovascular and Pulmonary Rehabilitation (AACVPR), and the American College of Cardiology (ACC), as well as several other professional associations and groups—all of which impose written expressions as to the standard of care.[27],[28],[29],[30] While each set of standards may be written to one degree or another by reference to a particular perspective, each greatly impacts the delivery of service, as well as the standard of care, owed to various patient populations. New standards have been developed by almost all of these organizations as of early 1991. Professionals practicing in these areas must be familiar with these standards and the developing effect of these standards on the provision of related services.

CONCLUSION

Legal concerns abound for those delivering exercise testing or prescription services. A familiarization with the legal concerns associated with these procedures as well as the standards of practice which impact same, can only assist the practitioner in avoiding patient/participant injury and claim, in addition to helping preclude a conflict with the legal system. Providers must stay abreast of professional developments in relevant areas and become familiar with what is expected of them in the course of carrying out their duties and responsibilities toward their patient population. Anything less may result in patient injury or death, and concomitant claims and suits. ❏

---

[27] ACSM, *GUIDELINES FOR EXERCISE TESTING AND PRESCRIPTION*, 4TH ED. (Philadelphia, PA: Lea & Febiger, 1991).

[28] AHA: Fletcher, et al., "Exercise Standards: A Statement for Health Professionals From the American Heart Association," *CIRCULATION* 82(6):2286-2322, 1990.

[29] AACVPR: *GUIDELINES FOR CARDIAC REHABILITATION PROGRAMS* (Champaign, IL: Human Kinetics, 1991).

[30] ACC: "Recommendations of the American College of Cardiology on Cardiovascular Rehabilitation," *CARDIOLOGY* 15(2):4-5, March 1986.

CHAPTER 7

•••••••••••••••••••••••••••••

UNDERSTANDING THE PHYSIOLOGICAL BASIS OF CARDIORESPIRATORY FITNESS*

by

James S. Skinner, Ph.D.

•••

Muscles involved in exercise produce a significant amount of energy by combining foodstuffs with oxygen. As the oxygen needs of your exercising muscles increase, your lungs supply more oxygen to the blood, perfusing them. Your heart, in turn, pumps more oxygenated blood to your working muscles. If a steady supply of oxygen is not produced to meet the energy demands of the activity, then an energy imbalance develops, blood lactate (LA) levels rise, blood pH decreases, and fatigue occurs. Your ability to engage in sustained high levels of physical activity without significant fatigue is determined by your body's ability to deliver oxygenated blood to your muscles, and the ability of your muscles to extract the oxygen from the blood and utilize it for the production of energy in the form of adenosine triphosphate (ATP). If you're really interested in having a fundamental knowledge of how your body works during different types of exercise, you need to understand both the basic concepts of energy production and the physiological adjustments made by your body to meet the increased energy requirements of exercising skeletal muscles.

BASIC CONCEPTS OF ENERGY AND ITS SOURCES

The energy that is required for the normal functioning (muscle contraction, conduction of nervous impulses, hormone synthesis, etc.) of every living cell in your body is produced by chemical reactions. These chemical reactions are either

---

*Note: Some of the material contained in this chapter is adapted from *Body Energy* by James S. Skinner, 1981 (Anderson World Inc., Mountain View, CA).

aerobic (occurring in the presence of oxygen) or anaerobic (without oxygen). You must continually produce energy or the various tissues and organs in your body will cease to function. It would be akin to pulling out the plug of an electric appliance.

To clarify the relationship between food consumption and energy production, you should think of your body as a factory. It must process different raw materials to make its final product—energy. This energy is used by every cell of your body. The three basic raw materials your body uses to produce energy are oxygen, carbohydrates (sugar and starches) and fat. These materials essentially are available in an unlimited supply. Since we live in a veritable sea of oxygen, an adequate supply is generally not a problem. When you eat food, you replenish the other raw materials your body needs to produce energy.

Under normal circumstances, your body does not directly use protein for energy production. Proteins provide much of the structural basis for cells and are a major component of enzymes (substances responsible for controlling various chemical reactions at the cellular level). If you consume more protein than your body needs, the excess will be converted into fat or carbohydrate.

Since the amount of energy required at rest is so small, your body doesn't consume much oxygen. Accordingly, your resting energy needs are easily met by your aerobic system. During the initial stages of exercise, however, the situation changes. When the work demands placed on your body increase, your body needs extra energy immediately. Unfortunately, the rate of aerobic energy production is sluggish (i.e., oxygen must be breathed in, transferred from your lungs to the blood, carried to your heart and then pumped to your muscles where it actually is needed). Thus, a delay exists in the delivery of oxygen from the outside. If a sudden demand for more energy arises, an emergency back-up system must exist that will permit your body to function until the aerobic "assembly line" speeds up its production. The anaerobic energy system serves this function.

A given amount of work requires a given amount of energy. The following descriptive time table illustrates how energy is produced during the initial stages of exercise and during mild exercise.

- When exercise first starts, only a limited supply of energy is present in the muscle for immediate use—during this phase, oxygen is not required.
- Either glycogen stored in the muscle or glucose transported by the blood from the liver can be used without oxygen to provide a limited supply of energy. Lactic acid is the by-product of this anaerobic reaction.
- Most of the lactic acid formed during an anaerobic reaction is released into the blood and transported to the liver, where it is converted back to glycogen and stored.
- As additional oxygen becomes available, the aerobic system is used more and more. After a few minutes, the aerobic system is able to supply all the energy needed for mild exercise.

- At this time, liver glycogen is converted to glucose and released into the blood to provide fuel for both systems (aerobic and anaerobic).
- Finally, adipocytes (fat cells) release more and more fat, the preferred fuel for the aerobic system.

If the exercise bout is intense, other events take place to ensure that adequate amounts of energy are provided for your working skeletal muscles. The production of energy during exercise of high intensity occurs as follows:

- The speed of the aerobic reactions increases to provide more energy— more carbon dioxide is also produced.
- The faster anaerobic system supplies increasing amounts of energy as the exercise becomes more intense. The intensity of the muscle contractions causes a compression of the small arteries and no oxygen, glucose or fat can enter the muscle cell. Thus, the majority of the carbohydrate needed comes from that which is already stored within the muscle itself.
- Eventually, more lactic acid is formed and increased amounts of lactic acid are released into the bloodstream. As lactic acid levels within the muscle increase, the efficiency of the aerobic chemical reactions are inhibited. When this occurs, inadequate amounts of energy can be produced aerobically. Accordingly, you have to either slow down (reduce the amount of energy needed) or rely more heavily on your anaerobic system.
- Only a small percentage of lactic acid is transformed back into glycogen in the liver; the majority remains in the blood and the muscles. Your body can accumulate and tolerate a limited amount of lactic acid. In all likelihood, it is the presence of lactic acid that causes you to breathe excessively, experience feelings of fatigue and heaviness in your muscles and forces you eventually to stop exercising.

To better understand the relative importance of the anaerobic and aerobic systems for energy production, refer to Figure 7-1. This figure provides an approximate idea of the maximal amount of energy a well-trained individual can produce over time, and how that energy is produced. For comparison purposes, the energy required at rest is given a value of one.

Although the stored energy can be used very rapidly, and individuals can perform a lot of work, these stockpiles are essentially exhausted after ten to twenty seconds. This partially explains why individuals cannot run 400 meters as fast as they can 100 meters, or why weight lifters can lift more in one lift than they can in three lifts without a pause.

The production of energy anaerobically is relatively high, peaking at around 40 to 50 seconds. It doesn't last long because you are limited by your body's tolerance of lactic acid. After 10 minutes, the amount of energy produced by this mechanism is very small.

After five to six minutes of continuous exercise, the majority of energy your body requires has to be produced aerobically. The longer the duration of exercise, the greater the importance of the aerobic system. Anything over ten minutes has to be performed aerobically, except for occasional, brief increases in work output.

Table 7-1. Relative importance of various energy-producing systems over time.

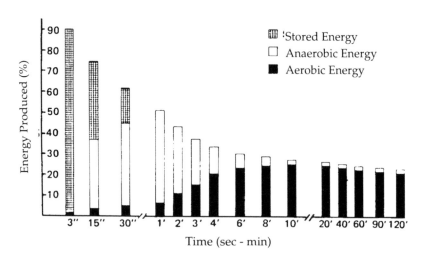

Used with permission from Body Energy by James S. Skinner, 1981 (Anderson World Inc., Mountain View, CA).

MAXIMAL OXYGEN UPTAKE

If you increase the intensity of exercise, a number of things happen in your body. A rise occurs in heart rate, respiration, and oxygen intake, as well as in the activity levels of other parts of your oxygen delivery and utilization (aerobic) systems. A point occurs, however, beyond which oxygen intake cannot increase, even though more work is being performed. At this point, you have reached a level that is commonly referred to as maximal oxygen uptake ($\dot{V}O_{2\ max}$). This is considered to be the best single indicator of cardiorespiratory fitness, since it involves the optimal ability of three major systems (pulmonary, cardiovascular, and muscular) of your body to take in, transport and utilize oxygen. Thus, the higher your level of maximal oxygen uptake, the greater your level of physical working capacity.

THE RELATIONSHIP BETWEEN THE PRODUCTION OF ENERGY AND THE INTENSITY OF EXERCISE

If the amount of work being performed is progressively increased, at some work output along the continuum as you approach your level of maximum capacity, your ability to produce energy aerobically will not be able to completely match your energy demands. For most sedentary people, this occurs at a work output requiring approximately half of their $\dot{V}O_{2\,max}$. In other words, below 50% $\dot{V}O_{2\,max}$, the "slower" aerobic system can provide all the energy that you need. Of course, your body does not switch over to the anaerobic system all at once, but gradually shifts gears to produce energy at a faster rate. A level between 50% and 70% $\dot{V}O_{2\,max}$ represents a transition phase for most people. Above 70% $\dot{V}O_{2\,max}$, your aerobic system does not produce energy fast enough causing you to rely more and more on your anaerobic system.

Figure 7-2 is a schematic diagram of the level of lactic acid in the blood relative to the intensity of exercise. The level of lactic acid is a rough indicator of the degree to which you are using the anaerobic mechanism. As the diagram illustrates, lactic acid will begin to rise slowly around 50% $\dot{V}O_{2\,max}$. Up to 70% of maximum, because the increase is not too great, your body can compensate with little trouble. Beyond 70% $\dot{V}O_{2\,max}$, however, as the buildup of lactic acid becomes more dramatic, you will start to get "winded." This explains why you can run at a certain pace (50% to 60% $\dot{V}O_{2\,max}$) with no problem, but become exhausted quickly after trying to run faster (80% to 90% $\dot{V}O_{2\,max}$).

Table 7-2. Lactic acid in the blood related to exercise intensity.

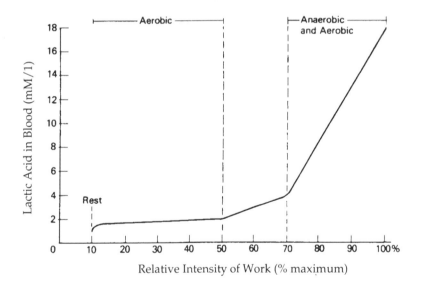

Used with permission from Body Energy by James S. Skinner, 1981 (Anderson World Inc., Mountain View, CA).

Depending on the intensity and duration levels of the activity, most sporting activities require both aerobic and anaerobic production of energy. For example, soccer players perform aerobic exercise when running for twenty to thirty minutes nonstop. Of course, if the activity did not depend on the aerobic system for energy, they would not be able to run for nearly so long. Occasionally, soccer players must sprint after the ball. During those high-intensity intervals, which exceed 70% of their $\dot{V}O_{2\,max}$, they are forced to draw upon their emergency, anaerobic sources. Anaerobic chemical reactions are primarily used in high-intensity exercise of relatively brief duration (e.g., sprinting short distances or heavy weight lifting), while aerobic chemical reactions are primarily involved in low-intensity, long-duration exercise activities such as walking, cycling, stair climbing, etc.

PHYSIOLOGICAL ADJUSTMENTS TO EXERCISE

The aerobic metabolism of fats and carbohydrates is the preferred and more efficient mode of energy production. It, however, can be limited by your body's ability to transport and deliver oxygen to, and the utilization of oxygen by, your working muscles. Several physiological adjustments are made during exercise. The primary objective of these adjustments is to provide an exercising muscle with oxygenated blood that can be used for the production of energy. Your endurance capabilities will be greatly influenced by the magnitude and direction of these changes.

CARDIAC OUTPUT

The amount of blood pumped per minute by your heart is termed your cardiac output ($\dot{Q}$). This measure is indicative of the rate of oxygen delivery to your peripheral tissues (e.g., exercising skeletal muscles). Cardiac output, which is the product of heart rate (HR) and stroke volume (SV), increases linearly as a function of work rate. At rest, $\dot{Q}$ is roughly five liters per minute (an average value for males), but can rise to 20-25 liters per minute during exercise in young, healthy adults. This exercise-induced increase of $\dot{Q}$ is due to alterations in both HR and SV.

HEART RATE

Heart rate, one of the two primary determinants of $\dot{Q}$, also rises linearly with work rate. The gradual withdrawal of vagal (parasympathetic nervous system) influences and the progressive increases in sympathetic nerve activity which occur during exercise are largely responsible for the observed increases in HR. At or near $\dot{V}O_{2\,max}$, HR begins to level off and is referred to as maximal heart rate. The equation "220 minus your age" (expressed in whole years) provides a rough estimate of your maximal heart rate (with a standard deviation of 10 to 12 beats per minute). As the equation implies, your maximal heart rate declines with age.

STROKE VOLUME

Stroke volume is the other primary determinant of $\dot{Q}$ and represents the amount of blood ejected from the heart during each beat. Unlike HR, SV does not increase linearly with work rate. SV increases progressively until a work rate equivalent to approximately 50-75% $\dot{V}O_{2\,max}$ is reached. Thereafter, continued increases in work rate cause little or no increase in SV. Exercise-induced increases in SV are believed to be the result of factors that are both intrinsic and extrinsic to the heart. According to the Frank-Starling law, a greater stretch is placed on the muscle fibers of the heart (due to a greater venous return of blood to the heart), resulting in a more forceful contraction of those fibers and consequently a greater SV. Extrinsic factors such as increased nervous (sympathetic) or endocrine (release of adrenal hormones epinephrine and norepinephrine) stimulation to the myocardium can also contribute to the increased SV that occurs during exercise.

BLOOD PRESSURE

Systolic blood pressure (SBP) represents the force developed by your heart during ventricular contraction. SBP increases linearly with work rate. In healthy adults, SBP tends not to exceed 220 mm Hg at maximal exercise levels (according to the American College of Sports Medicine, 250 mm Hg should be considered an end point for a maximal exercise test). Diastolic blood pressure (DBP) is indicative of the pressure in the arterial system during ventricular relaxation and reflects peripheral resistance to blood flow. It changes little from rest to maximal levels of exercise. Therefore, the pulse pressure (the algebraic difference between SBP and DBP) increases in direct proportion to the intensity of exercise. The pulse pressure is important since it reflects the driving force for blood flow in the arteries.

TOTAL PERIPHERAL RESISTANCE

The sum of all the forces that oppose blood flow in the systemic circulation is called the total peripheral resistance (TPR). Numerous factors can affect TPR including blood viscosity, vessel length, hydrostatic pressure, and vessel diameter. Vessel diameter is by far the most important of these factors, since TPR is inversely proportional to the fourth power of the radius of the vessel. If one vessel has one-half the radius of another and if all other factors are equal, the larger vessel would have 16 times (2^4) less resistance than the smaller vessel. As a result, 16 times more blood would flow through the larger vessel at the same pressure. This has important implications for exercise, since certain organs require more blood flow than others during physical activity. During exercise, resistance in the vessels supplying the muscle and skin is decreased (this implies that blood flow to these parts of the body is enhanced), while resistance in vessels supplying visceral organs (e.g., the liver, GI tract, kidneys) is increased (blood flow is reduced). These changes are almost entirely due to intrinsic factors (the increased metabolic demand of the muscle and the requirement of skin blood flow to facilitate heat dissipation). The TPR tends to decrease during progressive dynamic exercise, because vasodilation occurring in the muscle and skin seem to override the vasoconstriction which is occurring in the visceral organs.

ARTERIOVENOUS OXYGEN DIFFERENCE

The arteriovenous oxygen difference, as its name implies, is the difference between the oxygen content of the arterial blood and mixed venous blood. It is a reflection of the amount of oxygen extracted from your blood by your muscles. The oxygen content of venous blood can be reduced to one-half to one-third the resting levels by exercising muscles, indicative that your muscles are extracting a much higher proportion of the oxygen delivered to them in the arterial blood (approximately 85% of the oxygen in arterial blood can be removed during maximal exercise).

ENERGY IS THE KEY

The physiological adjustments of the cardiovascular and muscular systems are essential to determining your ability to sustain low resistance, dynamic physical activity (i.e., cardiorespiratory fitness level). These adjustments, as discussed in this chapter, support the increased energy requirements associated with exercise. The Fick equation ($\dot{V}O_2 = \dot{Q} *$ a-vO$_2$ difference) illustrates how your cardiovascular and muscular systems adjust to supply oxygen to exercising muscles. As the oxygen requirements of your muscles increase, your cardiovascular system responds by elevating HR and SV. Concurrently, your muscular system responds by extracting more oxygen from the blood. For the majority of individuals, oxygen uptake primarily is dependent upon the delivery of oxygen to, and utilization of oxygen by, the exercising muscles. ❏

BIBLIOGRAPHY •

1. Åstrand, P.O., Rodahl, K. *Textbook of Work Physiology*, 3rd Ed. New York, NY: McGraw-Hill, 1986.

2. Brooks, G.A., Fahey, T.D. *Exercise Physiology: Human Bioenergetics and Its Applications*. New York, NY: John Wiley & Sons, 1984.

3. Burke, E., Cerny, F., Costill D., et al. "Characteristics of skeletal muscle in competitive cyclists." *Med Sci Sports* 9:109-112, 1977.

4. Chapman, C.B., Mitchell, J.H. "The physiology of exercise." *Sci Am* 212(5):88-96, 1965.

5. Costill, D., Daniels, J., Evans, W., et al. "Skeletal muscle enzymes and fiber composition in male and female track athletes." *J Appl Physiol* 40:149-154, 1976.

6. Fox, E.L., Bowers, R.D., Foss, M.L. *The Physiological Basis of Physical Education and Athletics*, 4th Ed. Philadelphia, PA: W. B. Saunders Company, 1988.

7. Gollnick, P., Armstrong, R., Saubert, C., et al. "Enzyme activity and fiber composition in skeletal muscle of untrained and trained men." *J Appl Physiol* 33:312-319, 1972.

8. Komi, P., Rusko, H., Vos, J., et al. "Anaerobic performance capacity in athletes." *Acta Physiol Scand* 100:107-114, 1977.

9. Lamb, D.R. *Physiology of Exercise: Responses & Adaptations*, 2nd Ed. New York, NY: Macmillan, 1984.

10. Magel, J., Andersen, K.L. "Pulmonary diffusing capacity and cardiac output in young trained Norwegian swimmers and untrained subjects." *Med Sci Sports* 1:131-139, 1969.

11. Skinner, J.S. "Functional effects of physical activity." In *Physical Education and Sport: An Introduction*. Zeigler, E.F. (Ed). Philadelphia, PA: Lea & Febiger, 1982.

12. Skinner, J.S., Noeldner, S.P., O'Connor, J.S. "The development and maintenance of physical fitness." In *Sports Medicine*, 2nd Ed. Ryan, A.J., Allman, F.D. (Eds). New York, NY: Academic Press, 1989.

13. Thorstensson, A., Larsson, L., Tesch, P., et al. "Muscle strength and fiber composition in athletes and sedentary men." *Med Sci Sports* 9:26-30, 1977.

14. Wilmore, J.H., Costill, D.L. *Training for Sport and Activity*, Ed 3. Dubuque, IA: Wm. C. Brown Publishers, 1988.

CHAPTER 8

• •

UNDERSTANDING THE PHYSIOLOGICAL BASIS OF MUSCULAR FITNESS

by

James E. Graves, Ph.D.
and
Michael L. Pollock, Ph.D.

• • •

Muscular fitness is one of the primary parameters of physical fitness. It involves two basic components: muscular strength[1] and muscular endurance.[2] It is developed by placing a demand (overload) on the muscles of an individual. As the individual's body adapts to the demand, the individual becomes stronger or better able to sustain muscular activity, depending on the nature of the demand.

The process of overloading the muscular system is commonly referred to as resistance training.[3] Resistance training not only can develop muscular strength and muscular endurance, it can also improve the ability of the muscles to recover more quickly from the stresses imposed by physical activity. In addition, properly performed resistance training has been found to produce an increase in an individual's level of muscle mass, bone mineral density, and strength of connective tissue. All of these changes have been shown to have a positive effect on fitness and health—particularly as an individual ages.

Research has documented the fact that physical fitness declines with age. However, many of the detrimental age-related changes in physiological function

---

[1] Muscular strength refers to the ability to generate force at a given speed (velocity) of movement (Knuttgen and Kraemer, 1987).

[2] Muscular endurance refers to the ability to persist in physical activity or resist muscular fatigue (Baumgartner and Jackson, 1987).

[3] The term "resistance" training is used in this chapter to cover all types of "strength" or "weight" training including free weight, isokinetic, variable resistance, and isometric.

are due to decreased physical activity associated with aging and can be attenuated or even reversed with proper exercise training. Just as aerobic training is required for the development and maintenance of cardiorespiratory fitness, resistance training is required for the development and maintenance of muscular fitness.

The importance of resistance training for maintaining muscle mass was recently illustrated in a study of master athletes. The investigators measured the aerobic capacity and body composition of 24 master track athletes, 50 to 82 years of age, over a ten-year period. The results showed that when aerobic training was maintained, cardiorespiratory fitness remained unchanged over the course of the study. Percent body fat, however, increased significantly—even among those athletes who maintained their aerobic training. The change in percent fat was attributed to a reduction in fat-free weight (muscle mass), specifically in the upper body, and not an increase in fat weight. Three athletes who supplemented their aerobic training with either resistance training or cross-country skiing, were able to maintain their upper body muscle mass.

In recognition of the need for a well-rounded training program to develop and maintain muscular as well as cardiorespiratory fitness, the American College of Sports Medicine (ACSM) recently revised its original Position Stand on "The Recommended Quantity and Quality of Exercise for Developing and Maintaining Fitness in Healthy Adults" to include a resistance training component. The ACSM recommends resistance training of a moderate- to high-intensity, sufficient to develop and maintain muscle mass, as an integral part of an adult fitness program. One set of 8-12 repetitions of eight to ten exercises that conditions the major muscle groups at least two days per week is the recommended minimum.

In addition to the development and maintenance of muscular strength and muscle mass, the physiological benefits of resistance training include increases in bone mass and in the strength of connective tissue. These adaptations are beneficial for middle-aged and older adults, and in particular postmenopausal women who rapidly lose bone mineral density. Research has also shown that the following additional health benefits[4] are associated with resistance training:

- Modest improvements in cardiorespiratory fitness
- Reductions in body fat
- Modest reductions in blood pressure
- Improved level of glucose tolerance
- Improved blood lipid-lipoprotein profiles

Muscular fitness is required for successful performance in many sports. Thus, resistance training is common among recreational and professional athletes who wish to enhance athletic performance. Resistance training is also prescribed in rehabilitation programs designed to facilitate recovery from accidents and

---

[4] These health benefits have been most often associated with circuit weight training, a method of resistance training in which a series of exercises are performed in succession with only a minimal amount of rest allowed between exercises.

sport-related injuries. The effectiveness of resistance-training exercises in clinical rehabilitation is well documented.

An important benefit associated with resistance training is to reduce the risk of orthopedic injury. Strong muscles support and, thus, help protect the joints that they cross. It is also recognized that inadequate muscular strength can lead to serious musculoskeletal disorders that result in pain and discomfort and loss of income due to disability and premature retirement. The overall strengthening of the musculoskeletal system (muscle, bone and connective tissue) resulting from resistance training has been shown to reduce the risk of elbow and shoulder injuries in tennis players and swimmers. Resistance training may have an even greater importance for individuals participating in contact sports and in reducing the risk of injury due to accidents. Low back pain is a major medical problem in our society. Increasing muscular strength may reduce the risk of developing low back pain as well as reduce the symptoms of pain in low back pain patients. Thus, the adaptations to resistance training increase the potential for a greater quality of life. This chapter will address the basic physiological adaptations to resistance training and methods of assessing muscular fitness.

Physiological Adaptation To Resistance Training

Neural Adaptations

It was once believed that the ability of a muscle to generate force depended solely on the size of the muscle: as muscles increased in size (hypertrophy) they became stronger, and as they decreased in size (atrophy), they became weaker. It is now known that muscular strength is determined not only by the size of the muscles, but also by the ability of the nervous system to activate the muscles. In fact, there are a number of short-term resistance training studies that have demonstrated increases in muscular strength with no accompanying hypertrophy.

Skeletal muscles are innervated by motor neurons. Groups of individual muscle fibers that are innervated by the same motor neuron are called motor units. The amount of force generated during muscle contraction depends on two factors: the number of motor units that are fired and the frequency of motor unit firing. Firing frequency refers to the rate of firing or the number of nerve impulses per unit of time that the motor unit receives.

Neural adaptations to resistance training include both an increase in the number of motor units that can be fired at any given time and an increase in the frequency of motor unit firing. Increasing the number of motor units that are fired at a given time may be caused by an increase in the neural drive to the muscle and/or a removal of neural inhibition. Improved coordination among agonist muscles (muscles that work together to produce a specific movement) and removal of activation of antagonist muscles (muscles that produce force and movement in the opposite direction) may also contribute to an increased ability to generate greater muscular force following resistance training.

In young subjects, neural adaptations to resistance training predominate during the first four weeks of a training program, while morphological changes (hypertrophy) to the muscle itself predominate thereafter. In older subjects, neural adaptations are the primary mechanism for increased strength for a period of at least eight weeks. Because most studies typically involve training programs that last 8 to 20 weeks, much of the documented improvements in muscle strength are related to a combination of neural and morphological adaptations. There is relatively little information available on the specific mechanisms of muscular strength gains found during long-term training.

MORPHOLOGICAL ADAPTATIONS

An increase in muscle size is probably the most readily recognized adaptation to resistance training. Such an increase is often observed following as little as two months training. Two theories (hypertrophy vs. hyperplasia) have been advanced to explain the phenomenon of increased muscle size in response to overload stress. The majority of research supports the notion that greater muscle size results from the enlargement (hypertrophy), not proliferation (hyperplasia), of individual muscle fibers. Support for the hyperplasia hypothesis in humans comes from studies of certain athletes (e.g., swimmers, kayakers, body builders) who display hypertrophy of specific muscles even though fiber diameters are relatively small. It is unknown from these cross-sectional studies, however, how many fibers were present prior to training.

Studies on laboratory animals indicate that the number of muscle fibers is genetically determined. In addition, in order for hyperplasia to be an adaptive phenomenon the new fibers would have to become completely separate from the existing fibers and innervated. Such a situation has not been documented. Therefore, the general consensus is that the number of muscle fibers does not increase during postnatal growth and under normal training conditions, hyperplasia does not occur in humans.

The degree of skeletal muscle hypertrophy induced by resistance training depends on a number of factors which include the characteristics of the training program as well as the potential for the muscle to increase in size. Human skeletal muscle is made up of two distinct fiber types: Type I or slow-twitch (oxidative) fibers which have a high capacity for aerobic or endurance types of activities, and Type II or fast-twitch (glycolytic) fibers which are best suited for activities that require strength, speed, and power. Progressive heavy resistance training stimulates an increase in the cross-sectional area of both Type I and Type II muscle fibers although a greater degree of hypertrophy generally occurs in Type II fibers. The greater degree of hypertrophy found in Type II fibers is probably reflective of a greater involvement of these fibers with resistance training. Likewise, atrophy resulting from disuse occurs to the greatest extent in Type II fibers. There are no studies to indicate that resistance training increases the number of Type II fibers relative to Type I. Therefore, the potential for individuals to increase muscle size and muscle strength may be genetically predetermined by the number of Type II fibers they possess.

The increased cross-sectional area of muscle fibers is associated with an increase in the contractile proteins actin and myosin. The amount of protein in the muscle can increase by increasing protein production (synthesis) or by decreasing the rate at which proteins are broken down. Hypertrophy of Type II fibers occurs primarily through an increase in protein synthesis. Hypertrophy of Type I fibers occurs primarily through a decrease in protein breakdown.

Actin and myosin are organized within the muscle fiber in cylindrical units called myofibrils. Myofibrils increase in both size and number following resistance training. Increased myofibril cross-sectional area following resistance training results from an addition of actin and myosin filaments to the periphery of the myofibril. Similarly, atrophy following immobilization or disuse is associated with a loss of contractile protein from the periphery of the myofibril. Myofibrils increase in number by splitting into two or more daughter myofibrils.

The specific mechanism by which resistance training stimulates increased protein synthesis is unknown. There are currently two hypotheses which have been developed to explain the mechanism responsible for muscle hypertrophy. One hypothesis suggests that the tension developed during resistance exercise provides a signal that is read by the genetic machinery of the cell which in turn stimulates protein synthesis. This hypothesis is supported by the fact that little or no hypertrophy will occur during resistance training when the intensity is low. The second hypothesis involves the theory of breakdown and repair. It is thought that during each training session part of the muscle is broken down and that the repair process gradually builds the muscle up to a higher level. The breakdown and repair hypothesis is supported by studies that have identified skeletal muscle damage following heavy resistance exercise.

Because heavy resistance training is associated with an increase in fiber size but does not necessarily stimulate capillary or mitochondrial proliferation, capillary and mitochondrial density are often found to decrease. That is, resistance training does not change the capillary to fiber ratio but since the fibers have increased in size with no change in the number of capillaries, the capillary density is reduced. A training regimen consisting of a high number of repetitions with moderate loads, however, may induce capillary proliferation. Body builders who emphasize high repetition training systems have been found to have a greater capillary density than weight lifters (e.g., power lifters) who train with heavy loads and fewer repetitions. Although capillary and mitochondrial density may be reduced following resistance training, the activity of enzymes reflecting anaerobic metabolism remains unchanged. In addition, significant increases in resting concentrations of anaerobic energy stores such as muscle glycogen, and the high energy phosphates creatine phosphate and ATP have been observed. These adaptations improve the ability of individuals to continue to perform work with moderate to heavy loads (anaerobic capacity or muscular endurance). The morphological adaptations to heavy resistance training are illustrated in Table 8-1.

Table 8-1. Morphological Adaptations to Heavy Resistance Training.

Muscle Fiber Size	▲
Myofibril size	▲
Myofibril number	▲
Contractile Protein Content	▲
Fiber Type Composition	NC
Capillary Density	▼
Mitochondrial Density	▼
Aerobic Enzyme Content	NC or ▼
Anaerobic Enzyme Content	
Glycolytic	NC
Non-glycolytic	NC
Muscle Glycogen	▲
ATP and CP	▲
Lipid Content	NC
Myoglobin Content	▼
Connective Tissue	
Absolute amount	▲
Strength	▲

ATP = adenosine triphosphate; CP = creatine phosphate; ▲ = increase; ▼ = decrease; NC = no changes

ADAPTATIONS TO BONE AND CONNECTIVE TISSUE

Bone is a dynamic tissue that changes in density and form in response to the stresses placed upon it. Immobilization and weightlessness cause a rapid loss of bone mass. Physical activity, on the other hand, has a positive influence on bone mineral density but the rate of adaptation for bone is much slower than that of muscle. The influence of resistance training on bone is highly dependent on hormonal and nutritional conditions. For example, bone loss is common in estrogen deficient postmenopausal women. Estrogen replacement therapy is effective at minimizing this bone loss but only when a sufficient amount of dietary calcium is available.

Cross-sectional studies have shown that athletes who participate regularly in weight bearing or resistance training activities have greater bone densities than sedentary controls. Certain athletes who participate in unilateral sports (e.g., tennis and baseball players) exhibit bone hypertrophy in their dominant (playing) arm. The location and degree of hypertrophy are influenced to a great extent by the specific sport; for example, femoral and spinal bone density are highest in weight lifters and lowest in swimmers.

Although it is widely recognized that weight-bearing activities can increase bone mineral density, there are relatively few longitudinal studies involving resistance training. Conflicting results exist for the few longitudinal studies conducted on the influence of resistance training on bone density. Much of the discrepancy among results from different studies may be due to issues related to specificity of training and the length of training. It is quite evident that additional research is needed.

Connective tissue has an important role during exercise because it provides the basic structural framework and force conveying network for human movement. Most studies on the influence of exercise on connective tissue have used short term aerobic protocols on animal models. There are relatively few studies that have addressed the effects of resistance training on connective tissues.

Resistance training increases the maximum tensile strength of both tendons and ligaments. Strengthening connective tissue may reduce the likelihood of strains, sprains and other injuries associated with physical activity. Body builders have been found to have similar volume densities for collagen and other non-contractile tissue when compared to untrained controls. This finding suggests that the absolute amount of connective tissue within the muscle increases but because muscle cell size also increases, the proportion of muscle that is made up of connective tissue does not change. Thus, training induced increases in muscle fiber size are accompanied by corresponding increases in connective tissue.

The morphological adaptations to resistance training, as discussed in this section, include increases in the strength and mass of muscle, bone, and connective tissue. These adaptations reduce the risk of orthopaedic injury. While muscular strength can improve rather rapidly through neural mechanisms, noticeable changes to bone and connective tissue take longer to occur.

SPECIFICITY OF TRAINING

Strength increases resulting from resistance training are specific to the type of contraction used in training, the range-of-motion (ROM) through which training occurs, the velocity of contraction during training, and whether exercises are performed unilaterally or bilaterally. These examples of specificity of training are all at least partially attributed to neural adaptation; however, for specificity of contraction type and velocity of contraction there is evidence to suggest that resistance training also has specific effects on the contractile properties of the muscle. Each of these examples of specificity of resistance training will be briefly discussed.

There are two basic types of muscle activity: static and dynamic. In a static (commonly referred to as isometric) contraction the muscle attempts to shorten against a fixed or immovable resistance. Thus, there is no movement of the skeleton and the muscle neither shortens nor is forcibly lengthened. A dynamic contraction involves movement and can be either concentric where the force produced by the muscle is sufficient to overcome the resistance and shortening of the muscle occurs, or eccentric where the muscle exerts force, lengthens, and is overcome by the resistance.

Training a muscle group with dynamic actions (e.g., lifting weights) produces relatively large increases in dynamic muscle strength but only small increases in isometric contraction strength. Isometric training on the other hand, has been shown to improve isometric strength more so than dynamic strength. Studies from our laboratory, however, have shown similar improvements in isometric strength through a full ROM following both isometric and dynamic training when the dynamic training involved slow controlled repetitions through a full ROM. In addition to specificity involving isometric and dynamic modes of training, lifting weights has been shown to improve weight lifting strength to a greater extent than isokinetic (constant velocity) concentric contraction strength.

Increases in voluntary strength are specific to the ROM that is trained for both isometric and dynamic resistance training. A significant transfer of isometric strength within 20^0 of the training angle occurs following an isometric strength training program. At positions beyond 20^0 from the training angle, little transfer of isometric strength tends to occur. Thus, when isometric exercises are used to improve muscular strength, training should occur at multiple positions throughout the ROM. When training consists of dynamic muscle actions performed through a limited ROM, strength gains have been noted up to 50^0 away from the ROM used for training. However, improvements in the untrained ROM have been significantly less than those in the ROM in which training was conducted.

Strength training at slow speeds results in relatively large increases in the ability of the muscle to generate force at slow speeds but relatively small increases during contractions at faster speeds. Training at fast speeds results in specifically larger increases in strength at faster speeds. The carry-over of strength from high speed training to slow speed testing is somewhat greater than the carry-over from slow speed training to fast speed testing. However, it is not clear how much of an influence measurement (impact) artifact[5] associated with isokinetic testing has on these particular findings related to the speed of training.

REDUCED TRAINING

When resistance training programs are terminated, muscular strength and muscle mass can be rapidly lost. An important question related to long-term maintenance of muscular fitness is how much resistance training is required to retain strength. Can people reduce training frequency periodically and still maintain strength? Individuals participating in strength training programs must occasionally reduce or stop training for brief periods of time. Studies on endurance exercise suggest that aerobic capacity can be maintained during reduced training frequency and duration as long as intensity is maintained.

Results from a study conducted at our laboratory indicate that as long as training intensity is maintained, people can reduce training frequency to as little

---

[5] On an isokinetic dynamometer which provides a written recording of force output, an impact artifact is the initial spike that occurs during the concentric movement. This artifact (spike) does not correspond to force production by the muscle; rather, it represents the effect of the accelerating limb engaging the movement arm of the machine.

as one day per week for up to 12 weeks without a significant loss in strength. It may be important to note that the subjects in this reduced training study were initially untrained and had only trained from 12 to 18 weeks. Whether highly trained athletes can reduce training frequency to a similar extent or whether reduced training can be carried out for more than 12 weeks without a loss in strength are not known. Available evidences, however, suggest that missing a workout once in a while or having to reduce training frequency because of a busy schedule will not adversely affect muscular fitness. The important consideration is not to stop training altogether.

MEASUREMENT OF MUSCULAR STRENGTH

The primary function of skeletal muscle is to generate force. In most instances, forces generated by skeletal muscles are used to produce movement or for anatomical stabilization. The measurement of muscle force production is used to assess fitness, identify weakness, evaluate progress in rehabilitation programs, and to measure the effectiveness of resistance training. The maximum amount of force that a muscle or group of muscles generate can be measured by a variety of methods: cable tensiometers, dynamometers, strain-gauge devices, one-repetition maximal (1-RM) tests, or computer assisted force and work output determination. Each of these methods will be briefly described.

Regardless of the method chosen to assess muscular strength, certain conditions are required for accurate and reliable measurements of muscle force output. Body position must be stabilized to allow only the desired movement. In the case of measuring muscle force generation during an isometric contraction, the involved joint or joints at which movement would occur must be isolated. An example of the need for stabilization to isolate a specific group of muscles for functional assessment occurs during the measurement of lumbar extensor torque production. The lumbar extensors work in conjunction with the larger, more powerful, gluteus and hamstring muscles to extend the trunk. If the pelvis is free to move during lumbar extension, the pelvis will rotate as the gluteus and hamstring muscles contract. Pelvic rotation would then contribute to the observed torque. Thus, pelvic stabilization is required to accurately assess isolated lumbar extensor function.

Muscle force production varies through a ROM. The most descriptive measures of muscle function account for this fact. The term "strength curve" is used to describe a plot of the resultant force exerted versus an appropriate measure of the joint configuration. Because of acceleration at the beginning and deceleration at the end of all human movements, and the fact that dynamic strength is influenced by the speed of movement, dynamic strength tests are not appropriate for the quantification of muscle function through a ROM. In addition, if dynamic muscle actions are performed at fast speeds, kinetic forces may be recorded that give an inaccurate measure of true force production. Depending upon the specific exercise movement, these kinetic forces can be potentially dangerous, especially for orthopaedic patient populations because of the impact that occurs upon rapid deceleration. In our laboratory at the University of Florida, we have observed that isometric tests can safely and accurately quantify muscle force production through a ROM if multiple joint angles are measured.

A final consideration required for the accurate assessment of muscle force production is whether the mass of the involved body part will influence the measurement. For example, if the force generated by the quadriceps muscles during knee extension does not equal or exceed the mass of the lower leg, no measurable force would be observed. Thus, the mass of the lower leg detracts from observed force production of the quadriceps muscles during knee extension testing. This mass must be accounted for to accurately quantify force. Although there is some controversy concerning the need for correction of the influence of gravitational forces during testing because most bodily activities are not "corrected" for gravity, the actual force generated by specific muscles in certain positions may be greatly influenced by body mass. Thus, although one cannot neglect the fact that in normal daily activities muscles are influenced by body mass, standardization of the testing position and correction for gravitational forces are required for the accurate quantification of muscle force production. The need for stabilization, positional standardization, compensation for gravitational influences and measurement through a ROM have been recently discussed by Pollock et al. (in press).

MEASUREMENT DEVICES

The cable tensiometer is an instrument used to measure static strength by recording the tension applied to a steel cable. This instrument was originally designed to measure aircraft cable tension and was adapted and later refined to measure the strength of various muscle groups. One end of the cable is attached to a fixed object (e.g., a wall or the floor) and the other end is fitted with a bar, a handle, an ankle cuff, or some similar device to which force can be applied by a limb segment. In order for the measurement to accurately reflect muscle force production, the cable must be in the plane of movement and must make a 90° angle at its point of attachment to the body or body part. The tensiometer, which is placed along the length of the cable, measures cable tension when the subject applies force to the cable.

Because the force generating capacity varies through a ROM, establishing the proper angle of measurement is critical. A goniometer is usually used to set the joint angle for testing. The cable tensiometer strength test can accurately measure the static strength of virtually all major muscle groups. The device is highly reliable when used on normal subjects. However, the cable and attachments often stretch during testing which makes positional standardization difficult.

The dynamometer is an instrument used to measure static strength by recording the amount of force exerted. Two portable types of dynamometers are widely available—one for hand grip and one for back and leg strength. The most common type is the hand or grip dynamometer. Grip strength is measured as kilograms of force exerted by squeezing the hand dynamometer as hard as possible.

Dynamometers are popular for testing large numbers of people because they are easy to use and portable. Cumbersome set-up procedures that often accompany other types of muscle performance measurements are not necessary. Limitations of dynamometers include the fact that they can be used to measure only a few muscle groups and their reliability is not well established. In addition, isolation of specific muscle groups is not accomplished which makes standardization difficult.

Strain-gauge devices can be employed to measure static and dynamic muscle force capacity for a variety of muscle groups. Strain gauges are made of electroconductive material that is usually applied to the surfaces of finely machined metal parts. When a load (from a muscle contraction) is placed on the metal parts, the metal and the strain gauge attached to it deforms. The deformation of the strain gauge causes change in the electrical resistance of the gauge to a voltage or current passed through it. The change in voltage is related to the load and can be recorded on a strip chart, digital display, or volt meter. In most instances strain-gauges are used to measure static strain or compression by pushing or pulling on the device. Applications of strain gauges for dynamic strength measures, however, are commercially available (e.g., isokinetic machines). Strain gauge measurements are reliable but they have the same limitations as the cable tensiometer.

One-repetition maximum tests measure the greatest amount of weight that can be lifted one time for a specific weight-lifting exercise. These tests are usually limited to the amount of weight that can be lifted at the weakest position in the ROM and, therefore, do not assess muscle performance through a full ROM. Generally the test begins with an amount of weight that can be easily lifted. After a successful trial, a two to three minute rest period is allowed. Then the weight is increased by five to ten pounds (or more depending on the difficulty of the previous lift) and another trial is attempted. The 1-RM is the amount of weight for the last trial that can be successfully completed with good form and can usually be obtained in four to six trials. The 1-RM provides a measure of dynamic strength that can be applied to almost any weight lifting exercise. One repetition maximum tests are popular because they are easy to administer and can often be performed with the same equipment used for training. They are highly reliable although they do involve a factor of skill and subsequent tests may yield greater results due to practice. Thus, 1-RM tests may not be specific for muscle force production.

The application of computer technology and advancements in machine design have improved the accuracy and standardization of muscular strength testing. Electromechanical dynamometers have been developed for both static and dynamic measures of muscular strength. Some electromechanical dynamometers are capable of both static and dynamic strength measurements. Many electromechanical dynamometers employ a load cell to measure static strength. This method may be considered the electronic equivalent of the cable tensiometer. A major advantage of machines that use load cells, however, is the ease of making multiple measurements through a ROM. Cable tensiometer systems are usually cumbersome to adjust and, therefore, are usually used to provide a measure of static strength at only a single joint angle. Because strength varies through a ROM based upon the biomechanical arrangement of the muscles and bony levers of the skeletal system, single joint angle measures do not provide an indication of how strength varies through the ROM. Multiple joint-angle isometric tests are often employed to quantify full ROM static strength. Multiple joint-angle isometric tests have been shown to be highly reliable for a variety of muscle groups.

Some electromechanical instruments have been designed to measure dynamic muscular strength at a pre-set movement speed. In theory, these constant-velocity (isokinetic) dynamometers are thought to measure the maximum force that can be applied throughout the constant velocity movement. Because a period of acceleration is required to reach the pre-selected velocity of movement, and a period of deceleration is required at the end of the movement, isokinetic dynamometers cannot measure force production through a full ROM. In addition, oscillation in observed forces, called torque overshoot, can limit the accuracy of these devices. These torque overshoots represent impact forces between the moving body part and the measurement device. Manufacturers have attempted to overcome these measurement errors by various software controlled averaging systems (called dampening mechanisms) with limited success. While data averaging may be effective at presenting smooth force curves, it cannot eliminate potentially dangerous impact forces. Measurement error associated with isokinetic dynamometry has been discussed in detail. Unfortunately, in spite of their shortcomings, isokinetic dynamometers are a common method of strength assessment in many clinical and research settings.

Measurement Of Muscular Endurance

Almost all of the devices for measuring strength can also be used for assessing muscular endurance. Tests of muscular endurance should be designed to evaluate the ability of a muscle group to produce submaximal force for an extended duration. More specifically, the length of time a muscle contraction can be held or the number of repeated submaximal contractions a muscle group can make should be determined. Accordingly, similar to strength, muscular endurance can be assessed either statically or dynamically.

Measuring Muscle Endurance Statically

Two basic methods exist for assessing muscular endurance statically. One method involves having an individual perform a maximal static contraction and sustain that level of contraction for 60 seconds. The force being exerted by the muscle should be recorded at 10-second intervals. Accordingly, individuals who experience a slower rate of decline in force production are exhibiting a greater level of muscle endurance for that specific muscle group than those whose level of recorded force falls at a faster rate. The other method for statically assessing muscular endurance is to determine how long a given percentage of an individual's maximum voluntary contraction strength can be sustained.

MEASURING MUSCLE ENDURANCE DYNAMICALLY

A number of ways exist for determining muscular endurance dynamically. One way dynamic muscle endurance can be assessed is for an individual to perform the maximum number of repetitions possible using an absolute weight, a given percentage of maximum strength, or some set percentage of body weight. The endurance of a muscle group can be determined isokinetically through the performance of successive maximal repetitions. Isokinetic muscular endurance is measured as the number of repetitions completed before the torque production drops below 50% of the maximal torque value. Perhaps the most commonly used method for evaluating muscular endurance is calisthenic-type (e.g., sit-ups, push-ups, pull-ups, etc.) exercise testing. During such tests, the maximum number of times an individual can lift his or her own body weight is used as the measure of endurance. For individuals of below-average muscular fitness or above-average body weight, however, calisthenic-type exercises can often involve more of a measure of muscular strength than muscular endurance. ❑

BIBLIOGRAPHY •

1. American College of Sports Medicine. "Position stand: The recommended quantity and quality of exercise for developing and maintaining cardiorespiratory and muscular fitness in healthy adults." *Med Sci Sports Exerc* 22:265-274, 1990.
2. Baumgartner, T.A., Jackson, A.S. *Measurement for Evaluation in Physical Education and Exercise Science*. Dubuque, IA: Wm. C. Brown Publishers, 1987.
3. Fleck, S.J., Kraemer, W.J. *Designing Resistance Training Programs*. Champaign, IL: Human Kinetics Publishers, 1987.
4. Graves, J.E., Pollock, M.L., Carpenter, D.M., et al. "Quantitative assessment of full range-of-motion isometric lumbar extension strength." *Spine* 15(4):289-294, 1990a.
5. Graves, J.E., Pollock, M.L., Foster, D., et al. "Effect of training frequency and specificity on isometric lumbar extension strength." *Spine* 15(6):504-509, 1990b.
6. Graves, J.E., Pollock, M.L., Jones, A.E., et al. "Specificity of limited range of motion variable resistance training." *Med Sci Sports Exerc* 21(1):84-89, 1989.
7. Graves, J.E., Pollock, M.L., Leggett, S.H., et al. "Effect of reduced training frequency on muscular strength." *Int J Sports Med* 9(5):316-319, 1988.
8. Graves, J.E., Welsch, M., Pollock, M.L. "Exercise training for muscular strength and endurance." *Idea Today* 9(7):33-40, 1991.
9. Grimby, G. "Progressive resistance exercise for injury rehabilitation." *Sports Med* 2:309-315, 1985.
10. Jones, N.L., McCartney, N., McComas, A.J. (Eds). *Human Muscle Power*. Champaign, IL: Human Kinetics Publishers, 1986.
11. Knuttgen, H.G., Kraemer, W.J. "Terminology and measurement in exercise performance." *J Appl Sport Sci Res* 1(1):1-10, 1987.
12. Komi, P.V. (Ed). *Strength and Power in Sport*. Cambridge, MA: Blackwell Scientific Publications, 1992.
13. MacDougall, J.D., Wenger, H.A., Green, H.J. (Eds). *Physiological Testing of the High-Performance Athlete*. Champaign, IL: Human Kinetics Publishers, 1991.

14. Pollock, M.L., Graves, J.E., Carpenter, D.M., et al. "The lumbar musculature: testing and conditioning for rehabilitation." In *Rehabilitation of the Spine: Science and Practice*. Hockshulers, G.R., Colter, H., Carranza, C. (Eds). New York, NY: Springer-Verlag, (in press).

15. Pollock, M.L., Wilmore, J.H. *Exercise in Health and Disease: Evaluation and Prescription for Prevention and Rehabilitation*, 2nd Ed. Philadelphia, PA: W. B. Saunders Company, 1990.

16. Risch, S., Norvell, N., Pollock M., et al. "Lumbar strengthening in chronic low back pain patients: Psychological and physiological benefits." *Spine* (in press).

17. Stone, M.H., Fleck, S.J., Triplett, N.T., et al. "Health- and performance-related potential of resistance training." *Sports Med* 11(4):210-231, 1991.

Chapter 9

UNDERSTANDING CROSSROBIC™ TRAINING

by

Cedric X. Bryant, Ph.D., James A. Peterson, Ph.D.,
Lee Rawls, M.S., and Ronald J. Hagen, M.S.

• • •

*A*ctivities of daily living and most athletic events impose a combination of physical and metabolic demands on the human body. Climbing stairs, running to answer a phone, picking up a child, and mowing the lawn are just a few examples of how an individual, within a relatively brief period of time, may be forced to respond to an ever-changing set of very different physical/metabolic demands. Collectively, these demands may be grouped into four basic performance-related categories: endurance (aerobic and muscular), speed, strength, and power (speed x strength). In turn, these factors are "blended together" in different combinations and sequences depending on the physical task to be performed.

Traditionally, individuals who want to improve their level of physical fitness engage in an exercise program which develops each component of fitness or performance-related factor separately—one at a time. Little or no thought is typically given to the need for developing (in an integrated fashion) the metabolic pathways which provide the energy required to perform a particular task.

In order to elicit a training response involving not only the development of the aforementioned performance-related factors, but also the enhancement of the body's metabolic pathways, an individual must exercise on a modality which meets at least four criteria: provides precise control of the level of resistance an individual must overcome while exercising; offers a wide range of loads; provides precise control of the rate of speed (velocity) at which an individual exercises; and offers a wide range of velocities. It has been recognized for some period of time that no single machine meets all four of the design criteria essential for integrated physical and metabolic conditioning. The extent to which a particular exercise modality permits such a training response to occur tends to vary from modality to modality. For example, some types of exercise machines do not meet any of the four criteria, while other machines meet a few—but not all—of the necessary requirements.

The StairMaster® Crossrobics® 1650 LE™ CardioSquat™ conditioning system was conceived, designed, and manufactured as a direct result of the identified need to provide a means by which individuals can improve their functional capacity level in specific performance-related factors, as well as enhance their level of metabolic conditioning. The CardioSquat employs a patented mechanism that features a loading system which controls the resistance throughout the entire exercise ROM over a wide range of submaximal loads, while simultaneously maintaining precise control of the operating velocity at all points over a wide spectrum of velocities. A weight stack is used to allow an individual to precisely set the load against which the user chooses to exercise, while an electronic braking system is utilized to ensure that an individual exercises at the preselected exercise movement speed.

Depending upon how the two training variables (load and velocity) are manipulated, an individual can combine the physical and metabolic stressors of several different kinds of physical activities (e.g., running up stairs, sprinting to catch a plane or cab, lifting a heavy object, walking, etc.) into a single workout. This enhanced ability to stress the metabolic system in a manner that emphasizes the performance-related factors of endurance, speed, strength, and power to varying degrees during a single workout will have a substantial impact on an individual's functional capabilities.

Physical fitness is frequently defined in the literature as the capacity to engage in reasonably vigorous activities for an extended period of time. Collectively, this capacity involves the interaction of five separate components: aerobic fitness, muscular strength, muscular endurance, flexibility, and body composition. Traditionally, individuals who want to improve their level of physical fitness engage in an exercise program which develops each component of fitness separately—one at a time. Little or no thought is typically given to the need for developing (in an integrated fashion) the metabolic energy pathways which provide the energy required to perform a particular task.

Activities of daily living and most athletic events involve a combination of physical and metabolic demands on the human body. Climbing stairs, running to answer a phone, picking up a child, and mowing the lawn are just a few examples of how an individual, within a relatively brief period of time, may be forced to respond to an ever-changing set of very different physical/metabolic demands. Collectively, these demands may be grouped into four basic performance-related categories: endurance (aerobic and muscular) , speed, strength, and power (speed x strength). In turn, these factors are "blended together" in different combinations and sequences depending on the physical task to be performed. The ability of the body to meet the changing physical demands that are placed upon it without undue fatigue or risk of injury can be viewed collectively as an individual's functional fitness level.

The Evolution to Crossrobics®

Because of the tendency to focus on a single component of fitness while overlooking the necessity to concomitantly enhance the body's metabolic pathways in an integrated fashion, traditional approaches to conditioning and exercise training are severely limited in their ability to enable individuals to meet the constantly changing physical and metabolic demands of daily life. Not surprisingly, the resultant dilemma attendant to this limitation has caused many members of the medical and exercise science communities to reconsider their attitudes towards what constitutes an appropriate way to train. Ultimately, these changes in attitudes served as the catalyst for StairMaster® Sports/Medical Products, Inc. to set upon a course to develop a machine which fully enhances the functional capabilities of the exerciser. The efforts of StairMaster resulted in the development of Crossrobics—a concept of training (based upon a system of precisely controlling both load and velocity while exercising) which has evolved over a period of at least two decades.

One of the earliest indications of the critical need for a revolutionary new concept of training was provided by a series of high-intensity training studies that was conducted at the United States Military Academy in the mid-1970s. These studies examined the effects of performing circuit strength training in a manner which attempted to develop both aerobic fitness and muscular fitness simultaneously. The findings of those research efforts indicated that training more than a single component of physical fitness at the same time has the potential for substantial benefits above and beyond the changes which might have otherwise occurred had the components been developed separately. Not only did the subjects undergoing the experimental training achieve substantial improvement on all of the strength assessment measures, they also improved on several commonly accepted indicators of aerobic fitness (e.g., RPE, resting pulse rate, heart rate response to a submaximal work bout, etc.). More importantly, the subjects incurred a significant degree of improvement on each of the performance-related dependent variables. For example, the subjects decreased their average two-mile run time by over ninety seconds. By all traditional standards, the extent of the improvement achieved on the performance-related items exceeded the level which might have been expected given the results on the conventional measures of aerobic fitness. At the time, the investigators hypothesized that the combined training regimen had a substantial—yet somewhat inexplicable—effect on the ability of the metabolic systems of the subjects to provide energy to their muscles as needed. Despite the fact that a strong argument could be made for the potential benefits of high intensity training which combines both aerobic and strength training into a single workout, such an approach to conditioning was essentially dismissed at the time as being too impractical, too inconvenient, and too intense for most individuals.

Eventually, in the mid-1980s the search for a better way to train resulted in the development of the StairMaster® 5000™ ergometer (and its successors—the StairMaster 6000® ergometer, the StairMaster 4000 PT® and the StairMaster Stepmill® 7000 PT™ exercise systems). Mechanical stair climbing machines, these

StairMaster products provided an exercise environment in which an individual could safely develop both aerobic fitness and lower body muscular strength. Furthermore, the resultant popularity of these machines served to strongly indicate that exercising on these products had adequately addressed the design factors of practicality, convenience, and user comfort.

What the engineers of these machines had not been able to adequately resolve was how to precisely control resistance over a wide range. The load an individual must handle while exercising on these StairMaster products is limited to the body weight of the user. On the other hand, the engineers were able to control the speed of the exercise movement pattern during the exercise bout. Velocity is precisely controlled over a wide range on these machines by means of an electronic braking system which determines how fast the pedals will move/fall.

One of the earliest attempts to rectify the loading limitations of mechanical stair climbing machines involved individuals wearing weighted vests while using the StairMaster 6000. Wearing the vests was hypothesized to simulate the physiologic and metabolic demands imposed on fire fighters wearing their turn-out suits in actual fire fighting situations. The results of these efforts showed that individuals who wore the vests were able to significantly increase the conditioning intensity of the exercise bout. Similar to the high intensity circuit training protocol followed in the West Point studies, however, wearing weighted vests while exercising proved to be both inconvenient and impractical.

Furthermore, researchers found that individuals could decrease the energy cost (i.e., workout intensity) of an exercise bout on a StairMaster machine by off-loading (i.e., supporting a portion of their body weight on the handrail or the front of the machine). Although the ability to vary the load while exercising has merit, off-loading in this manner is simply not an effective means to accomplish such an objective because it isn't precise and it isn't safe. The degree to which a user off-loads while exercising on a mechanical stair climbing machine tends to vary, not only from workout to workout, but also from individual to individual. Off-loading also compromises the functional movement pattern that is inherent in properly using a machine. In addition, depending upon how an individual off-loads while exercising, the resultant body position may subject the user to an undue risk of injury.

In the 1990s, the need to reconsider the way people approach exercise has become even more apparent. For example, many experts have become convinced that aerobic exercise alone is simply not sufficient for developing an optimal level of fitness. An individual can possess a heart and lungs which work efficiently and yet (due to losses in strength) be unable to effectively perform certain activities of daily living. Unfortunately, with each passing year (after age 30), an individual can expect to lose more strength. These losses are significant in individuals who do not engage in exercise specifically designed to enhance their levels of muscular fitness. In other words, individuals need to be both muscularly fit and aerobically fit in order to have the functional capacity needed to perform their activities of daily living.

Another example of the transition that attitudes towards exercise have undertaken in recent years is the significant change in the process of orthopaedic rehabilitation. The traditional approach of rehabilitating an injured lower limb by performing exercises in joint isolation (e.g., by doing knee extensions) has been rejected by many medical professionals in favor of rehabilitating injuries in a more functional manner. Commonly referred to as closed chain exercise or closed kinetic chain exercise, the functional approach to treating lower extremity injuries involves having an individual exercise in a manner in which all the joints of the lower body (hip, knee, and ankle) are required to interact with each other as they would in a real-life environment.

The value of rehabilitating lower body injuries with closed chain exercise can be more clearly understood when the effects of the resultant interactions between the joints are considered. For example, properly performed closed chain exercises result in a pattern of muscular excitation that elicits a co-contraction of the quadriceps and hamstrings across the knee. This co-contraction stabilizes and enhances the integrity of the knee joint by eliminating the anterior shear forces about the knee joint. In addition, the synchronization which occurs between the musculature and the associated structures (tendons, ligaments, nerves) of the three joints not only expedites the healing process, but also heightens the level of the functional capability of the limb receiving treatment.

The focus on function has not been restricted to the rehabilitation process. In recent years, a number of renowned exercise science experts, as well as medical professionals, have become outspoken advocates of the necessity of having exercise prepare an individual to handle the demands of daily life. Consistent with this more functional view of exercise is the fact that not only must individuals develop specific performance-related factors, but also their ability to respond to the energy demands of their working muscles. Accordingly, not only does substantial value exist in having an individual's musculoskeletal and neurological systems operate in synchrony, but also in having an individual's various metabolic energy pathways interface in a manner appropriate to the constantly changing physical stressors of real life. This process of metabolic interfacing can perhaps best be termed as "integrated metabolic conditioning." (Note: Refer to page 91 for a discussion of the adaptations which can occur as a result of this process.)

At first glance, however, the concept of integrated metabolic conditioning might appear to contradict the almost universally accepted theory of specificity which suggests that aerobic athletes should train aerobically and that anaerobic athletes should train anaerobically. In reality, however, integrated metabolic conditioning is very consistent with the theory of specificity. Because very few activities are purely aerobic or anaerobic, individuals who want to improve their level of functional capabilities should include both kinds of training in their exercise programs. The best means of accomplishing this objective is engaging in conditioning activities which constantly switch back and forth from one energy pathway to another.

Finally, another factor which has contributed to the ever-changing attitudes of the exercise science and medical communities towards exercise in the past two decades has been the trend towards prescribing exercise in terms of the minimum effective dosage to produce a training effect. In many aspects of exercise, research has shown that "more is not better." On the other hand, current societal time constraints encourage people to get as much as they can, as quickly as they can with regard to exercise. Consequently, many individuals frequently incorporate efficiency as one of their selection criteria when choosing a personal exercise regimen. The focus on efficiency also appears to extend to most health and fitness clubs. Not surprisingly, personnel who manage these facilities which serve as the primary exercise environment for millions of Americans often view efficiency of exercise as one of the most effective ways of maximizing their limited spatial resources.

In response to the aforementioned factors, StairMaster Sports/Medical Products, Inc. made an unbounded commitment to developing an exercise machine that addresses the physiologic and metabolic demands attendant to the dynamic equilibrium of daily life—the StairMaster® Crossrobics® 1650 LE™ CardioSquat™. Such a commitment was not without great cost, however. A substantial outlay of resources, almost two million dollars and involving tens of thousands of man hours, was devoted to the effort to design and manufacture a machine which will enable an individual to achieve a superior, functional training response. The cumulative result of this commitment is a product which incorporates the scientific findings of a number of disciplines, including biomechanics, physics, medicine, psychology, exercise science, and biomechanics. The net result is the CardioSquat—the standard by which all other exercise modalities will be judged.

BIOENERGETICS:
A THEORETICAL BASIS FOR CROSSROBIC™ CONDITIONING

Human beings require energy to move and function. All bodily cells have the ability to convert foodstuffs (carbohydrates, fats, and, in certain instances, proteins) into a biologically usable form of energy (i.e., adenosine triphosphate—ATP). This process of energy conversion is referred to as bioenergetics. A basic comprehension of what energy is and how the human body acquires, stores, transforms, and uses it is essential to understanding how individuals are able to perform various occupational, recreational, and athletic tasks. In fact, muscular contraction becomes impossible when foodstuffs are not converted into ATP. As a result, physical work would cease. Fortunately, the human metabolic system is capable of supplying the cells of the body with energy on a nearly continuous basis. The energy for all biologic work is produced by three distinct metabolic pathways (ATP-PC, anaerobic glycolysis, and aerobic respiration). Two of these metabolic pathways (ATP-PC and anaerobic glycolysis) are termed anaerobic because energy production occurs without oxygen. The aerobic respiration pathway is termed aerobic because energy production occurs in the presence of oxygen. These metabolic pathways operate under varying conditions, at different rates, and for different durations. Collectively, the three metabolic pathways help determine an individual's ability to effectively perform power-type, speed-type, and endurance-type activities. To optimally prepare an individual for daily life, leisure time, and athletic activities requires a basic understanding of the ATP-PC, anaerobic glycolysis, and aerobic respiration metabolic pathways and their interactions with each other.

ATP: The Primary Energy Source

The immediate source of energy for muscular contraction is a high-energy phosphate compound called ATP. ATP is by far the most important energy-carrying molecule in a cell. In fact, muscular contraction becomes impossible when sufficient amounts of ATP are not available. As a result, without ATP, physical work would cease.

Adenosine and three simpler components called phosphates comprise the ATP molecule. The process of producing energy involves an enzyme called ATPase which is responsible for breaking down ATP to adenosine diphosphate (ADP) and a free, inorganic phosphate (Pi). During the process, energy that an individual can use to perform work is released.

In order to be able to work or exercise for prolonged periods of time, a constant supply of ATP must be made available to the muscle cells. Muscle cells, however, are able to store only limited amounts of ATP. Thus, the cells must be capable of resynthesizing (remaking) ATP for reserve energy sources. Fortunately, metabolic pathways capable of producing ATP exist in the muscle cells. The muscle cells can produce ATP by any one of three metabolic pathways. ATP can be formed via the ATP-PC pathway, the anaerobic glycolysis pathway, and the aerobic respiration pathway.

ATP-PC Pathway

Phosphocreatine (PC) is a chemical compound stored within the muscles, whose chemical bonds (similar to ATP) contain a great deal of energy. When phosphocreatine's chemical bonds are broken, energy is released which can be used to resynthesyze ATP from ADP and Pi. This process is a single step chemical reaction in which one compound (PC) is broken down to form another (ATP). Since this process involves such a simple chemical reaction, it occurs very rapidly and yields energy at a very high rate (i.e., relatively large amounts of ATP are produced in a short period of time). In fact, ATP-PC metabolic pathway has the highest rate of energy production and is the primary fuel source for short-term, high-intensity activities (e.g., sprinting, weight lifting, etc.). Due to the fact that the ATP-PC metabolic pathway can produce energy very rapidly and does not require oxygen to do so, it is always the first energy pathway that an individual calls upon for energy. A major drawback of this pathway, however, is that it cannot continuously produce energy for little more than 10 seconds due to the fact that, similar to ATP, only limited quantities of PC are stored within the muscles.

ANAEROBIC GLYCOLYSIS PATHWAY

A second metabolic pathway capable of rapidly producing ATP via the breakdown of carbohydrates within the cell through a series of chemical reactions is known as anaerobic glycolysis. The carbohydrate which is stored within the muscle cells is known as glycogen. Glycogen is, simply, a long string of glucose (sugar) molecules. Glycolysis involves the breakdown of a single glucose molecule into two molecules of pyruvic acid. Two molecules of ATP are produced with the energy released from the splitting of each glucose molecule. This process is referred to as being anaerobic because it does not require oxygen. Collectively, the entire process of splitting glucose and producing ATP in the absence of oxygen is called anaerobic glycolysis.

It should be noted that the two ATP molecules produced via anaerobic glycolysis represent approximately 5% of the potential ATP yield (i.e., relative to what would occur if oxygen were available and the glucose were completely broken down to carbon dioxide and water). Besides its relatively low energy yield, anaerobic glycolysis results in the formation of lactic acid from pyruvic acid. The buildup of lactic acid in the bloodstream and the muscle cells has several detrimental effects. High concentrations of lactic acid can irritate nerve endings thereby causing pain. In addition, elevated levels of lactic acid lower cellular pH (i.e., increase cellular acidity levels) resulting in the inhibition of many of the chemical reactions needed for energy production. The human body can tolerate only limited amounts of accumulated lactic acid. It is the accumulation of lactic acid that is generally believed to cause an individual to breathe excessively, experience feelings of fatigue and heaviness in his or her muscles, and eventually forces an individual to stop exercising.

Despite its adverse effects, lactic acid should not be viewed solely as a performance-limiting factor. The production and clearance (removal) mechanisms for lactic acid clearly play a positive role in exercise performance, since they can contribute to energy production by resynthesizing ATP. This factor is particularly true during and following high intensity work bouts. Furthermore, across the power output (exercise intensity)-duration curve, the body does not exclusively choose one metabolic pathway over another (e.g., ATP production via anaerobic glycolysis only). At any given point in time, the exercising or working muscles simply use whatever energy is readily available to meet the demands.

For the majority of physical activities, a blend of all energetic pathways is the most likely occurrence. In fact, lactic acid production (via anaerobic glycolysis) occurs simultaneously with aerobic respiration. The relative contribution of each system varies dramatically according to the physiological demands being imposed by the task. All other factors being equal, the body selects the most efficient metabolic pathway (i.e., aerobic respiration) to meet these demands when-

---

*Acetyle Co-A can also be formed by the breakdown of fats or amino acids, then pass into the mitochondria of the cell, where it is eventually metabolized in the presence of oxygen—similar to carbohydrates, the end products are ATP, carbon dioxide, and water.

ever possible. Consequently, the rate of ATP resynthesis can be maximized while the detrimental effects of lactic acid accumulation are minimized.

Thus, it should be quite apparent that short-term activities (i.e., less than two minutes) do not always signify a predominance on the part of the anaerobic metabolic pathways. A vast majority of activities (both athletic and daily-life) are not sustained maximal efforts. In fact, when maximal efforts are necessary, they are often interspersed with multiple periods of recovery. As a result, lactic acid accumulations remain low. In reality, because an individual's body is constantly trying to resynthesize ATP aerobically, anaerobic glycolysis simply serves to help meet an individual's metabolic demands (i.e., bridge the gap) until that person's aerobic energy-producing mechanisms "catch up."

AEROBIC RESPIRATION PATHWAY

The third and final metabolic pathway capable of producing ATP is called aerobic respiration. As implied by its name, the aerobic respiration pathway utilizes oxygen to form ATP, primarily from the breakdown of carbohydrates and fats. The catabolism (breakdown) of glycogen aerobically starts exactly the same way as it does anaerobically—a single glucose molecule is broken down into two pyruvic acid molecules. Unlike anaerobic glycolysis, however, the pyruvic acid is not converted into lactic acid. Instead, it is converted to acetyl Co-A* which then enters into two complex series of chemical reactions (the Kreb's cycle and the electron transport system). These reactions produce energy (ATP), carbon dioxide, and water as their end products.

A major advantage of aerobic respiration is that it results in the production of relatively large amounts of energy in the form of ATP. The maximal amount of energy that can be produced via aerobic respiration is largely determined by the collective efforts of the lungs, heart and circulatory system to deliver oxygen to the cells. Unfortunately, this process is quite complex and time-consuming.

Because of the time lag associated with oxygen transport and delivery, the aerobic respiration metabolic pathway cannot produce energy rapidly enough to meet the demands of high speed, high strength, or high power activities (e.g., sprinting, heavy resistance training, or jumping). Aerobic respiration can, on the other hand, more than adequately handle the energy demands of mild-to-moderate intensity exercise of extended durations (e.g., walking, jogging, swimming long distances, etc.).

INTERACTION OF THE METABOLIC PATHWAYS

All physical activities can be viewed as being on an energy continuum. At one end of the continuum are highly anaerobic activities (high power output) such as sprinting and heavy lifting. At the other end of the spectrum are highly aerobic activities (low power output) like endurance runs and extremely long sets of an exercise at a relatively low level of intensity. The ATP-PC pathway supplies most of the energy for activities near the highly anaerobic end of the continuum. The aerobic respiration pathway, on the other hand, provides the major portion of the energy for activities near the highly aerobic end of the continuum. Anaerobic glycolysis is responsible for supplying the vast majority of the energy for activities that fall in the mid-range of the continuum (e.g., a half-mile run and multiple sets of resistance training involving a moderate-to-high number of repetitions at a moderate-to-high level of resistance).

Although one of the three metabolic pathways may serve as the primary energy source for a given physical activity (e.g., ATP-PC for lifting a heavy object or sprinting up stairs; anaerobic glycolysis for a quarter-mile run or a 100-meter swim; aerobic respiration for walking in a mall or running a marathon), all three pathways contribute to the supply of ATP needed to perform a particular activity. All three metabolic pathways are in action during any and all activities (refer to Figure #1). In other words, the ATP-PC pathway also operates while the body is at rest and the aerobic respiration pathway functions during a 40-yard sprint. This process does not, however, represent the only type of interaction that occurs between the respective metabolic pathways. For example, most real-life situations require the metabolic system to respond to steady-state type energy demands (which are principally supplied by the aerobic respiration pathway) mixed with intermittent anaerobic challenges (which are supplied primarily by either the ATP-PC pathway or anaerobic glycolysis, depending upon the duration of the physical stressor). The interaction between the three metabolic pathways reinforces the conclusion that the concept of integrated metabolic conditioning is consistent with the theory of specificity. Being able to stress the metabolic system in a way that is consistent with what occurs in real life will pay the greatest dividends in terms of enhancing an individual's physical working capacity in the most efficient manner possible.

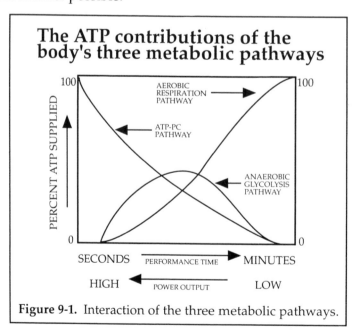

Figure 9-1. Interaction of the three metabolic pathways.

ADAPTATIONS TO INTEGRATED METABOLIC CONDITIONING

One of the primary basic objectives of conditioning is to cause or induce adaptations to enhance an individual's performance capabilities. A specific exercise overload (stress) must be applied to elicit the desired training adaptation—a process which is frequently referred to as the SAID principle (specific adaptation to imposed demands). When applied to conditioning, the SAID principle refers to adaptations in both the metabolic and physiologic systems depending upon the type of and the manner in which the overload is imposed. According to the precepts of the SAID principle, conditioning programs that stress the metabolic system in an integrated or blended fashion bring about specific changes in all three metabolic pathways. The specific metabolic adaptations which result from such conditioning include:

- Increases in resting levels of ATP, PC, free creatine, and glycogen (anaerobic substrate) with the muscle.
- Increases in the amount and activity of specific enzymes that control anaerobic glycolysis.
- Increases in lactic acid clearance or removal capacity.
- Increases in lactic acid tolerance.
- Increases in the capacity of skeletal muscle mitochondria to synthesize ATP aerobically via aerobic respiration.
- Increases in the size and number of mitochondria.
- Increases in the amount and activity level of oxidative (aerobic) enzymes.
- Increases in skeletal muscle myoglobin content.
- Increases in the muscle's ability to mobilize and utilize fat as an energy source.
- Increases in the muscle's ability to metabolize carbohydrates.

Collectively, these metabolic training adaptations allow individuals to more effectively and efficiently produce energy (ATP) both anaerobically and aerobically. At the minimum, these adaptations lead to the following:

- Enable individuals to more rapidly produce energy.
- Enable individuals to more quickly recover from anaerobic bursts of work.
- Enable individuals to more readily switch the emphasis between metabolic (anaerobic and aerobic) pathways.

The net result is that such individuals will be better able to meet the metabolic demands and, in turn, the physical demands they encounter in life (i.e., they will become more functionally fit).

OPERATIONAL CONSTRUCTS OF CROSSROBIC™ TRAINING

In order to elicit a training response involving not only the development of the aforementioned specific performance-related factors, but also the enhancement of the body's metabolic pathways, an individual must exercise on a modality which meets at least four fundamental criteria:

- Precisely controls the level of resistance an individual must handle while exercising.
- Offers a wide range of loads during the exercise bout.
- Precisely controls the rate of speed at which an individual exercises.
- Offers a wide range of velocities during the exercise bout.

Precise control of load. A machine must ensure that the level of resistance (load) that an individual must handle while exercising must be precisely controlled. There are two aspects which must be addressed to provide such control. First, the load that an exerciser selects must be accurate. Second, the machine must require the user to exert a controlled amount of force throughout the entire ROM.

Wide range of loads. A machine must ensure that an individual has the opportunity to choose from a wide range of possible loads.

Precise control of velocity. A machine must ensure that the rate of speed at which an individual is exercising is precisely controlled. There are two aspects which must be addressed to provide such control. First, the velocity that an exerciser selects must be accurate (i.e., the machine does not vary from the preselected speed). Second, the machine must ensure that the user exercises at the preset velocity or adjusts the speed to continue exercising.

Wide range of velocities. A machine must ensure that an individual has the opportunity to choose from a wide range of possible velocities.

IDENTIFYING THE NEED FOR A BETTER WAY TO TRAIN

A review of the characteristics of existing exercise modalities conducted early in the 1990s indicated that no single machine meets all four of the design criteria essential for integrated metabolic conditioning. The extent to which a particular exercise modality permits such a training response to occur tends to vary from modality to modality. For example, three types of exercise machines—rowers, simulated ski machines, and dependent step-action stair climbers—do not meet any of the four criteria. On the other hand, some machines were found to meet a few—but not all—of the necessary requirements.

A treadmill, for example, precisely controls the velocity the exerciser moves over a relatively wide range of velocities. It does not, however, satisfy the load-related criteria. Because users can off-load part of their body weight while exercising on a treadmill by holding onto either the side rails or the front support bar (if it has one), the treadmill does not offer precise control of the load. In addition, unless the user wears a weighted vest while exercising, the load on a treadmill is limited to the user's body weight. Yet another factor contributing to a treadmill's inability to precisely control load is that the load on a treadmill directly interacts with the velocity of the exercise—the greater the exercise velocity, the greater the load.

Other conventional exercise machines were also found to be incapable of eliciting the metabolic interfacing necessary for truly functional conditioning. Exercise cycles, for example, fail to precisely control either velocity or load. While most exercise cycles permit a wide range of speeds, the speed is controlled by the user not the machine. The user is not required to keep up with the machine. Exercise cycles are also very limited in their ability to either precisely control the load or provide a wide range of loads. Several of the more popular exercise cycles (e.g., Lifecycle®, Cybex®, etc.) use an electronic braking system to provide the load. A system where voltage is converted into resistance is very imprecise. Another disadvantage of using an electronic braking system to set the load is the fact that, in many instances, the resistance level is affected by the velocity of the exercise (i.e., the load changes as the velocity changes). Furthermore, the level of resistance (load) at a given setting can vary from machine to machine and from workout to workout.

An exerciser can obtain a wide range of loads on a multi-station weight training machine, but will be unable to precisely control the selected load. The level of control the user will have while exercising on such a machine will be diminished by both inertia (initially to get the weight stack moving) and momentum (subsequently to stop the weight stack from continuing to move away from the user). In addition, multi-station weight stack machines neither precisely control the velocity of the exercise movement nor offer a wide range of velocities (exercise velocities on weight training equipment typically need to be slow to ensure safety and effectiveness) to the user.

Of all the conventional exercise modalities, the StairMaster® 5000™, the StairMaster 6000®, the StairMaster Stepmill® 7000 PT™, and the StairMaster 4000 PT® come closest to allowing users to achieve integrated metabolic conditioning in a safe, efficient exercise environment. These machines do an excellent job of precisely controlling velocity. These machines drive the user to maintain the preselected speed. Users who fail to keep up with the chosen velocity are given a very distinguishable cognitive cue—either the user gradually sinks towards the bottom of the revolving staircase or the pedals sink to the floor. These machines also offer a relatively wide range of possible velocities. Unfortunately, as was previously discussed in the section on the evolution of Crossrobics, these machines cannot precisely control the load an individual must handle while exercising. This lack of precise control of load is due, in large part, to the ability of the user to off-load while exercising. In addition to lacking precise control of load, each of these machines provides a very narrow range of loads (e.g., unless the user wears a weighted vest—or a similar device—while exercising, the loading capacity of each of these StairMaster products is limited to the body weight of the user).

Given the extensive documentation of the ability of the 4000 PT to improve, not only the endurance (both aerobic and muscular) level, but also the lower body strength level of the user, the positive impact that a 4000 PT can have on an individual's functional fitness level is readily apparent. Nonetheless, a critical question arose out of the aforementioned review of whether or not conventional equipment was capable of eliciting an integrated metabolic conditioning training effect: What would be the effect of taking the 4000 PT one step further and designing a machine which precisely controlled load over a wide range of resistance levels, as well as being able to precisely control velocity over a wide range of exercise movement speeds? In response to that question, StairMaster® Sports/Medical Products, Inc. developed the StairMaster Crossrobics 1650 LE CardioSquat conditioning system.

THE STAIRMASTER CROSSROBICS® 1650 LE™ CARDIOSQUAT™ CONDITIONING SYSTEM

The CardioSquat was conceived, designed, and manufactured as a direct result of an identified need to provide a means by which individuals can improve their functional capacity level in specific performance-related factors, as well as enhance their level of metabolic conditioning. Table 9-1 provides a comparative overview of the need for and benefits of the CardioSquat. Unlike conventional exercise modalities, the CardioSquat features a Crossrobic™ loading system which addresses each of the four criteria which are essential for achieving a functional training response.

The key element in the way the CardioSquat incorporates the four operational constructs for Crossrobic training into an integrated system is control—control for a purpose. The machine is designed to require users to exercise in a manner which is most beneficial for them biomechanically, muscularly, and metabolically. Among the ways that the CardioSquat achieves this objective are the following:

Precise control of load. The CardioSquat ensures that the load is precisely controlled during the exercise through the combined interaction between its weight stack and its electronic braking mechanism. This interaction requires the user to apply a level of force while exercising that exactly opposes the load of the weight stack. A prerequisite for precisely controlling the load in this fashion is a very low momentum environment.

Wide range of loads. The CardioSquat provides each user with a wide range of loading levels to ensure that the exerciser has the opportunity to develop a diverse array of performance-related factors (e.g., speed, endurance, strength, and power). Such a range enhances the capability of each user to design an exercise program (prescription) that is appropriate to the exerciser's needs and interests.

Precise control of velocity. The CardioSquat ensures that the velocity is precisely controlled while exercising by combining an electronic braking system with a weight-stack loading system. The braking system establishes the speed at which the user must move the pedal arms. The weight stack provides the exerciser with

Table 9-1. A comparative overview between the StairMaster® Crossrobics® 1650 LE™ CardioSquat™ and selected types of conventional training equipment.

	DESIGN CRITERIA				PERFORMANCE-RELATED FACTORS				Integrated Metabolic Conditioning
	Precise Velocity	Wide Velocity	Precise Load	Wide Load	Speed	Endur-ance	Strength	Power	
StairMaster® Crossrobics® 1650 LE™ CardioSquat™	Y	Y	Y	Y	Y	Y	Y	Y	Y
StairMaster® 4000 PT®	Y	Y	SL	N	Y	Y	Y	VL	SL
Dependent Step-Action Stair Climber	N	N	N	N	VL	Y	VL	VL	VL
Exercise Cycle	N	Y	VL	VL	SL	Y	VL	VL	VL
Multi-station Weight Training Machine	N	N	SL	Y	VL	SL	Y	Y	VL
Rowing Machine	N	N	N	N	SL	Y	SL	SL	SL
Simulated Ski Machine	N	N	N	N	VL	Y	VL	VL	VL
Treadmill	Y	Y	SL	N	Y	Y	VL	VL	SL

KEY: Y = Yes N = No SL = Somewhat Limited VL = Very Limited

instantaneous, cognitive feedback regarding how well the user is actually keeping up with the selected velocity. If the pedal arms are moving too slowly, the weight stack falls. On the other hand, if the individual is exercising at a rate which exceeds the chosen velocity, the weight stack will rise to the top of the guide rods. The requirement to keep the weight suspended while exercising helps "drive" the user to maintain the preselected velocity.

Wide range of velocities. The CardioSquat provides each user with a wide array of movement exercise speeds—ranging from very slow to very fast—in order to provide an exercise environment in which the individual has the capability of being able to stress the various metabolic pathways within a single workout. When combined with the wide range of loading options, such a diversity in velocity choices provides the exerciser with the capability of rapidly (and precisely) changing the training focus of the workout.

The Crossrobic Loading System

The first piece of exercise equipment to meet the criteria required to classify it as a Crossrobic conditioning system is the StairMaster Crossrobics 1650 LE CardioSquat conditioning system. The CardioSquat employs a patented loading system which controls the resistance throughout the entire exercise ROM over a wide range of submaximal loads, while simultaneously maintaining precise control of the operating velocity at all points over a wide spectrum of velocities. A weight stack is used to allow an individual to precisely set the load against which the user chooses to exercise, while an electronic braking mechanism is utilized to ensure that an individual exercises at the preselected exercise movement speed.

Depending upon how the two training variables (load and velocity) are manipulated, an individual can combine the metabolic stressors of several different kinds of physical activities (e.g., running up stairs, sprinting to catch a plane or cab, lifting a heavy object, walking, etc.) into a single workout. This enhanced ability to stress the metabolic system in a manner that emphasizes the performance-related factors of endurance, speed, strength, and power to varying degrees during a single workout can have a substantial impact on an individual's functional capabilities.

As might be expected, training on the CardioSquat significantly improves an individual's functional capacity by inducing systemic adaptations that increase endurance, speed, strength, and power (refer to Figure 9-2). Being able to rapidly and continuously change the training emphasis during a workout results in a metabolic conditioning effect that not only enhances an individual's ability to perform speed, endurance, power, and strength-related tasks, but also an individual's ability to switch rapidly between these kinds of activities without experiencing a noticeable decrement in performance. This conditioning response is the most unique and perhaps one of the most significant adaptations that results from Crossrobic training.

While it can certainly be argued that it is possible for an individual to train for endurance, speed, strength, and power using several different exercise modalities, it would be incorrect to assume that such training would produce the same adaptations as those that occur as a result of exercising regularly on a CardioSquat. The metabolic conditioning specific to switching from endurance to speed or strength to power is best achieved by requiring the body to make such adjustments. The physical stressors of daily life should be viewed as a dynamic equilibrium consisting of long-term aerobic energy production and short, intermittent bursts of intense anaerobic activity. Throughout the course of a day, an individual's steady-state metabolism is disrupted by activity demanding instantaneous high energy. Therefore, a combination of speed, endurance, power, and strength is needed to meet the physical challenges posed by daily living. Similarly, the demands of athletics require a continuous blending or fluctuation between aerobic and anaerobic energy production. The CardioSquat is the only (single) machine available that allows an individual to train any or all four performance-related factors while simultaneously enhancing the entire metabolic en-

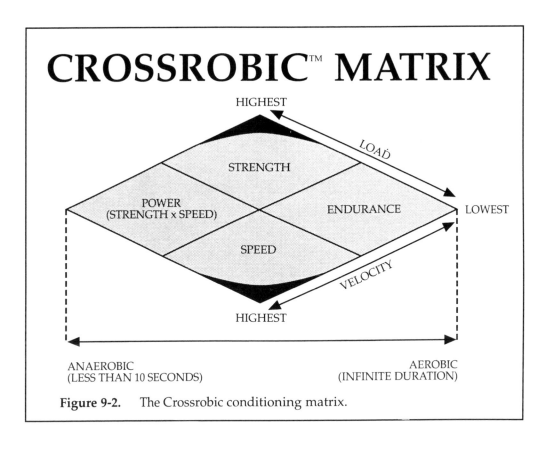

Figure 9-2. The Crossrobic conditioning matrix.

ergy production continuum. Clearly, no other exercise machine has the capacity to improve an individual's physical working capacity to the extent that a CardioSquat can.

THE UNIQUE FEATURES AND BENEFITS OF THE STAIRMASTER® CROSSROBICS® 1650 LE™ CARDIOSQUAT™

•*Involves a maximal amount of the muscle mass in the lower extremities.* The CardioSquat is designed to involve a maximum level of muscle mass of the lower extremities. Electromyographical (EMG) data reveal that the CardioSquat elicits significant involvement of the three major muscle groups of the lower extremities—gluteals, quadriceps, and hamstrings. Metabolic studies have shown that maximal oxygen uptake measured on a CardioSquat falls somewhere between the values obtained on a treadmill or a StairMaster® Stepmill® 7000 PT™ exercise system and a cycle ergometer (oxygen uptake increases in direct proportion to the amount of muscle mass involved in the activity).

•*Emphasizes the hamstring and gluteal muscles.* The CardioSquat was designed so that the hip extension muscles provide the driving force for the exercise motion. Figure 9-3 shows that the hip joint moves through a greater range than the knee joint during the first 37 degrees of pedal motion. The knee joint starts to predominate only during the last 20% of pedal motion. Since most of the muscular force is applied during the first part of the exercise motion and the driving force is coming from the hip joint, one would expect the hamstrings and gluteals to be the most active muscle groups. EMG data show this to be the case (refer to Figure 9-4). Also, the pedal forces during the last 10 degrees are low and the resulting knee stress is minimized.

•*Provides a safe exercise environment.* During exercise on the CardioSquat, the antagonist hamstring and quadriceps muscle groups exhibit peak EMG activity at the same time (refer to Figure 9-5). This co-contraction of the hamstrings and quadriceps acts to stabilize the knee joint and limits shear stress. The arc-shaped movement pattern of the pedal arms (refer to Figure 9-6) ensures that the line of force application coincides with the long axis of the shin. This muscular recruitment pattern also helps to reduce shear stress at the knee joint. Furthermore, whenever a muscle group becomes disproportionately stronger than its antagonist, the weaker muscle is more susceptible to injury. It is widely accepted that the underlying cause of most hamstring injuries is the muscular imbalance between relatively strong quadriceps and relatively weak hamstrings. Emphasizing all the major muscle groups of the lower extremity not cnly stabilizes the knee joint, but can also help to prevent injury and enhance functional capacity.

•*Encourages a functional movement pattern.* By requiring you to keep its weight stack suspended, the CardioSquat directs you towards a functional movement pattern which simulates actions of your lower extremities during weight-bearing

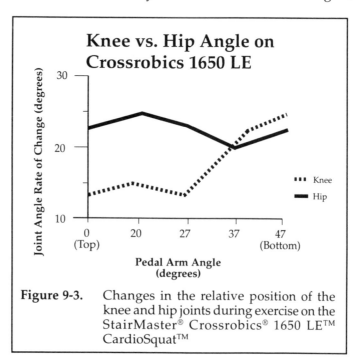

Figure 9-3. Changes in the relative position of the knee and hip joints during exercise on the StairMaster® Crossrobics® 1650 LE™ CardioSquat™

activities. The pattern and nature of muscular excitation indicate that the CardioSquat requires the following muscular actions which are similar to normal ambulation: (1) quadriceps/hamstrings co-contraction across the knee joint, (2) synergistic involvement of the muscles and joints (i.e., they support and oppose each other as they do in real life), and (3) significant range of motion of your hip, knee, and ankle joints. These observations and findings suggest complete involvement of the lower extremities and a natural pattern of muscular activation during exercise on the CardioSquat.

•*Encourages full range exercise movements.* The CardioSquat not only allows but encourages you to exercise your hip and knee joints through a complete range of motion (refer to Figure 9-5). The design of the CardioSquat ensures that your mechanical efficiency increases in direct proportion to your exercise range of motion. In other words, exercising through a complete range of motion makes it easier for you to keep the weight stack suspended—particularly at the more challenging exercise intensities. Few, if any, exercise products encourage you to use them properly (i.e., through a full range of motion). When your muscles are exercised through a full range of motion, your level of joint flexibility is at least maintained and, in many instances, improved. Exercising through a full range of motion also provides your muscles with a more effective training stimulus, since a demand is being placed on them over the entire distance through which they move and function. Performing less than full range exercise movements has limited practical value, since many daily life activities and most athletic tasks require the application of force over distances that are frequently neglected with less-than-full range exercise.

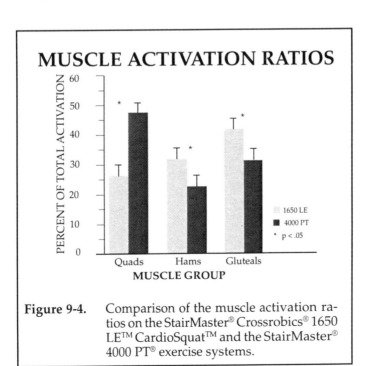

Figure 9-4. Comparison of the muscle activation ratios on the StairMaster® Crossrobics® 1650 LE™ CardioSquat™ and the StairMaster® 4000 PT® exercise systems.

•*Provides controlled, targeted stress to the musculoskeletal system.* By varying the exercise range of motion, you can control and target the stress applied by the load (weight) to specific joint areas/muscle groups. For example, limiting the exercise range of motion (i.e., taking shorter strokes near full extension) results in a more concentrated focus on the quadriceps while simultaneously co-contracting the hamstring and gluteal muscles. This capability has enormous implications for orthopaedic rehabilitation, given the fact that the quadriceps muscles can be stressed without compromising the integrity of the knee joint. The CardioSquat also stresses your muscles, bones, ligaments, and tendons in a safe and appropriate manner, so that they adapt positively to the physiological demands placed on them by becoming stronger and more dense.

•*Features variable weight loading.* Through the use of a weight stack, the CardioSquat precisely and accurately controls the amount of resistance (load) that your muscles must overcome while performing the exercise movement. Your ability to control the load is fully independent of the exercise velocity (speed) you select. In addition to precisely and accurately controlling the exercise load (weight), the CardioSquat allows you to select from a relatively wide range of loads (30-120 pounds). The higher the weight selected, the greater the strength demand placed on the musculature of your lower body throughout the exercise range of movement. This feature enables you to reap the combined benefits of weight-loading and aerobic exercise without the impact trauma of weight-bearing exercise.

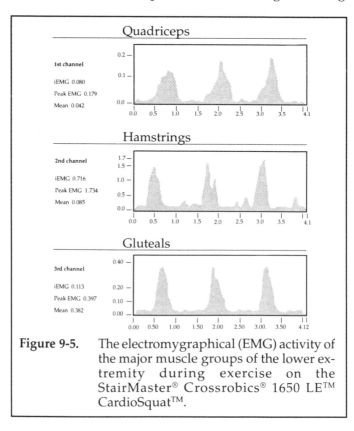

Figure 9-5.   The electromygraphical (EMG) activity of the major muscle groups of the lower extremity during exercise on the StairMaster® Crossrobics® 1650 LE™ CardioSquat™.

•*Features variable velocity levels.* The CardioSquat uses an electronic braking mechanism that controls the pedal arm velocity. The exercise velocities can range from very slow to very fast, and are controlled entirely independent of the load you select (no interaction exists between the selected velocity and load). This feature allows you to quickly shift the training emphasis from speed, power, strength or endurance.

•*Simulates the demands of a wide range of physical activities.* By achieving fully independent control of both load and velocity, over very wide ranges, the CardioSquat allows you to simulate and control the physiologic/metabolic demands of essentially any activity. Accordingly, the CardioSquat is the ideal conditioning device for developing functional fitness since it can so effectively simulate the physiologic/metabolic demands of a vast array of activities.

•*Promotes successful weight management.* The CardioSquat helps you to attain and to maintain your ideal body weight (the weight at which you are not at risk for obesity-related diseases and at which your functional abilities are not impaired). An analysis of the available data (refer to Table 9-2) indicates that, in general, the combination of a conventional aerobic exercise program with calorie reduction does little to preserve lean body mass during weight reduction. The less lean body mass you have, the lower your resting metabolic rate. As a result, it is more likely that you will regain some or all of the weight you may have lost.

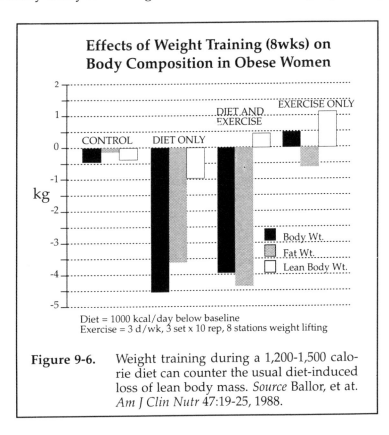

Figure 9-6.   Weight training during a 1,200-1,500 calorie diet can counter the usual diet-induced loss of lean body mass. *Source* Ballor, et at. *Am J Clin Nutr* 47:19-25, 1988.

On the other hand, if you engage in exercise designed to improve your muscular fitness level at the same time you are losing weight, you enhance the likelihood that you will be able to sustain your level of lean body mass (refer to Figure 9-6). The CardioSquat, with its unique ability to blend aerobic conditioning with strength training, can provide you with the optimum exercise for weight management. Exercising on the CardioSquat allows you to expend a sufficient number of calories and simultaneously preserve or increase your lean body mass.

•*Offers a vast array of prescription options.* Each of the seven preset program options has twenty intensity levels. Within each intensity level, you can exercise at fourteen distinct velocities. In addition, the manually operated self-pace program operates with fourteen increments over the entire range of velocities. By manipulating the variable velocity options and variable weight loading choices (30-120 pounds), you have over two thousand (2,000) different exercise prescription alternatives from which to choose. With this vast array of prescription options, you can design your workouts such that you exercise across the entire Crossrobic conditioning matrix (refer to Figure 9-2). The wide variety of choices which this feature offers you, gives you the ability to (finely) adjust your exercise dose as needed or desired and should also help enhance your level of exercise adherence. ❏

Table 9-2. Review of studies where subjects on reducing diets were randomly assigned to aerobic exercise and nonexercise groups.

Changes in Body Weight for an Exercise Group vs. Dieting Sedentary Group

Reference	Diet (kcal/da)	Exercise (hrs/week)	Length of Study (weeks)	Body Wt. (lbs.)	Fat Wt. (lbs.)	Lean Wt. (lbs.)
Nieman (1988)	1268	3.8	5	NS	NS	NS
Hagan (1986)	1200	2.5	12	-5.5	-3.3	-2.2
Van Dale (1987)	767	2.7	12	NS	NS	NS
Hill (1987)	800	5.0	5	NS	-3.7	+2.9
Phinney (1988)	720	7.0	4	NS	NA	NA
Katch (1988)	1200	2.5	20	NS	NS	NS
Van Dale (1989)	800	4.0	14	8.6	7.5	NS
Hammer (1989)	800/1450	3.8	16	NS	NS	NS
Warwick (1981)	800	14.0	3.5	NS	NA	NA
Lennon (1985)	1500	3.0	12	NS	NS	NS

NS = Not significant
NA = Information not available

BIBLIOGRAPHY •

1. Armstrong, R. "Biochemistry: Energy liberation and use." In *Sports Medicine and Physiology*, Strauss, R. (Ed). Philadelphia, PA: W.B. Saunders Company, 1979.

2. Åstrand, P.O., Rodahl, K. *Textbook of Work Physiology*, 3rd Ed. New York, NY: McGraw-Hill, 1986.

3. Atha, J. "Strengthening muscle." *Exerc Sports Sci Rev* 9:1-73, 1981.

4. Ballor, D.L., Katch, V.L., Becque, M.D., Marks, C.R. "Resistance weight training during caloric restriction enhances lean body weight maintenance." *Am J Clin Nutr* 47:19-25, 1988.

5. Basmajian, J.V., De Laca, C.J. *Muscles Alive: Their Functions Revealed by Electromyography*, 5th Ed. Baltimore, MD: Williams & Wilkins, 1985.

6. Ben-Ezra, V., Verstraete, R. "Stair Climbing: An alternative exercise modality for firefighters." *J Occup Med* 30(2):103-105, 1988.

7. Bessman, S., Carpender, C. "The creatine phosphate shuttle." *Ann Rev Biochem* 54:831-62, 1985.

8. Brooks, G.A. "The lactate shuttle during exercise and recovery." *Med Sci Sports Exerc* 18(3):360-368, 1986.

9. Brooks, G.A., Fahey, T.D. *Exercise Physiology: Human Bioenergetics and Its Applications*. New York, NY: John Wiley & Sons, 1984.

10. Burke, E.J. "Work physiology and the components of physical fitness in the analysis of human performance." In *Toward An Understanding of Human Performance*, 2nd Ed., Burke, E.J. (Ed). Ithaca, NY: Mouvement Publications, 1980.

11. DeCarlo, M., et al. "Electromyographic and cinematographic analysis of the lower extremity during closed kinetic chain (StairMaster 4000 PT) exercise." *Isokin Exerc Sci* 2(1):24-29, 1992.

12. Dudley, G.A. "Metabolic consequences of resistive-type exercise." *Med Sci Sports Exerc* 20(5 Suppl.):158-161, 1988.

13. Fisher, G.A., Jensen, C.R. *Scientific Basis of Athletic Conditioning*. Philadelphia, PA: Lea and Febiger, 1990.

14. Fleck, S.J., Kraemer, W.J. *Designing Resistance Training Programs*. Champaign, IL: Human Kinetics Publishers, 1987.

15. Fox, E.L. "Differences in metabolic alterations with sprint versus endurance interval training programs." In *Metabolic Adaptation to Prolonged Physical Exercise*, Howald, H., Poortmans, J. (Eds). Basel, Switzerland: Birkhauser Verlag, 1975.

16. Fox, E.L. "Energy sources during rest and exercise." In *Encyclopedia of Physical Education, Fitness, and Sports*, Stull, G.A. (Ed). Salt Lake City, UT: Brighton Publishing Company, 1980.

17. Fox, E.L. "Physical training: Methods and effects." *Orthop Clin N Am* 8(3):53-598, 1977.

18. Fox, E.L. "Physiological effects of training." *Encyclopedia of Physical Fitness*. New York, NY: John Wiley and Sons, 1979.

19. Fox, E.L. *Sports Physiology*. Philadelphia, PA: W.B. Saunders Company, 1984.

20. Fox, E.L., Bowers, R.D., Foss, M.L. *The Physiological Basis of Physical Education and Athletics*, 4th Ed. Philadelphia, PA: W.B. Saunders Company, 1988.

21. Fox, E.L., et al. "Intensity and distance of interval training programs and changes in aerobic power." *Med Sci Sports* 5(1):18-22, 1973.

22. Fox, E.L., et al. "Metabolic responses to interval training programs of high and low power output." *Med Sci Sports* 9(3):191-196, 1977.

23. Fox, E.L., Mathews, D. *Interval Training: Conditioning for Sports and General Fitness*, 4th Ed. Philadelphia, PA: W.B. Saunders Company, 1974.

24. Fox, E.L., McKenzie, D.C., Cohen, K. "Specificity of training: Metabolic and circulatory responses." *Med Sci Sports* 7:83, 1975.

25. Fox, E.L., Robinson, S., Wiegman, D.L. "Metabolic energy sources during continuous and interval running." *J Appl Physiol* 27:174-178, 1969.

26. Fox, S.I. *Human Physiology*, 3rd Ed. Dubuque, IA: Wm. C. Brown Publishers, 1990.

27. Gollnick, P.D., King, D.W. "Energy release in the muscle cell." *Med Sci Sports* 1:23-31, 1969.

28. Gray, G.W., Peterson, J.A., Bryant, C.X. "Plane sense: Closed chain exercise." *Fit Manag* 8(5):30-33, 1992.

29. Hagan, R.D., Upton, S.J., Wong, L., Whittam, J. "The effects of aerobic conditioning and/or caloric restriction in overweight men and women." *Med Sci Sports Exerc* 18:87-94, 1986.

30. Hammer, R.L., Barrier, C.A., Roundy, E.S., Bradford, J.M., Fisher, A.G. "Calorie-restricted low-fat diet and exercise in obese women." *Am J Clin Nutr* 49:77-85, 1989.

31. Hermansen, L. "Anaerobic energy release." *Med Sci Sports* 1:32-38, 1969.

32. Hill, J.O., Sparling, P.B., Shields, T.W., Heller, P.A. "Effects of exercise and food restriction on body composition and metabolic rate in obese women." *Am J Clin Nutr* 46:622-630, 1987.

33. Holloszy, J.O., Booth, F.W. "Biochemical adaptations to endurance exercise in muscle." *Ann Rev Physiol* 38:273-291, 1976.

34. Holloszy, J.O., Coyle, E. "Adaptations of skeletal muscle to endurance exercise and their metabolic consequences." *J Appl Physiol* 56:831-38, 1984.

35. Hultman, E., Bergstrom, J., McClennan-Anderson, N. "Breakdown and resynthesis of phosphocreatine and adenosine triphosphate in connection with muscular work in man." *Scand J Clin Invest* 19:56-66, 1967.

36. Hunt, D.C., et al. "Effect of training on physical work capacity at the fatigue threshold in the elderly." *Med Sci Sports Exerc* 24(5 Suppl.):S14, 1992.

37. Jequier, E., Flatt, J. "Recent advances in human bioenergetics." *News in Physiol Sci* 1:112-14, 1986.

38. Karlsson, J. "Lactate and phosphagen concentrations in working muscle of man." *Acta Physiol Scand* (Suppl. 358):1-72, 1971.

39. Karlsson, J., Saltin, B. "Lactate, ATP, and CP in working muscles during exhaustive exercise in man." *J Appl Physiol* 29:598-602, 1970.

40. Katch, V., Becque, M.D., Marks, C., Moorehead, C., Rocchini, A. "Basal metabolism of obese adolescents: Inconsistent diet and exercise effects." *Am J Clin Nutr* 48:565-569, 1988.

41. Komi, P., Rusko, H., Vos, J., Bihko, V. "Anaerobic performance capacity in athletes." *Acta Physiol Scand* 100:107-114, 1977.

42. Lamb, D.R. *Physiology of Exercise: Responses & Adaptations*, 2nd Ed. New York, NY: Macmillan, 1984.

43. Lehninger, A.L. *Bioenergetics*, 2nd Ed. New York, NY: W.A. Benjamin, 1971.

44. Lennon, D., Nagle, F., Stratman, F., et al. "Diet and exercise training effects on resting metabolic rate." *Int J Obes* 9:39-47, 1985.

45. Luttgens, K., Wells, K.F. *Kinesiology: Scientific Basis of Human Motion*, 7th Ed. Dubuque, IA: Wm. C. Brown Publishers, 1989.

46. Margaria, R. *Biomechanics and Energetics of Muscular Exercise*. Oxford, England: Oxford University Press, 1976.

47. McArdle, W.D., Katch, F.I., Katch, V.L. *Exercise Physiology: Energy, Nutrition, and Human Performance*. Philadelphia, PA: Lea & Febiger, 1991.

48. Nieman, D.C., Haig, J.L., De Guia, E.D., et al. "Reducing diet and exercise training effects on resting metabolic rates in mildly obese women." *J Sports Med* 28:79-88, 1988.

49. Palmitier, R.A., An, K.N., Scott, S.G., Chao, E.Y. "Kinetic chain exercise in knee rehabilitation." *Sports Med* 11(6):402-413, 1991.
50. Peterson, J.A. "The effects of high intensity weight training on cardiovascular function." Exercise Physiology and Athletic Ability and Its Relevance to Athletic Ability. In *Physical Activity and Human Well-Being*, Landry, F., Orban, W.A.R. (Eds), 1977.
51. Peterson, J.A., Bryant, C.X. (Eds). *StairMaster Fitness Handbook: A User's Guide to Exercise Testing and Prescription*. Indianapolis, IN: Masters Press, 1992.
52. Phinney, S.D., LaGrange, B.M., O'Connell, M., Danforth, E. "Effects of aerobic exercise on energy expenditure and nitrogen balance during very low calorie dieting." *Metabolism* 37:758-765, 1988.
53. Poortmans, J.R. (Ed). *Biochemistry of Exercise*. Baltimore, MD: University Park Press, 1968.
54. Shelbourne, K.D., Nitz, P. "Accelerated rehabilitation after anterior cruciate ligament reconstruction." *Am J Sports Med* 18(3):292-299, 1990.
55. Shelbourne, K.D., Wilckens, J. "Current concepts in anterior cruciate ligament rehabilitation." *Orthop Rev* 19(11):957-964, 1990.
56. Skinner, J.S., Noeldner, S.P., O'Connor, J.S. "The development and maintenance of physical fitness." In *Sports Medicine*, 2nd Ed., Ryan, A.J., Allman, F.D. (Eds). New York, NY: Academic Press, 1989.
57. Smidt, G.L. "Biomechanical analysis of knee flexion and extension." *J Biomechanics* 6:79-92, 1973.
58. Solomonow, M., et al. "The synergistic action of the anterior cruciate ligament and thigh muscles in maintaining joint stability." *Am J Sports Med* 15(3):207-213, 1987.
59. Stegemann, J. *Exercise Physiology: The Physiologic Bases of Work and Sport*, 2nd Ed. Chicago, IL: Year Book Medical Publishers, Inc., 1977.
60. Van Dale, D., Saris, W.H.M. "Repetitive weight loss and weight regain: Effects on weight reduction, resting metabolic rate, and lipolytic activity before and after exercise and/or diet treatment." *Am J Clin Nutr* 49:409-416, 1989.
61. Van Dale, D., Saris, W.H.M., Schoffelen, P.F.M., Ten Hoor, F. "Does exercise give an additional effect in weight reduction regimens?" *Int J Obes* 11:367-375, 1987.
62. Warwick, P.M., Garrow, J.S. "The effect of addition of exercise to a regime of dietary restriction on weight loss, nitrogen balance, resting metabolic rate and spontaneous physical activity in three obese women in a metabolic ward." *Int J Obes* 5:25-32, 1981.

CHAPTER 10

• •

UNDERSTANDING THE PSYCHOLOGICAL BASIS OF EXERCISE

by

Debra J. Crews, Ph.D.
and
Elizabeth Hart, M.A.

• • •

*A*n intrinsic interaction between your mind and your body exists during all daily activities, including exercise. The relationship between psychological state and exercise is cyclical, such that your psychological state prior to exercise can influence your physiological response to exercise and the performance outcome. Similarly, exercise is known to influence your psychological state both during and after exercise. Psychological state is usually defined as the mental and emotional processes at a given point in time. Such a definition involves several factors, including affect, mood, stress reactivity, anxiety, depression, cognitive functioning, self-perception, personality characteristics and addictive behaviors. This chapter is divided into two main parts. The first section discusses the influence of *psychological state on exercise*. The other primary section addresses the effects of *exercise on specific psychological states*.

Over the years, research in this area has generally involved an interdisciplinary approach between psychology and exercise science. As a result, in the past two decades the field of exercise psychology has evolved as an effective force in the effort to obtain more accurate information on the relationship between exercise and the mind-body connection. This chapter presents an overview of several of the important research findings concerning this relationship. The critical information within each main section and sub-section is summarized at the end of each particular segment with a special "points to remember" discussion. Viable mechanisms to explain the reason exercise influences each psychological state are also summarized within each section.

PSYCHOLOGICAL INFLUENCES ON EXERCISE

Your psychological state can have a profound effect on your ability to perform physically. Unfortunately, the importance of your psychological state, as it relates to physical performance, is sometimes ignored. For example, it is highly unlikely that if your fitness is assessed in a structured situation such as an exercise facility, a cardiac rehabilitation program, or a laboratory situation that your present psychological state and how it may influence your test results are taken into account. By the same token, how the effectiveness of a particular training regimen might be influenced by specific psychosocial variables on a given day or over a given period of time is also frequently overlooked.

Three categories of psychosocial variables have been identified which influence either the physiological response to exercise or the exercise performance outcome. All variables are grouped into one of three basic classifications: affect/mood, perceptions, and cognitions.

Affect is defined as a state of mind or body, an emotion or feeling related to an idea or object. It tends to be more of an immediate and intense psychological experience. In contrast, mood is an enduring, less intense emotional state representing a predominant or prevailing feeling.

Perception involves the use of senses, awareness, and comprehension to understand objects, qualities, etc. Hypnosis and personality characteristics are two factors that alter an individual's perception and have been found to influence exercise behavior.

The third category—cognitions—refers to the process of knowing. Examples of variables in this classification include memory, judgment, and perception. Exercisers use specific cognitive strategies at various stages of training to enhance their performance outcome. These strategies, which are commonly referred to as coping techniques, include the use of biofeedback in some cases.

Affect/mood. Research has shown that affect/mood influences both your physiological responses during exercise and your performance outcome. One major study was designed in such a way that the conditions of anger, happiness, sadness, and fear using imagery were compared with conditions of relaxation and control while subjects completed a stepping task. Researchers in this investigation found that heart rate (HR) and systolic blood pressure (SBP) were the main reactors during exercise and that anger, fear, and happiness produced more step climbing in less time compared with the control condition. The HR of subjects in this study actually doubled during the anger and exercise conditions. On the other hand, the sadness and relaxation conditions produced lower performance outcomes than the control condition. Sadness also exhibited an inhibitory effect on the HR and diastolic blood pressure (DBP) responses to exercise.

Researchers in other studies have also discovered that affect/mood influences physiological and performance responses. For example, happiness has been shown to produce greater grip strength responses than sadness. In another study, daily variations in running economy (i.e., the oxygen cost of exercise at a given work load) were found to be highly related to overall mood state—specifically, tension (i.e., running economy decreases as tension increases). This particular response, for example, may affect a cardiac rehabilitation patient in an angry state or a sad state who as a result of this specific affect/mood may experience significantly different HRs during training.

Perception. Noted exercise psychologist, William Morgan, has demonstrated through a series of studies that exercisers working at a constant workload will exhibit varying physiological responses during an altered state of consciousness (i.e., hypnosis). For instance, exercisers who are led to believe that they are lifting a heavier weight than they actually are, or are cycling up a hill when they are on level terrain, will have greater oxygen demands and changes in ventilation, respectively.

Type A behavior, which is separately addressed in a latter section of this chapter, has been associated with a more positive perception of exercise at low-to-moderate intensity work and a more negative affect at high intensity work levels than found among individuals with Type B personalities. This finding suggests that your psychological state prior to exercise can influence your perception of the exercise. Accordingly, many researchers conclude that any physiological information monitored during exercise can be influenced at a subconscious level by the exerciser's pre-existing psychological state. Furthermore, they contend that this physiological information is somehow altered prior to reaching the conscious level of awareness in the cerebral cortex of the brain. As a result, these researchers assert that it is highly likely that it is important for an exerciser to attain a positive psychological state prior to exercising in order to receive the greatest benefit from the exercise bout.

In addition to considering the effects of psychological factors on exercise, it is also important to note the effect of exercise on your perception of the exercise as well. The most common measure of perceived effort during exercise is the rating of perceived exertion (RPE). Exertion or RPE has been defined by several exercise scientists as the integration of various *physiological* sensations. A strong argument could be advanced that RPE would be more appropriately defined as the integration of various *psychosocial* influences and *physiological* sensations. RPE, using this definition, would involve both physiological cues (two-thirds) and psychological cues (one-third). Psychological cues are believed to have a greater influence during low and moderate intensity exercise, while physiological cues dominate RPE assessment at high-intensity work levels. Among the various psychosocial factors which are associated with a decrease in RPE are: extroversion, hypnosis, dissociation, anxiety, gender of the exercise tester, and athletic experience.

RPE was originally structured to provide scores which were almost linearly related to HR (RPE x 10 = HR). In a few studies, however, ventilation and lactate levels have been found to have a closer relationship with RPE scores than HR. Such findings suggest that some degree of caution is necessary when you're using RPE to determine training intensity. The intensity of the exercise bout should be assessed by at least one additional physiological measure, as well as through the use of RPE, since several psychological factors have been shown to influence RPE.

Cognition. The three categories within cognition which have been shown to influence exercise include: mental strategies (e.g., association, dissociation), coping strategies (e.g., stress management, relaxation), and biofeedback (information provided to an individual regarding a physiological response during exercise).

The two mental strategies which have received the greatest attention are association and dissociation. Association refers to an attentional focus on bodily responses during exercise. In contrast, dissociation refers to an attentional focus on anything other than bodily responses. It appears that beginning exercisers benefit most from dissociative techniques. Advanced exercisers encounter a similar experience when they participate in a novel task. Novice exercisers seem to benefit most from distraction, or dissociation, since they are not familiar with the pain or discomforts of starting an exercise program, and, thus, have not devised appropriate coping strategies for dealing with the pain.

Experienced exercisers participating in an exercise mode familiar to them benefit most from an associative style. Individuals who exercise on a regular basis in a familiar activity learn the coping techniques necessary for controlling their pain and discomfort. Focusing on bodily responses during exercise evokes the cues needed for eliciting the appropriate coping technique. It is important to note, however, that during an exercise bout, you use both associative and dissociative strategies, and that your adherence to one strategy does not usually exceed 80% of the total time you exercise. Exercise psychologists caution exercisers to keep in mind the fact that the existing research suggests that these two mental strategies do not adequately encompass all of the thoughts you use to control your responses while exercising. Unfortunately, however, they conclude that until which time more precise definitions and conclusive classifications are identified and tested, these two strategies offer the best basis for explaining how you cognitively attempt to influence your response to exercise.

Stress management is probably the coping strategy most commonly used during exercise. Stress management includes relaxation, visualization, imagery, biofeedback, and cognitive restructuring (e.g., changing self-talk patterns). Research has shown that oxygen cost decreases during the first half of an aerobic exercise bout for individuals who employ stress management techniques. Other studies have found that the use of relaxation techniques has resulted in enhanced running performance. Researchers conclude that such performance changes are probably the consequence of improvements in running economy which result from the reduction in the tension level experienced by the exercisers.

Several biofeedback studies have examined the effects of manipulating a specific physiological response during exercise to determine what changes occur in the energy cost of exercise or in the performance outcome. Recent research suggests, however, that such studies have substantial methodological limitations. The majority of these studies, for example, have used a single physiological response measure to alter the cost or the performance result of an exercise bout. The use of multiple physiological measures, however, has been found to be more effective in producing changes in exercise economy and performance. Studies employing multiple physiological measures have shown that programs using biofeedback may have to be conducted over a relatively longer period of time to produce substantial changes in the energy cost levels of the exercisers. Furthermore, researchers surmise that any changes in the performance outcome of an exercise bout are likely to be subsequent to changes in energy economy levels.

POINTS TO REMEMBER:
- Anger, fear, and happiness produce greater physiological responses during exercise and better performance outcomes, while sadness inhibits these responses.
- Anxiety has been shown to increase the energy cost of exercise on a given day.
- Your psychological state prior to exercise can influence the ratings of effort you experience during exercise.
- RPE should be used in conjunction with a physiological measure since many psychological factors influence RPE.
- Novice exercisers effectively use dissociative strategies, while experienced exercisers effectively use associative strategies while exercising on a mode familiar to them.
- Stress management techniques can reduce the oxygen cost of exercise.
- Biofeedback training can effectively alter a physiological response pattern. Multimeasure biofeedback training, however, appears to be the most effective way to reduce the oxygen cost of exercise and ultimately, to improve performance.

THE EFFECTS OF EXERCISE ON SPECIFIC PSYCHOLOGICAL STATES

Among the many benefits often attributed to exercise is the perception that exercise improves your ability to perform certain tasks and to think more clearly. In fact, many corporations, for example, have made substantial investments in exercise facilities at least partially on the belief that their employees who use these facilities will be, not only healthier, but more productive as a result of the opportunity to exercise on a regular basis. The possible effect of exercising on cognitive functioning gives rise to several questions. First, do individuals think better or perform tasks more efficiently if they exercise on a regular basis? More specifically, does their cognitive functioning improve during and/or after exercise? At least two factors should be considered when attempting to answer this question. First, what type of exercise influences cognitive functioning? Second, what aspects of performance are influenced by exercise?

Research findings suggest that exercise does influence cognitive functioning. How it affects your ability to think and perform certain tasks appears to depend on certain features attendant to the general type of exercise in which you engage—for example, how often and how long you exercise. Acute (i.e., a single exercise bout) exercise, for example, differs widely from chronic (i.e., repeated exercise bouts over time) exercise in the way it affects cognitive functioning. When examining cognitive performance during or immediately after exercise, it appears that an exercise bout of high intensity and short duration enhances performance. In addition, as the intensity of an exercise bout is reduced, its duration may be lengthened (within limits) without incurring a concomitant decrement in performance. On the other hand, exercising a relatively longer period of time that produces fatigue has been shown to have a debilitating effect on cognitive performance. Tasks involving speed rather than accuracy have been shown to be enhanced by an acute bout of exercise. Moderate difficulty tasks are most likely to improve with exercise rather than tasks which are at either end of the spectrum (e.g., too easy or too difficult).

Chronic exercise has been associated, both during and following physical activity, with levels of higher intelligence and enhanced memory. It is not clear whether intelligent people choose to exercise or whether exercise affects intelligence. It also appears that exercise enhances memory recall. Such a finding has very important implications—particularly for older populations.

The mechanism by which exercise may influence cognitive functioning has received considerable attention by researchers. One theory which has been advanced suggests that increases in core temperature, which accompany exercise, may speed specific catalytic events in the body which facilitate cognitive functioning and performance. Core temperatures, for example, may be elevated for as long as 90 minutes after you stop exercising. Credence to this theory has been provided by investigators who have been able to show that exercise in which core temperature changes are blocked inhibits improvements in cognitive performance via altered brain wave patterns. Another possible explanation for the relationship between exercise and cognitive functioning has been termed by researchers as the "hardware" alteration. This interpretation suggests that the density of blood vessels in your cerebral cortex increases as the result of exercise, while the number of synapses associated with a particular motor activity increases as you learn the activity. The temperature and the structural changes interact with each other in such a way to produce improved cognitive functioning.

POINTS TO REMEMBER:
- Short duration, high intensity exercise facilitates cognitive functioning (specifically speed), both during and after exercise.
- Exercise of a moderate duration and a moderate intensity also facilitates cognitive performance both during and after exercise. The effects are larger for moderate difficulty tasks.
- Longer duration, low intensity exercise enhances your ability to think clearly and perform certain motor functions until you become fatigued. Fatigue inhibits cognitive functioning and performance.

EXERCISE INFLUENCES ON STRESS REACTIVITY

Many individuals who lead an active lifestyle often believe that exercise reduces the stresses which arise during daily living. Stress is an emotional response which occurs when the demands of a situation exceed an individual's perceived capabilities to handle that situation in an appropriate manner. What these exercisers may be perceiving is that exercise reduces the extent of their response to the self-defined stressors in their life. As a result, they subsequently spend less time in a "stressful" state. The potential impact of such a consequence can be significant. For example, some evidence exists to support the contention that decreasing the extent and the time for which you are suffering from stress elicits a concomitant reduction in your level of cardiovascular risk and improves your immunological competence (e.g., your resistance to infection and disease).

The basic assumption by which exercise is believed to have a positive effect on stress suggests that your physiological response to exercise is somewhat similar to your physiological response during stress. Accordingly, exercise may train your body to more effectively cope with the daily stressors you encounter. On the other hand, a few subtle differences exist between your physiological response to exercise as compared to psychological stress. One of the more obvious differences lies in the source of where in your body the physiological response is initiated. On one hand, the demands of exercise elicit increases in primarily sympathetic activation from the periphery of your body (e.g., your muscles). On the other hand, your response to psychological stress is initiated from the central command center of your brain. The common factor in your physiological reaction to both exercise and psychological stress is the response of your adrenal system. Research findings in this area suggest that your adrenal receptor sensitivity is altered by exercise, thus reducing your physiological response to stress.

Despite the subtle differences which exist between your physiological responses to exercise and stress, the available data indicate that you will experience an overall reduction in your stress level as a result of exercise. Most of the research on this subject has attempted to identify the effect of chronic aerobic exercise on stress reactivity by comparing fit with unfit individuals. Fit subjects have been found to exhibit both a reduced reactivity to stress and an enhanced ability to recover to their pre-stress emotional state following a bout of stress.

Only a limited amount of research has been conducted which has examined the effects of an acute bout of exercise on stress. Unfortunately, these studies have produced equivocal results depending on the amount of time which has elapsed between when an exercise bout occurred and when the stressor was present. For example, a group of researchers from Wake Forest University were able to demonstrate a reduction in HR and SBP reactivity when the subjects were allowed a 30-minute recovery period following their exercise session. In addition, these researchers found that higher intensity exercise produced a greater reduction in HR and SBP response to psychosocial stressors than did low intensity exercise.

Finally, anaerobic exercise should not be ignored as a potential means of reducing stress. At least one group of investigators have reported findings that indicate that anaerobic exercise reduces stress reactivity more effectively than aerobic exercise.

Several theories have been advanced to explain the possible basis regarding why stress reactivity is reduced following exercise. The "time-out hypothesis" suggests that time away from the stressor reduces stress. Yet, this hypothesis does not explain why higher intensity exercise elicits greater reductions in stress reactivity than lower intensity exercise. The "opponent process theory" suggests that the physical stress of exercise may produce an opposing response (e.g., reduced stress) following exercise. Dienstbier's "sympathetic toughness concept" proposes that repeated exposure to physical stress (e.g., exercise) may train your body to be less affected by certain demands on it and recover more quickly from psychosocial stress.

The finding that exercise can have a positive effect on stress reactivity has several potential implications for other health benefits, such as reduced cardiovascular risk and enhanced immunological function. Considerable research has confirmed that your level of stress is a significant causal factor in both coronary heart disease and immune system response. Accordingly, the ability of exercise to decrease your level of stress reactivity can have a corresponding positive influence not only on how well you handle stress, but also on the effect of that stress on your exposure to certain diseases. A lower blood pressure response reduces your level of cardiovascular risk, which subsequently diminishes the likelihood that you will suffer from coronary heart disease. The research findings concerning the possible effect that exercise has on immune function are equally promising. Data is available which show that aerobic exercise has a positive effect on natural killer cell activity, thereby enhancing immunological competence.

POINTS TO REMEMBER

- Acute aerobic exercise with adequate recovery time reduces stress reactivity among conditioned individuals. These effects are greater following high intensity exercise.
- Chronic aerobic exercise reduces both stress response and your ability to recover from stress.
- Anaerobic exercise appears to reduce stress reactivity.
- Exercise which reduces stress may also reduce cardiovascular risk and enhance immunological competence.

EXERCISE INFLUENCES ON ANXIETY, MOOD STATE, AND DEPRESSION

People often report that they "feel better" after exercising. "Feeling better" may represent many responses to exercise, including physiological responses (increased energy), perceptual responses (enhanced self-esteem), and affective responses (reduction of negative thoughts and feelings).

Exercise psychologists are particularly interested in these responses to exercise since they may help to explain individual motives for exercise involvement and adherence. This section of the chapter explores the influence of exercise on emotion or, as it is more commonly referred to in the exercise literature— "affect." Specifically, the influence of exercise on anxiety, general mood state and depression is addressed.

Anxiety and General Mood State. A recent scientific review of the effects of exercise on anxiety and mood combined the results from a variety of investigations. Researchers involved in this effort concluded that exercising can improve both anxiety and mood over baseline levels. The type of comparison group used, the type of exercise performed, and the intensity and duration of the exercise bout were all found to influence this relationship. For example, some of the investigations compared the effect of an exercising group to a non-exercising group and found that exercise reduced anxiety and improved mood levels. Other studies compared participants to each other before and after exercising and still found that a reduction in anxiety and an improvement in mood levels resulted. Other investigators compared an exercising group to a placebo control group (e.g., yoga, relaxation). In these research efforts, exercise was found to be somewhat better in improving mood state than the placebo control treatment.

The findings of these studies suggest that the effects of exercise on anxiety are dependent on whether the anxiety is short-term ("state anxiety") or more chronic ("trait anxiety"). Exercise does not reduce state anxiety to a greater degree than "other activities." These results lend some support to the "time-out" hypothesis regarding why stress levels are reduced following exercise—a theory which suggests that exercise may serve simply as a distraction from your daily worries.

Long-term exercise appears to reduce trait anxiety to a greater extent than shorter-term exercise. This reduction is commonly linked to the "training" effect that accompanies long-term exercise participation. Many researchers have shown that exercise itself represents a physiological stressor. Accordingly, regular exposure to exercise subsequently reduces your body's negative response to exercise. In turn, after an appropriate period of time, regular exercise elicits specific positive reactions which "toughen" it, thereby enabling it to respond in a more appropriate manner to other subsequent stressors (e.g., physiological and/or psychological).

The duration and intensity of exercise have been found to influence anxiety and mood state. It appears that exercise needs to be performed at least 20 minutes at an intensity of greater than 70% HR-max to be associated with reduced anxiety and improved mood. Exercise bouts lasting longer than 30 minutes have not been shown to result in greater changes. Increasing intensities of exercise, however, have been associated with a more positive mood state and reduced anxiety. A few studies have explored anxiety and mood responses to exercise intensities as high as 90%. The findings from these studies indicate that exercising at extremely high intensity levels may have a negative effect on both anxiety and mood state. Reductions in anxiety and mood improvements have been reported to continue for at least 30 minutes, and perhaps as long as six hours, after the exercise bout has actually ceased. The type of exercise performed is yet another factor which appears to influence whether an anxiety reduction or mood state improvement occurs. The majority of the research performed in this area has focused on aerobic exercise—the type of activity which has been shown to have the most positive affect on anxiety and mood state levels. Unfortunately, relatively little is known about the effects of anaerobic exercise on anxiety and mood state.

Exercise Influences on Depression. Exercise has long been advocated as a possible positive factor in the treatment of depression. Early research on the subject suggested that higher levels of depression existed primarily in individuals who exhibited lower levels of fitness. As a result, it was erroneously believed that only poorly fit people could diminish their feelings of depression by exercising and that the general population would not receive a similar benefit. Eventually, however, researchers rightfully concluded that such research had several significant design limitations. For example, information which explained the degree of depression or the type of exercise intervention in the study was frequently not reported in the summary of the research findings.

Recently, many studies have shown that both acute and chronic exercise significantly decrease depression. Contrary to other findings, these results suggest that the antidepressant effect of exercise may begin in the first session of exercise. In addition, these studies have found that exercise is a better antidepressant than relaxation or other "enjoyable" activities, and is as effective in decreasing depression as psychotherapy. It is important to note, however, that considerable evidence exists which indicates that exercise when combined with psychotherapy is a more effective alternative than exercise alone in reducing depression. Finally, decreases in levels of depression have been observed across a variety of subject characteristics, including age, gender, and degree of depression. In terms of reducing depression, exercise has been found to be effective across all age groups, for both men and women, and for varying degrees of depression. Contrary to the earlier assumptions, this finding indicates that exercise will have a positive effect on the level of depression among the general population, not just the deconditioned person.

A variety of explanations have been advanced regarding the antidepressant effects of exercise. The reasons offered generally fall into one of two categories: psychological or physiological. The psychological factors which have been proposed include cognitive-behavioral changes, social interaction factors and the "time-out" hypothesis.

PSYCHOLOGICAL BASIS OF EXERCISE
• • •

The cognitive changes that may occur as a result of exercise include an increased level of self-confidence and self-esteem that often results when you meet the challenges of a task that you perceive to be somewhat difficult (e.g., exercise). In turn, your ability to master one set of challenges often enables you to be better prepared to deal with different challenges in other areas of your life—all of which may lead to a decrease in your sense of depression.

The belief that social interaction factors can have a positive effect on depression levels implies that contact with others may lead to decreases in depression. Some researchers suggest that the social aspects of exercise may be more influential at the onset of an exercise program, since the rewards of exercise are primarily external and have not been internalized at this point. Such a conclusion, however, was not supported by the findings of a recent study which discovered that exercise programs conducted in the home led to greater decreases in depression than those in either community center or university settings. As was discussed in a previous section in this chapter, the "time-out" hypothesis suggests that exercise may simply offer a distraction from daily worries and problems.

The physiological factors which have been advanced to explain the antidepressant effects of exercise include an increase in cardiovascular fitness, biochemical changes and the release of endorphins. It is highly unlikely, however, that the antidepressant effect of exercise which occurs during the first few weeks of exercise is due to training-induced improvements in cardiovascular fitness (which have not occurred to any substantial extent for most individuals at this particular point in the training regimen). While it is possible that the initial increases in cardiovascular fitness you experience play some role in decreasing chronic depression, the acute effects of exercise may be better explained by the occurrence of specific biochemical alterations in your body. Depressed individuals are thought to have decreased secretions of specific neurotransmitter metabolites which are thought to increase during exercise . As a result, exercise is believed to stimulate the release of these substances, which in turn reduces depression. The release of endorphins (endogenous opiates) are also frequently cited as the mechanism for the alteration of mood state. While increases in endorphin levels have been observed in the blood of humans, they have not been found in the brain. Although euphoric feelings have been linked to endorphin release, until research determines whether endorphins cross the blood-brain barrier, any hypothesis regarding their mood altering properties remains speculation.

Points to Remember
- Exercise needs to be performed for a period lasting at least 20 minutes, at an intensity level of at least 70% HR-max, in order to reduce anxiety and improve mood state.
- Chronic, rather than acute, exercise may be needed to decrease depression.
- Exercise appears to reduce depression in a variety of populations, but the precise mechanism for its antidepressant effect has not, at this point, been identified.

EXERCISE INFLUENCES ON PERSONALITY CHARACTERISTICS

Your personality represents the unique product of your stable and enduring behaviors. In recent years, exercise psychologists have shown an increased interest in exploring the influence that exercise may have on an individual's personality. In particular, individual behaviors that may be related to health risk have received increased attention. The Type A behavior pattern (TABP) is perhaps the most widely studied of these personality characteristics, since it has been linked to coronary heart disease.

The Type A personality is characterized by a strong sense of time urgency, impatience, hostility, aggressiveness, and competitiveness. These characteristics are thought to influence cardiovascular reactivity and neuroendocrine responses, both of which are related to coronary heart disease. It is generally accepted that aerobic exercise lessens cardiovascular reactivity to psychosocial stress. As a result, researchers are interested in the effect that exercise has on Type A individuals, since these individuals often exhibit exaggerated cardiovascular responses to both exercise and stress.

In a recent study which investigated the effect of aerobic exercise on cardiovascular reactivity in Type A middle-aged men, exercise was found to be a promising intervention strategy. In addition, the cardiovascular benefits of aerobic exercise have been found to decrease diastolic blood pressure, heart rate and total peripheral resistance in borderline hypertensive Type A men.

Modifications in the characteristic TABP may also result from engaging in regular exercise. One study found that the basic TABP was modified to a limited extent in Type A females after only 10 weeks of participating in an aerobic exercise program. Some researchers caution, however, that even though some research findings lend support for exercise as a promising intervention in reducing TABP, additional factors must also be considered. First, the majority of Type A intervention research has focused on aerobic exercise. As a result, relatively little is known about the effects of anaerobic exercise. Also, much of the early Type A research utilized a Type A measurement tool (the Jenkins Activity Survey) whose reliability as a predictor of the relationship between TABP and coronary heart disease has recently come into question. In the past few years, the Structured Interview technique has become the preferred assessment tool in this area. The findings of studies using this tool suggest that TABP may not be as directly related to coronary heart disease as was originally thought. Finally, specific components of the Type A personality may be more strongly related to coronary heart disease than the collective (global) measure. In particular, the element of hostility has been identified as one of the personality components most highly linked to coronary heart disease. Interestingly, mood states such as depression and anxiety have been found to be equally valid predictors of coronary heart disease as the collective TABP. Accordingly, a strong argument can be advanced that it may be necessary to reduce specific components of the Type A personality to reduce coronary risk.

EXERCISE INFLUENCES ON SELF PERCEPTIONS

A commonly held notion in much of the popular literature suggests that positive perceptions of your body may be related to positive feelings about your self. Given the ingrained nature of this belief, it is quite possible that your self-perceptions may be influenced by your involvement in an exercise program. Early studies conducted in this area reported that participation in exercise programs was associated with improved self-esteem scores. Recent research, however, suggests that self-esteem is a global characteristic that is multidimensional in nature, representing a variety of subcomponents. For example, on one hand, you may have a high degree of esteem specific to your role as a parent; on another hand, you may have a low degree of esteem specific to your body. As a result, it is not all that unlikely that individuals with similar self-esteem scores may differ tremendously on the individual components that collectively comprise their global index of self-esteem.

In addition, the subcomponents of self-esteem may be further divided into more specific dimensions. For example, some researchers suggest that the physical component of self-esteem involves several dimensions. Several researchers have surmised that physical self-esteem is composed of physical self-efficacy, physical competence, and physical acceptance. Others, while also supporting the multidimensional nature of physical self-esteem, propose that physical self-esteem encompasses different factors, including perceptions of sport competence, bodily attractiveness, physical strength and muscular development, and physical conditioning.

When the hierarchical nature of self-esteem is taken into consideration, many exercise psychologists believe that exercise may have more of an immediate effect on the lower levels (specific subcomponents) of self-esteem. In turn, such a consequence has obvious implications regarding how and when physical self-esteem is influenced and, ultimately, global self-esteem. For example, researchers have found that at least 20 weeks of consistent exercise may be needed to observe significant changes in global self-esteem. It appears that the more specific the dimension of self-esteem, the more situationally specific it is in regard to change. Therefore, while participating in an exercise regimen may increase your perceptions of your physical self-attractiveness, it may not have a similar effect on your perception of your sport competence.

Unfortunately, the literature of the relationship between exercise and self-perception is currently somewhat vague and inconclusive. Considerable research does exist, however, to support the contention that the degree of importance an individual places on the physical dimension of self-esteem influences the degree to which exercise participation will influence global self-esteem. In addition, research indicates that factors other than improvements in your level of aerobic fitness may influence the relationship between your exercise participation and your level of physical self-esteem. Changes in your body weight, eating patterns and physical appearance may influence the degree to which your involvement in an exercise program affects your sense of physical self-esteem. Obviously, in this instance, other types of exercise (e.g., resistance training) may also influence particular dimensions of your sense of self-esteem. Attempts to explain the possible influence of exercise on self-esteem have also involved considering whether the sense of accomplishment (that comes when you successfully encounter a challenge) or the opportunity to have positive social interaction with others is consequential.

Finally, research findings indicate that negative physical self-perceptions can also influence whether an individual engages in an exercise program. For example, some individuals will actually avoid exercise (especially in a group setting) if they perceive that others hold a negative opinion of their bodies.

POINTS TO REMEMBER
- The physical self-esteem subcomponent of global self-esteem may be the aspect which is most directly influenced by exercise participation.
- The physical self-esteem subcomponent is divided into specific dimensions which may be differentially affected by various modes of exercise (e.g., running, resistance training).
- The perceived importance you hold for the physical dimension of self-esteem is an important consideration regarding the influence that exercise has on your sense of self-esteem.
- Individuals with a negative opinion regarding the way other individuals will perceive their bodies may avoid participating in physical activities that would otherwise be quite beneficial for them.

EXERCISE AND ADDICTION

Addictive behaviors are often related to poor self-esteem, depression, or high anxiety. Because exercise has been shown to influence these mood states, several efforts have been undertaken in recent years to study exercise as a possible treatment intervention for addictive behaviors. The possible influence of exercising on alcoholism, in particular, has received considerable attention in the past few years. The initial efforts to study the influence of exercise on alcoholism have focused on identifying what physiological changes can be attained by alcoholics who exercise on a regular basis. These studies have attempted to determine whether individuals with a drinking problem could attain improved fitness levels comparable to those achieved by nonalcoholic populations.

A limited amount of research has also attempted to identify the psychological changes in addictive individuals that may result from exercise participation. A reduction in the level of behavioral dysfunction exhibited by these individuals, specifically a decrease in both anxiety and depression, has been reported along with an increase in overall physical fitness . Significant decreases in state anxiety, trait anxiety and depression in alcoholics who exercise on a regular basis have also been observed.

Without question, exercise as a treatment intervention for alcoholism offers some promising findings. Exercise psychologists warn, however, that similar to other research findings in this particular field of specialization, some caution should be taken when interpreting the results of studies involving the possible relationship between exercise and alcoholism. Other alternative explanations should also be considered. For example, participating in an exercise program may enhance the receptivity of an alcoholic to standard psychotherapy intervention. In addition, engaging in a structured leisure-time activity, such as exercise, may cause alcoholics to reorganize the way they spend their leisure time—a process which may in itself serve to discourage past addictive behaviors. Finally, an increased level of fitness may enable an alcoholic to deal more effectively with a specific stress, which, in turn, may reduce the individual's dependence on alcohol.

Interestingly, exercise participation itself may become an addictive behavior. Some researchers suggest that exercise participation should be viewed as a "positive addiction." In other words, the pursuit of the energy and enthusiasm that accompany physical activity is a healthy addiction. Unfortunately, individuals who become dependent on exercise may experience frustration, hostility and guilt when deprived of the opportunity to be physically active. In fact, in one study, the investigators looked at what would happen if individuals were offered money to abstain from exercise for a month. Somewhat surprisingly (depending on your point of view), many habitual exercisers refused to stop participating for the specified length of time regardless of the monetary incentive. Research has also shown that individuals who experience negative feelings when missing a run scored significantly higher on a measure of "commitment to running" than those who do not. Even short-term variations from running schedules have often been found to have a negative effect on habitual runners.

Researchers have developed the following diagnostic criteria you can review to see if you have a "dependency" on exercise:

- you regularly engage in strenuous exercise (greater than four days per week for at least 30 minutes),

- you suffer from a dysphoric or anxious mood or self-depreciating thoughts when you're unable to exercise as much as planned,
- you alter your normal priorities to the extent that exercise is placed above other activities, with resultant social or occupational consequences,
- you hold irrational expectations regarding the amount of exercise you need to maintain a desired body shape or a perceived level of aerobic fitness,
- you persist with your exercise behavior in the face of certain negative physical consequences, emanating from such factors as injuries, bad weather, or unsafe exercise conditions.

If you recognize a strong similarity between your attitudes and lifestyle and the aforementioned criteria, keep in mind that while exercise may serve as an effective intervention in the treatment of addictive behaviors such as alcoholism, it may become an addictive behavior in your case. In other words, for some, one addiction replaces another. In the initial stages of treatment it may be useful to replace a negative addiction with a positive addiction. Every effort should be made, however, to preclude a positive addiction from being transformed into an addiction with negative consequences.

POINTS TO REMEMBER
- Exercise participation may offer a promising treatment intervention for alcoholism.
- Participation in exercise may enhance an alcoholic's receptivity to standard psychotherapy programs.
- Exercise may offer a positive leisure time activity that replaces past addictive behaviors (e.g., drinking).
- Exercise itself may become addictive leading to abnormal exercise dependence.

THE MIND-BODY CONNECTION

Exercise—particularly aerobic exercise—has been shown to have a positive effect on your state of mind. By the same token, your psychological state has been found to greatly influence what you get out of exercising, including how your body responds physiologically to the demands of the exercise, how much you enjoy the exercise bout, and how your attitudes are shaped regarding the value of exercise (a very component of exercise adherence).

As the field of exercise psychology continues to grow and to expand its efforts to learn more about the mind-body relationship to exercise, the psychological benefits and behavioral consequences of engaging in a sound exercise program will become even more apparent. Eventually, it is not unlikely that exercise prescriptions will address psychological objectives, as well as physiological concerns. Even though exercise psychology is still in its relative infancy, its future is extraordinarily promising. ❏

BIBLIOGRAPHY •

1. Booth-Kewley, S., Friedman, H.S. "Psychological predictors of heart disease: A qualitative review." *Psychol Bull* 101:343-362, 1987.
2. Carmack, M.A., Martens, R. "Measuring commitment to running: A survey of runner's attitudes and mental states." *Sport Psychol* 1:25-42, 1979.
3. Crews, D.J., Landers, D.M. "A meta-analytic review of aerobic fitness and reactivity to psychosocial stressors." *Med Sci Sport Exerc* 19:114-120, 1987.
4. Dientsbier, R.A. "Arousal and physiological toughness: Implications for mental and physical health." *Psychol Rev* 96(1):84-100, 1989.
5. Fiatarone, M.A., Morley, J.E., Bloom, E.T., et al. "Endogenous opioids and the exercise-induced augmentation of natural killer cell activity." *J Lab Clin Med* 112:544-552, 1988.
6. Fox, K.H., Corbin, C.B. "The physical self-perception profile: Development and preliminary validation." *J Sport Exerc Psychol* 11:408-430, 1989.
7. Frankel, A., Murphy, J. "Physical fitness and personality in alcoholism: Canonical analysis of measures before and after treatment." *J Studies Alcohol* 35:1271-1278, 1974.
8. Greist, J.H., Klein, M.H., Eischens, R.R., et al. "Running as a treatment for depression." *Comp Psychiatry* 20:41-54, 1979.
9. Hart, E.A., Leary, M.L., Rejeski, W.J. "The measurement of social physique anxiety." *J Sport Exerc Psychol* 11:94-104, 1989.
10. Kavanagh, D., Hausfeld, S. "Physical performance and self-efficacy under happy and sad moods." *J Sport Psychol* 8:112-123, 1986.
11. Lo, C.R., Phil, D., Johnston, D.W. "The self-control of the cardiovascular response to exercise using feedback of the product of the interbeat interval and pulse transit time." *Psychosom Med* 46:115-125, 1984.
12. Matthews, K.A. "Coronary heart disease and type A behaviors: Update on and alternative to the Booth-Kewley and Friedman (1987) quantitative review." *Psychol Bull* 104:373-380, 1988.
13. Morgan, W.P. "Psychogenic factors and exercise metabolism: A review." *Med Sci Sports Exercise* 17:309-316, 1985.
14. Morgan, W.P., Pollock, M.L. "Psychologic characterizations of the elite distance runner." *Ann NY Acad Sci* 301:382-403, 1977.
15. North, T.C., McCullagh, P., Tran, Z.V. "Effect of exercise on depression." *Exerc Sport Sci Rev* 18:379-415, 1990.
16. Palmer, J., Vacc, N., Epstein, J. "Adult inpatient alcoholics: Physical exercise as a treatment intervention." *J Studies Alcohol* 49(5):418-421, 1988.
17. Pandolf, K.B. "Advances in the study and application of perceived exertion." *Exerc Sport Sci Rev* 11:118-158, 1983.
18. Petruzzello, S.J., Landers, D.M., Hatfield, B.D., et al. "A meta analysis on the anxiety reducing effects of acute and chronic exercise: Outcomes and mechanisms." *Sports Med* 11:143-182, 1991.
19. Reeves, D.L., Justesen, D.R., Levinson, D.M., et al. "Endogenous hyperthermia in normal human subjects: I. Experimental study of evoked potentials and reaction time." *Physiol Psychol* 13:258-267, 1985.
20. Rejeski, W.J. "Perceived exertion: An active or passive process?" *J Sport Psychol* 7:371-378, 1985.
21. Rejeski, W.J., Gregg, E., Thompson, A., et al. "The effects of varying doses of acute aerobic exercise on psychophysiological stress responses in highly trained cyclists." *J Sport Exerc Psychol* 13(2):188-199, 1991.
22. Rosenberg, M. *Conceiving the Self.* New York, NY: Basic, 1979.

23. Roskies, E., Seraganian, P., Oseasohn, R., et al. "The Montreal type A intervention project: Major findings." *Health Psychol* 5:45-69, 1986.

24. Salazar, W., Landers, D.M., Petruzzello, S.J., et al. "Effects of exercise on intellectual function: A meta analysis." Paper presented at the North American Society for the Psychology of Sport and Physical Activity. Monterey, CA, June 1991.

25. Schwartz, G.E., Weinberger, D.A., Singer, J.A. "Cardiovascular differentiation of happiness, sadness, anger, and fear following imagery and exercise." *Psychosom Med* 43:343-364, 1981.

26. Solomon, R.L., Corbit, J.D. "An opponent-process theory of motivation: II. Cigarette addiction." *J Abnormal Psychol* 81(2):158-171, 1973.

27. Sonstroem, R.J., Morgan, W.P. "Exercise and self-esteem: Rationale and model." *Med Sci Sports Exerc* 21:329-337, 1989.

28. Tomporowski, P.D., Ellis, N.R. "Effects of exercise on cognitive processes: A review." *Am Psychol* 99:338-346, 1986.

29. Williams, T.J., Krahenbuhl, G.S., Morgan, D.W. "Mood state and running economy in moderately trained male runners." *Med Sci Sports Exerc* 23:727-731, 1991.

30. Ziegler, S.G., Klinzing, J., Williamson, K. "The effects of two stress management training programs on cardiorespiratory efficiency." *J Sport Psychol* 4:280-289, 1982.

CHAPTER 11

• •

UNDERSTANDING CLOSED CHAIN EXERCISE*

by

*Gary Gray, P.T., James A. Peterson, Ph.D.,
and Cedric X. Bryant, Ph.D.*

• • •

"The magic is not in the medicine, but in the patient's body—in the *vis medicatrix natural*, the recuperative or self-corrective energy of nature. What the treatment does is to stimulate natural functions or to remove what hinders them."

C. S. Lewis
from *Miracles*

*T*he aforementioned words of the late, renowned theologian and philosopher, C. S. Lewis, offer partial insight into a fundamental change which has begun to occur recently in the way medical professionals view the type of exercise necessary for effective rehabilitation of orthopaedic conditions. Traditionally, exercise has been perceived in a very structured way by the medical community. This perception involves introducing exercise into the rehabilitation process on a restricted basis after a suitable (extended) period of time. Stabilize one part of the body (primarily while in a non-weight bearing position), and then exercise another part. This is an approach which has often been characterized by its proponents with such phrases as . . . "conservative" . . . the "proven" alternative . . . the "right" thing to do.

Regrettably, while the traditional approach to orthopaedic rehabilitation certainly appears to have been compatible with the comfort zone of those who relied on it, a growing body of both research and empirical evidence supports the conclusion that it is neither the "right thing to do" nor the "proven alternative." The traditional approach does not, in the words of C. S. Lewis, "stimulate natural functions." Rather, it requires the body to exercise in a very unnatural, non-functional manner.

---

* Note: Some of the material contained in this chapter is adapted from "Plane Sense," an article which appeared in *Fitness Management* 8(5):30-33, 1992.

Not only does non-functional exercise limit the degree of success which can be attained in the healing process, in many instances, it may even be counterproductive (injurious) to the entire rehab effort. Considerable evidence suggests that all other factors being equal, the more functional the exercise, the more effective the healing process.

CLOSED CHAIN VS. OPEN CHAIN EXERCISE

A strong argument can be made that the most practical way of evaluating the therapeutic effectiveness of exercise is to examine the relative position of the body during the exercise. Your body can be viewed as a chain. Your limbs (legs and arms) serve as the opposite ends of the chain. If either set of limbs is involved in supporting your weight (e.g., a squatting exercise in which your legs are bearing the weight of your body; a push-up in which your arms are partially shouldering the weight of your body), the physical endeavor is referred to as an example of a "closed chain exercise." The end segment of the chain is closed (e.g., fixed).

If the end segment of the chain (your limbs) is not fixed (i.e., free—not supporting the weight of your body), the exercise is termed an "open chain exercise." For numerous reasons, closed chain exercises are much more functional and effective in facilitating the healing process than open chain exercises.

The Greek philosopher Aristotle provided a potential basis for comprehending the nature of closed chain exercise by stating, "The animal that moves makes its change of position by pressing that which is beneath it." This simple statement contains two elements which should be considered: the interaction between an animal (man) and its environment; and the way in which an animal organizes the pressing.

Closed chain exercise provides a natural way of exercising which involves functional movements. Functional movement is important because directly and indirectly it requires your body (joints, muscles, neurological system) to operate as it does normally. As you exercise, your joints, muscles, and neurological system are required to react to each other as they do in real life. Muscles vary the degree to which they support and oppose each other depending on which (axial) cardinal plane(s) they happen to be in at any specific moment in time. In functional movement, joints incur different natural stresses, depending on the plane of movement, the velocity of the movement, and the type of loading to which they are exposed. Of equal importance, functional movement facilitates normal proprioceptive feedback. Your neurological system interacts with your musculoskeletal system in a coordinated fashion that produces safe and natural movement patterns.

One of the intrinsically important rules of rehabilitation is to create an environment for optimal healing. Closed chain exercise provides the means for individuals to safely engage in constructive rehabilitation activities within a healing environment that focuses on the way bodies actually work.

CLOSED CHAIN EXERCISE

• • •

Open chain exercises, on the other hand, involve isolated movements which impose artificial stresses (i.e., non-natural) on the body. The body is simply incapable of responding to such stresses in a functional way. As a result, the healing process is severely impeded—if not stopped.

Table 11-1 presents a comparative overview between open and closed chain rehabilitation techniques on twelve critical factors. A review of the differences between the two techniques strongly suggests that the substantial growth in the use of closed chain exercises in orthopaedic rehabilitation programs is well justified. Such a review also suggests that when individuals seek advice on how to rehabilitate an injury, they should be encouraged to engage in closed chain exercises as opposed to open chain.

Table 11-1. A Comparison Between Open and Closed Chain Rehabilitation Techniques for the Knee.

	Open Chain Exercise	**Closed Chain Exercise**
End Segment	Free	Fixed
Axis of Motion	Distal to the joint	Both proximal and distal to the joint
Muscle Contraction	Primarily concentric	Concentric, eccentric, and isometric
Movement	Isolated	Functional
Load	Artificial and sometimes abnormal	Normal physiological load through the skeletal system
Velocity	Sometimes predetermined; unsafe at upper limits	Variable according to exercise requirements
Stress/Strain	Biomechanically inconsistent within soft tissues	Biomechanically consistent within the soft tissues
Stabilization	Afforded through artificial means	Synergistic muscle contractions
Planes	Occurs in only one of the three cardinal planes	Occurs in all three cardinal planes, consistent with the motion of the joint & structures
Proprioception	Facilitates probable foreign and erroneous proprioceptive feedback	Facilitates normal proprioceptive feedback mechanisms
Rehabilitation Techniques	Limited to the design of the equipment being used	Unlimited potential
Rehabilitation Reaction	Non-integrated open and many times isolated event	Integrated chain reaction

THE VALUE OF CLOSED CHAIN EXERCISE

The inherent value of closed chain exercise can be more clearly understood when the logic of noted endocrinologist Hans Selye's theory of stress adaptation is applied to the question of what type of exercises will have the most positive effect on the healing process. Selye found that the human body will gradually adapt to the stresses imposed upon it. If an individual imposes an artificial stress, the body adapts to that stress. Subsequently, when the body resumes functioning in a normal manner, the artificially-induced adaptation will be of minimal value. In all likelihood, if pain was present before the bout of open chain exercises, the pain will still exist if the body has otherwise failed to heal itself naturally over a specific period of time.

The validity of Selye's conclusions is even more apparent when the process of knee rehabilitation is considered. The knee is one area of the body which is commonly injured during participation in fitness and sport activities. Many fitness professionals erroneously advise an individual with knee pain to do leg extension exercises. In the first place, the cause of the individual's pain may originate in some other part of the body and have nothing to do with the muscles adjacent to the knee. Even if the pain was associated with some deficiency involving the muscles and attendant tissues and structures of the knee, having the individual perform an isolated exercise through a single plane of motion would make little, or no, sense. Rather, the individual should be counselled to perform closed chain exercises (e.g., unweighted step-ups, partial squats, exercise on an independent step-action, mechanical stair climbing machine, etc.).

The value of performing closed chain exercises is based on the concept that physiologically and biomechanically the human body is an extraordinarily complex entity in which the different parts interact according to the stresses imposed upon them in whatever position a particular structure is in at a given time. These positions vary from body area to body area, from moment to moment within any physical movement.

Biomechanists use the three basic cardinal planes (refer to Figure 11-1) of the body (frontal, sagittal, and transverse) as reference points. Unlike open chain exercise which isolates a part of the body during exercise to a single plane, closed chain exercise takes advantage of the fact that the human body constantly moves in a triplane mode. At any given moment, forces (stresses) are being imposed on the body in all three planes. Any effort to rehabilitate the body which is not based on this reality can be counterproductive to the healing process.

A CLEAR CHOICE

For reasons probably best appreciated by manufacturers of testing equipment which assess selected physiological and performance variables while individuals are performing open chain exercise, the question of which type of exercise—open chain vs. closed chain—is most appropriate for the rehabilitation process has traditionally been couched as an issue involving the conservative approach versus the aggressive approach. Aggressive has been unfairly perceived as taking undue risks, while the conservative approach has been viewed as the safe alternative. Neither categorization is justifiable. A more equitable way of looking at the entire matter is to examine the merits of a non-functional approach versus a functional approach. Artificial vs. natural. Make-do vs. can-do. Careful examination of the issue of open versus closed chain exercise would leave little doubt regarding which is the more functional method of rehabilitation. Closed chain exercise clearly makes good sense, as well as "plane sense." ❏

Figure 11-1. Schematic representation of the primary cardinal reference planes.

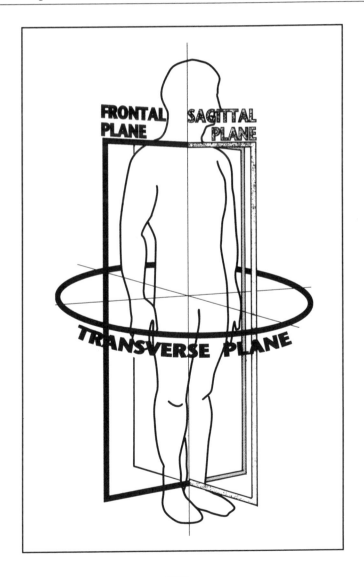

BIBLIOGRAPHY •••••••••••••••••••••••••••••••••••••••

1. American Academy of Orthopaedic Surgeons. Symposium on the Athletic Knee: Surgical Repair and Reconstruction. St. Louis, MO: The C. V. Mosby Company, 1980.
2. Cailliet, R. *Knee Pain and Disability*. Philadelphia, PA: F. A. Davis Company, 1973.
3. Davies, G.J. et al. "Mechanisms of Selected Knee Injuries," *Phys Ther* 60:1590-1595, 1980.
4. Enoka, R.M. *Neuromechanical Basis of Kinesiology*. Champaign, IL: Human Kinetics Publishers, 1988.
5. Evans, F.G. (Ed). *Studies in the Anatomy and Function of Bones and Joints*. New York, NY: Wiley-Interscience, 1979.
6. Feagin, J.E. (Ed). *The Crucial Ligaments*. New York, NY: Churchill Livingstone, Inc., 1988.
7. Gray, G. *Chain Reaction*. (Unpublished Manual). Adrian, MI: Wynn Marketing, 1992.
8. Grieve, G. *Common Vertebrae Joint Problems*. New York, NY: Churchill Livingstone Inc., 1981.
9. MacConaill, M.A., Basmajian, J.V. *Muscles and Movements: A Basis for Human Kinesiology*. Baltimore, MD: Williams and Wilkins, 1969.
10. Maigne, R. *Orthopedic Medicine*. Springfield, IL: Charles C. Thomas, Publisher, 1976.
11. Mangine, R.E. (Ed). *Physical Therapy of the Knee*. New York, NY: Churchill Livingstone, 1988.
12. Mercier, L.R., Pettid, F.J. *Practical Orthopedics*. Chicago, IL: Year Book Medical Publishers, Inc., 1980.
13. Nordin, M., Frankel, V.H. *Basic Biomechanics of the Musculoskeletal System*. Philadelphia, PA: Lea and Febiger, 1989.
14. Rasch, P.J. *Kinesiology and Applied Anatomy*. Philadelphia, PA: Lea and Febiger, 1989.
15. Zuidema, G.D. (Ed). *The Johns Hopkins Atlas of Human Functional Anatomy*, 2nd Ed. Baltimore, MD: The Johns Hopkins University Press, 1980.

CHAPTER 12

....

ASSESSING
HEALTH-RELATED &
FUNCTIONAL FITNESS

by

Paul M. Vanderburgh, Ed.D.
and
William J. Considine, P.E.D.

• • •

*A*ssessing your physical fitness level should be an integral part of any structured exercise program. By measuring each specific fitness component, you can determine the current status of your fitness "profile"—in other words, depending upon how you weigh, the results of your assessment efforts, you can ascertain how fit you are. What you do with that determination can help you in several ways. At the least, it can serve as the basis for prescribing a personalized conditioning program for yourself. Furthermore, periodic testing will enable you to monitor the progress of your conditioning regimen and make adjustments in your training program as needed. The results of a fitness assessment which uses valid measures can also provide you with a "snapshot" of your fitness-associated risks for various diseases and age-related problems in later life. Finally, and perhaps most importantly, you can use the results of such fitness testing to make appropriate lifestyle changes to enhance your current and future quality of life as well as the quantity (longevity) of your life.

Physical fitness testing, however, is not a process that is without critical issues that need to be considered. For example, before you can decide how to assess physical fitness, you have to determine what factors or measures to test. A fundamental first step that must be undertaken in such a task involves examining what is meant by the term "physical fitness."

Over the years, attempts to define physical fitness have largely taken a somewhat narrow focus. Almost every working definition of physical fitness has subjectively portrayed "fitness" as being the collective by-product of several basic components of fitness—each of which is a distinct entity unto itself. For proponents of this approach, the process of fitness assessment is fairly straightforward—simply assess each component separately. Identify a valid test for each fitness element, and then conduct the test. All factors considered, that's the easy part of this approach. Knowing what the results mean once you administer the various tests is the difficult part. One of the major limitations of this approach involves the inability to objectively weigh the various component "scores" into a single, meaningful measure.

Despite the problems with assessing physical fitness by evaluating each component independently, this approach continues to be the most popular method for determining how fit someone is. A review of the literature indicates that a number of valid test batteries exist to assess the health-related components of fitness: cardiorespiratory fitness (aerobic fitness), muscular strength, muscular endurance, flexibility, and body composition. The health-related components of fitness are those factors which have an impact on long-term health. As opposed to performance-related components (i.e., motor skills such as power, agility, coordination, kinesthetic awareness, balance, and speed) which are important for performing athletic-type activities but have little to do with long-term health, the relative status of your health-related fitness components can have a significant effect on the quality, and probably the quantity, of your life.

Certainly, the quality of your life is affected by your capacity to perform activities of daily living (ADLs) without undue risk of fatigue or injury. Collectively referred to as "functional fitness," this capacity is a by-product of the synergistic environment in which each component of fitness exists. Considerable evidence supports the concept that performing ADLs always involves the simultaneous interaction of the various components. Simply stated, every activity you do—at home, work, or play—involves the integration of each of the basic components of fitness. For example, at a minimum, carrying groceries up several flights of stairs involves both cardiorespiratory endurance and muscular endurance.

As a consequence, in recent years some experts have advocated assessing functional fitness as opposed to evaluating each component of fitness separately. Unfortunately, to date no one has advanced (let alone validated) a feasible, objective method for assessing functional fitness. Until which time such a method has been identified, exercise scientists will continue to discuss and assess the various components of fitness separately for the simple reason that such an approach is the easiest to implement and to explain.

For discussion purposes, the remainder of this chapter has been divided into two main sections: assessing health-related fitness and assessing functional fitness. The section on the assessment of health-related fitness will include an overview of each of the five basic components of fitness and the most common tests for measuring a particular component. The section on the assessment of functional fitness will present a brief discussion of the complex issues involved in such measurement.

Assessing Health-Related Fitness

Aerobic Fitness

Aerobic fitness—sometimes referred to in the scientific literature as cardiorespiratory fitness—is commonly defined as the coordinated ability of the pulmonary system (lungs), cardiovascular system (heart and blood vessels), and the metabolic pathways within the muscular system to take in, deliver, and utilize oxygen. All factors considered, the more oxygen you can take in, deliver, and utilize, the more aerobically fit you are. The most widely accepted measure of aerobic fitness is your level of maximal oxygen uptake ($\dot{V}O_{2\,max}$). A reflection of the greatest rate at which you can consume oxygen while exercising, $\dot{V}O_{2\,max}$ can be assessed in either a laboratory or a non-laboratory setting. When conducted in a laboratory, $\dot{V}O_{2\,max}$ testing usually involves the direct measurement of the gases you expire while exercising during either a maximal or near-maximal effort. An analysis of the expired oxygen and carbon dioxide levels provides a very accurate measurement of $\dot{V}O_{2\,max}$. It is also possible to evaluate your $\dot{V}O_{2\,max}$ level in a laboratory setting without collecting gases by identifying the highest work load you can achieve while exercising before the onset of undue fatigue.

In a non-laboratory setting, assessing your $\dot{V}O_{2\,max}$ level involves predicting your $\dot{V}O_{2\,max}$ on the basis of either how well you perform on a specific performance measure (e.g., how fast or how far you walk or run within specific limits) or how you respond (e.g., your heart rate) to submaximal exercise. Deciding whether to be tested in a laboratory or a non-laboratory setting and which assessment procedure to use is largely dependent upon the level of testing accuracy that is required, why the testing is being done, what testing resources (personnel and equipment) are available, and what (if any) unique characteristics you might have that would preclude or lend themselves to a specific mode of assessment.

Safety First

Prior to taking any exercise test (laboratory or non-laboratory), all individuals should be required to take certain precautionary steps. At the minimum, they should complete a health/medical questionnaire, have their resting blood pressure and resting heart rate measured, and complete an informed consent form. At the present time, one of the most widely used health/medical questionnaires is the Physical Activity Readiness Questionnaire (PAR-Q), a relatively simple, yet quite valid query form for screening individuals prior to their undergoing exercise testing (refer to chapter 3). The PAR-Q has been used extensively in the exercise science and fitness communities to determine whether an individual is an acceptable candidate for an exercise test. A "yes" answer to any of the seven questions on the PAR-Q disqualifies an individual from taking part in an exercise test until he or she obtains appropriate medical clearance.

Assessing Aerobic Fitness in a Laboratory

Within a laboratory setting, $\dot{V}O_{2\,max}$ is usually either directly measured or predicted using indirect means. The direct analysis of expired gases during a maximal exercise (stress) test yields the most accurate determination of $\dot{V}O_{2\,max}$. Unfortunately, this procedure requires extensive equipment: (1) an exercise testing modality, whose workloads are easily quantifiable, can be incrementally increased, and are highly reproducible, such as a treadmill, a cycle ergometer, or an independent step-action stair climbing machine; (2) a metabolic system for measuring and analyzing expired gases (oxygen and carbon dioxide); and (3) an electrocardiogram for monitoring the electrical activity and heart rate of the subject during the exercise test. Accordingly, the direct measurement of $\dot{V}O_{2\,max}$ is usually conducted only in research or clinical settings, since it tends not only to be time-consuming and costly (in terms of equipment), but it also requires specially trained personnel to administer.

ASSESSING AEROBIC FITNESS IN A NON-LABORATORY SETTING

Since laboratory testing is not a particularly feasible method of assessing aerobic fitness for the vast majority of health/fitness practitioners, several non-laboratory tests to predict $\dot{V}O_{2\,max}$ have been developed. The two types of tests which are most commonly used to predict $\dot{V}O_{2\,max}$ are performance-based measures (e.g., walking and running) and tests that use your heart rate response to a submaximal exercise bout as the primary predictor.

Performance-based measures—walking tests. In recent years, the Rockport One-Mile Fitness Walking Test has gained wide popularity as an effective means for estimating aerobic fitness. The primary task involved in this assessment procedure is to have an individual walk one mile as fast as possible, preferably on a track or a level surface. Immediately upon completion of the test, the individual's heart rate is taken using a 15-second pulse count and recorded. The time that it took the individual to cover the one-mile distance is also recorded. Both measurements are then entered into the following equation:

$$\dot{V}O_{2\,max} \text{ (in ml/kg/min)} = 132.853 - (0.0769 \times BW) - (0.3877 \times A) + (6.315 \times G) - (3.2649 \times T) - (0.1565 \times HR)$$

Where:		
BW	=	body weight in pounds
A	=	age in years
G	=	gender: 0 = female, 1 = male
T	=	time for the one-mile walk in minutes and hundredths of a minute (e.g., 15 minutes and 45 seconds would be expressed as 15.75)
HR	=	heart rate taken at the end of the one-mile expressed in beats per minute

Performance-based measures—running tests. Two of the most widely used running tests for assessing aerobic fitness are the Cooper 12-minute walk-run test and the 1.5-mile run test for time. The primary objective in the 12-minute walk-run test is to cover the greatest amount of distance in the allotted time period; while in the case of the 1.5-mile run test, the individual being tested attempts to run the distance in as short a period of time as possible. For both of the running tests, normative data are available to provide a reasonably accurate estimate of the aerobic fitness level of the individual who has been tested (refer to Tables 12-1 and 12-2). One of the most positive features of these tests is that they are very easy to administer. On the other hand, such performance-based tests have a few substantial limitations. For one thing, an individual's level of motivation and pacing ability can have a profound impact on that person's test results. Of greater potential importance, a certain degree of risk exists during such testing, since individuals are encouraged to put forth a maximal effort.

Table 12-1. Normative Data for 12-Minute Walk/Run (M = men; W = women)

12-Minute Run (miles)					
				Age (years)	
Fitness		13-19	20-29	30-39	40-49	50-59
Very Poor	M	<1.30	<1.22	<1.18	<1.14	<1.03
	W	<1.00	<0.96	<0.94	<0.88	<0.84
Poor	M	1.30-1.37	1.22-1.31	1.18-1.30	1.14-1.24	1.03-1.16
	W	1.00-1.18	0.96-1.11	0.95-1.05	0.88-0.98	0.84-0.93
Fair	M	1.38-1.56	1.32-1.49	1.31-1.45	1.25-1.39	1.17-1.30
	W	1.19-1.29	1.12-1.22	1.06-1.18	0.99-1.11	0.94-1.05
Good	M	1.57-1.72	1.50-1.64	1.46-1.56	1.40-1.53	1.31-1.44
	W	1.30-1.43	1.23-1.34	1.19-1.29	1.12-1.24	1.06-1.18
Excellent	M	1.73-1.86	1.65-1.76	1.57-1.69	1.54-1.65	1.45-1.58
	W	1.44-1.51	1.35-1.45	1.30-1.39	1.25-1.34	1.19-1.30
Superior	M	>1.87	>1.77	>1.70	>1.66	>1.59
	W	>1.52	>1.46	>1.40	>1.35	>1.31

Table 12-2. Normative Data for 1.5 Mile Run (M = men; W = women)

1.5-Mile Run (mins.)					
				Age (years)	
Fitness		13-19	20-29	30-39	40-49	50-59
Very Poor	M	>15:31	>16:01	>16:31	>17:31	>19:01
	W	>18:31	>19:01	>19:31	>20:01	>20:31
Poor	M	12:11-15:30	14:01-16:00	14:44-16:30	15:36-17:30	17:01-19:00
	W	16:55-18:30	18:31-19:00	19:01-19:30	19:31-20:00	20:01-20:30
Fair	M	10:49-12:10	12:01-14:00	12:31-14:45	13:01-15:35	14:31-17:00
	W	14:31-16:54	15:55-18:30	16:31-19:00	17:31-19:30	19:01-20:00
Good	M	9:41-10:48	10:46-12:00	11:01-12:30	11:31-13:00	12:31-14:30
	W	12:30-14:30	13:31-15:54	14:31-16:30	15:56-17:30	16:31-19:00
Excellent	M	8:37-9:40	9:45-10:45	10:00-11:00	10:30-11:30	11:00-12:30
	W	11:50-12:20	12:30-13:30	13:00-14:30	13:45-15:55	14:30-16:30
Superior	M	<8:37	<9:45	<10:00	<10:30	<11:00
	W	<11:50	<12:30	<13:45	<13:45	<14:30

Source: Cooper, 1982. *The Aerobic Program for Total Well-being.* New York, NY: M. Evan & Co.

Tests that predict $\dot{V}O_{2\,max}$ based on heart rate response to exercise. The primary aim of assessment techniques that predict $\dot{V}O_{2\,max}$ based on heart rate is to determine the slope of an individual's heart rate response to exercise and use that slope to estimate $\dot{V}O_{2\,max}$ (refer to Figure 12-1). The YMCA submaximal cycle protocol is an excellent example of a test that predicts $\dot{V}O_{2\,max}$ based on heart rate response to exercise.

Figure 12-1. Predicting $\dot{V}O_{2\,max}$ from a series of submaximal HR responses.

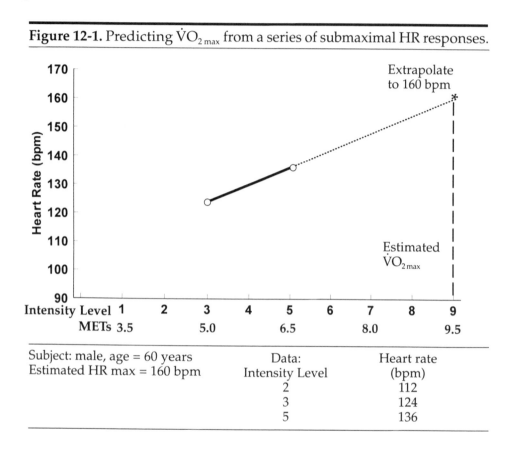

Subject: male, age = 60 years	Data:	Heart rate
Estimated HR max = 160 bpm	Intensity Level	(bpm)
	2	112
	3	124
	5	136

In order to determine the slope of an individual's heart rate response to exercise, the heart rate needs to be measured at two or more submaximal exercise work levels. The degree of accuracy of predicting $\dot{V}O_{2\,max}$ from submaximal exercise heart rates is subject to certain limitations. For example, it should be noted that all submaximal fitness tests make several assumptions:

- That a steady-state heart rate is obtained for each exercise workload.
- That a linear relationship exists between heart rate, oxygen uptake, and workload.
- That the maximal heart rate for a given age is uniform.
- That the mechanical efficiency of the physical activity performed (i.e., oxygen uptake at a given workload) is the same for everyone.

It should be kept in mind that any one or all of the above mentioned assumptions may not be met during a submaximal exercise test. If for any reason one of the assumptions is not met, then errors in predicting $\dot{V}O_{2\,max}$ will occur.

Unfortunately, it is often quite difficult to meet all of the requirements for the four listed assumptions. For example, exercising at a given workload for only a few minutes can involve an insufficient amount of time for many individuals to achieve a true steady-state. To ensure that a steady-state has been achieved, the heart rate should be measured after two minutes of exercise at a given workload and again after the third minute of exercise at that workload. These two heart rates should then be compared. If a difference of more than five beats per minute between the two is found, the subject should continue to exercise at one-minute intervals at the same workload until two successive heart rates differ by less than five beats per minute.

It is also important that the submaximal heart rates obtained be between 115 and 150 beats per minute, because it is within this heart rate range that a linear relationship tends to exist between heart rate and oxygen uptake or workload for most adults. When the heart rate is less than 115, many external factors (e.g., talking, laughing, apprehension, etc.) can greatly influence heart rate. Once the heart rate reaches a level between 115 and 150, external factors no longer influence heart rate, and a linear relationship exists. As the heart rate rises above 150, the heart rate-oxygen uptake relationship becomes curvilinear.

The third assumption involves maximal heart rate. Maximal heart rate is the greatest heart rate that can be measured when an individual is exercising to the point of volitional fatigue (i.e., exhaustion) during a graded exercise test. Several equations have been developed to estimate the average maximal heart rate for humans:

- Maximal heart rate = 220 - age (low estimate)
- Maximal heart rate = 210 - (0.5 x age) (high estimate)
- Maximal heart rate = 226 - age (estimate for older individuals)

Maximal heart rate can, however, vary greatly among different individuals of the same age. One standard deviation is + 12 bpm, which means that two-thirds of the population varies an average of plus or minus 12 heart beats from the average given by a prediction equation. If an individual's age-predicted maximal heart rate is higher than that person's true maximal heart rate, then his/her estimated $\dot{V}O_{2\,max}$ will be an overestimation of the correct or actual value.

The final assumption addresses the issue of mechanical efficiency. Because oxygen uptake at any given work rate can vary by approximately 15% between different individuals, individuals vary in the amount of oxygen they require to perform a certain exercise workload. Some individuals are more efficient at performing a given task than others. As a result, the average oxygen consumption associated with a given workload may vary significantly from one person to another. Thus, $\dot{V}O_{2\,max}$ predicted by submaximal exercise tests tends to be overestimated for those who are mechanically efficient and underestimated for those who are inefficient.

The point to remember is that submaximal exercise testing, though not as precise as maximal exercise testing, is not without advantages. For example, the results of such testing can provide a fairly accurate reflection of an individual's fitness status without the cost, risk, effort (on the part of the subject), and time involved in max testing. If an individual is given repeated submaximal exercise tests and that person's heart rate response to a fixed workload is found to decrease over time, it is reasonably safe to conclude that the individual has made improvements in aerobic (cardiorespiratory) fitness, irrespective of the accuracy of the $\dot{V}O_{2\,max}$ prediction.

Submaximal exercise testing on the StairMaster® 4000 PT® exercise system. Although motor-driven treadmills and cycle ergometers are the most commonly used exercise testing modes, the StairMaster 4000 PT offers the health/fitness professional the same control and reproducibility of exercise workloads as do the more traditionally used ergometers. As a result, the 4000 PT can be used for exercise testing. A suggested submaximal exercise testing protocol which can be used with the StairMaster 4000 PT is presented in Figure 12-2. (Note: The subject to be tested should employ the manual control program while exercising.)

Figure 12-2. Submaximal Exercise Testing Protocol for the StairMaster® 4000 PT® Exercise System.

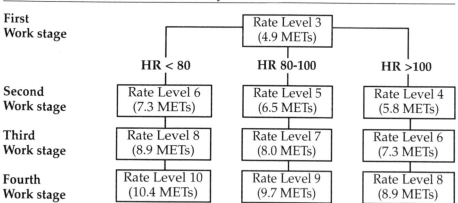

Instructions:
1. Set the first work stage at rate level 3.
2. If the heart rate measured after three minutes is
   • less than (<) 80 bpm, set the second work stage at rate level 6,
   • between 80-100 bpm, set the second work stage at rate level 5,
   • greater than 100 bpm, set the second work stage at rate level 4.
3. Set the third and fourth (if needed) work stages according to the rate levels in the columns below the second work stages.
4. It is important that you obtain at least two steady-state heart rates between approximately 115-150 bpm.

After allowing the subject a three-to-five minute warm-up (in addition to a period for stretching), the initial work stage should be set at rate level 3 (4.9 METs). The subject should exercise at this initial workload for three minutes. Once this work stage is completed and the exerciser's heart rate is obtained, the StairMaster 4000 PT rate level is increased to the next or second work stage based upon the subject's heart rate response. This procedure is continued until at least two heart rates between 115 and 150 bpm are obtained. The exercise test leader should watch for common signs or symptoms of exertional intolerance: dizziness, nausea, ataxia (unsteadiness), angina (chest pain), dyspnea (labored breathing), claudication (intermittent leg pain), mental confusion, pallor or cyanosis, severe fatigue or distress. An individual's $\dot{V}O_{2\,max}$ can be estimated by using the following formula:

$$\dot{V}O_{2\,max} \text{ (in METs *)} = b(MHR - HR2) + WL2, \text{ where}$$

$$b = (WL2 - WL1)/(HR2 - HR1)$$

WL1 = the first submaximal exercise rate level producing a heart rate between 115-150 bpm in METs
WL2 = the second submaximal exercise rate level producing a heart rate between 115-150 bpm in METs
HR1 = the steady-state heart rate recorded at WL1
HR2 = the steady-state heart rate recorded at WL2
MHR = maximal heart rate

The proper use of a submaximal testing protocol for the StairMaster 4000 PT can be best illustrated by the following example. If the heart response of an individual to the first work stage (Rate Level 3) is 92 bpm, then Rate Level 5 (6.5 METs) and Rate Level 7 (8.0 METs) would be selected for the second and third work stages. Assuming that the subject's heart rate responses at Rate Level 5 and 7 were 120 and 144 bpm, respectively, the test could be terminated since the two obtained heart rates are within 115-150 bpm. The first step in predicting the $\dot{V}O_{2\,max}$ of this individual would be the computation of the slope (b) of their heart rate response.

$$b = \frac{(WL2 - WL1)}{(HR2 - HR1)} = \frac{(8.0 - 6.5)}{(144 - 120)} = \frac{1.5}{24} = 0.0625$$

The slope (b) defines the rise in $\dot{V}O_2$ per change in heart rate. In this example, for each increased beat in heart rate, oxygen uptake increases by 0.0625 METs. If the individual tested was a 40-year-old woman, then her estimated

---

* 1 MET = 3.5 ml O_2/kg/min (amount of oxygen consumed at rest)

maximal heart rate [210 minus (0.5 age)] would be 190 bpm. $\dot{V}O_{2\,max}$ could be predicted by the following equation:

$$
\begin{aligned}
O_{2\,max}\ (METs) &= \quad b \quad (MHR - HR2) + WL2 \\
&= \quad 0.0625\ (190 - 144) + 8.0 \\
&= \quad 2.9 + 8.0 \\
&= \quad 10.9
\end{aligned}
$$

According to the normative data (refer to Table 12-3), this woman would be classified as having an "average" level of aerobic fitness.

MUSCULAR FITNESS

Given the critical role that your muscular system plays in enabling you to perform activities of daily living (at home, work, and play) without undue risk of fatigue or injury, the importance of your muscles being capable of doing what you want them to do when you need it to be done cannot be overemphasized. Collectively, this capacity is frequently referred to as muscular fitness.

Traditionally, however, most exercise scientists have contended that muscular fitness should be viewed as being comprised of two distinct components of physical fitness: muscular strength and muscular endurance. Muscular strength can be defined as the ability of a muscle or a muscle group to exert maximum force. Muscular endurance, on the other hand, can be defined as the ability of a muscle or a muscle group to exert submaximal force for an extended period of time. Accordingly, the first step in assessing muscular fitness involves identifying which muscle-related component of physical fitness you wish to measure—muscular strength or muscular endurance.

Regardless of which component of muscular fitness is to be tested, a number of factors* must be taken into consideration, including:

1. *The devices commonly employed to assess muscular fitness all have design features and usage requirements that make the test results less than 100% reliable.* For example, if the device has a pad on it that you push against, the extent to which you depress the pad will effect the measurement obtained. By the same token, if the procedures for using the device require that your body must be in an exact angular position, it can be very difficult to assume a position that mandates a particular joint angle each and every time you are tested. Both examples serve to confirm the fact that measuring muscular fitness is

---

* Editors' Note: Much of this discussion concerning the potential problems involved with muscular fitness testing is based on information presented in *Advanced Fitness Assessment and Exercise Prescription*, Vivian H. Heyward, pp. 114-116; used with the permission of the publisher, Human Kinetics Publishers.

not a process that involves unequivocal precision. As a result, knowing the design limitations of the device you are using in the assessment process, as well as the potential problems that might occur with any deviation in the protocol for using the device, will enable you to be better prepared to interpret the results that are obtained.

2. *Muscular strength and muscular endurance are specific to the muscle or muscle group, the type of muscular contraction (static or dynamic—concentric, eccentric, isokinetic), the speed of muscular contraction (slow or fast), and the joint angle being tested (static contraction).* Accordingly, the results of any one test are specific to the specific parameters of the procedure used to obtain the measurement. No single test exists for evaluating total body muscular strength or muscular endurance.

3. *The test items used to measure either muscular strength or muscular endurance should be selected with care.* Assessment batteries which are designed to measure muscular strength should not include maximum repetition tests. By the same token, the most appropriate tests for measuring muscular endurance are those which are proportional to the body weight or the maximum strength level of the individual being tested.

4. *Because muscular fitness is often directly related to both the total body weight and the amount of lean muscle mass of the individual being tested, the test results should be expressed in relative terms.* The value of expressing muscular fitness test results in relative terms is particularly worthwhile when comparing one individual to another or one group to another.

5. *Because most muscular fitness tests require a maximum effort by the individual being tested, (as much as possible) care should be taken to control those factors that might affect maximum performance.* Among the factors that could influence how well an individual performs are: time of day, sleep, medication, motivation level, energy level, and emotional state. Steps should also be undertaken to ensure that the maximal effort being exerted does not subject the individual to an undue level of exertion.

6. *Caution should be taken when comparing the results of the muscular fitness testing to normative data.* Much of the normative data relating to muscular fitness is either out-dated or, to a degree, invalid or unreliable.*

---

* Editors' Note: A critical need exists for additional normative data for both muscular strength and muscular endurance. Compared to the other basic components of physical fitness, the two muscle-related components have received relatively minimal attention by the exercise science community.

Muscular fitness is typically assessed using either tests that employ specific devices for measuring muscular strength and muscular endurance or calisthenic-type tests. Most of the testing (but not all) that employs devices is conducted in a laboratory, rather than a field setting, because the devices often require trained personnel to use and are relatively expensive. Calisthenic-type tests, on the other hand, can be performed in a non-laboratory setting. This type of testing usually requires little or no equipment, can be performed almost anywhere, enables more than one person to be tested at the same time, and involves bodily movements which are somewhat more functional in nature.

Tests for measuring muscular fitness which involve devices. A number of devices for measuring muscular fitness have been developed, including dynamometers, cable tensiometers, electromechanical and hydraulic devices, and resistance machines. Deciding which (if any) device to use can involve several factors, including the cost and availability of the apparatus, the level of expertise required to use the device, the muscle or muscle group to be tested, the type of information desired, and for what purpose the findings will be used.**

Calisthenic-type tests for measuring muscular fitness. In certain situations, calisthenic-type tests may offer a more appropriate means for assessing muscular fitness. Calisthenic-type tests involve measuring, in terms specific to the muscle-related component being assessed, how (quantitatively) well you can perform calisthenic-type exercises (e.g., push-ups, chin-ups, pull-ups, dips, sit-ups, etc.). When you measure dynamic muscular strength by a calisthenic-type test, you determine the maximum amount of weight that you can lift, in excess of your body weight, for one repetition of the (exercise) movement. On the other hand, assessing dynamic muscular endurance through the use of calisthenic-type tests involves determining the maximum number of repetitions of each (calisthenic-type) exercise you can perform. Because calisthenic-type testing for muscular endurance is quite popular with several organizations (e.g., the U.S. military, the President's Council on Physical Fitness, etc.), some normative data relating to the results from this type of testing exists.

Field tests for measuring muscular strength. Unquestionably, the most widely used field test for evaluating muscular strength is the one-repetition maximum (1-RM) test. This test has traditionally been used to assess dynamic strength by determining how much weight an individual can lift for a single repetition. This approach to measuring muscular strength usually involves performing a battery of three or four exercises that are representative of the body's major muscle groups. For example, performing a bench press or an incline press is frequently used to assess the strength of the torso (upper body) muscles, while a squat or a leg press is typically performed to ascertain hip-leg (lower body) strength.

Similar to almost every attempt to quantify muscular endurance, conducting the test is often more easy than knowing how to accurately interpret the re-

---

* Author's Note: For more information refer to chapter 8 for a comprehensive overview of the devices most commonly employed to measure muscular fitness.

sults of your testing efforts. Once you've obtained your 1-RM results, you face a dilemma in deciding what, if anything, do the data mean. For example, are they an accurate reflection of how much work you actually performed in the weight room? Do they provide you with a reliable means for evaluating the effectiveness of your strength training efforts or your current strength level? Do they give you a logical means for comparing your strength level to another person's? All factors considered, for each of the aforementioned issues, the answer is, at best, questionable.

How much work you actually perform in the weight room and how strong you actually become are affected by a number of genetic factors which are beyond your control. Collectively, these genetic factors make muscular fitness and the assessment of muscular fitness a relative matter. In other words, what you do in the weight room is relative to your genetic capabilities. Accordingly, demonstrating a specific strength achievement is relative to such factors as the length of your arms, the proportion of fast-to-slow twitch fibers you have, the ratio of muscle length to tendon length, the insertion point of the muscle on the skeletal lever involved, your level of neuromuscular efficiency, etc.

In addition to the restraints that genetic factors impose on 1-RM testing, a more serious limitation with this approach to assessing strength is the fact that such testing can be dangerous. Safety can become a major concern if you attempt to exceed the physiological capacity of your body or if your lifting techniques expose you to undue risk of injury. Attempting to perform a 1-RM lift with a relatively heavy weight can place an inordinate level of stress on your muscles, bones, and connective tissues. Unfortunately, the trial-and-error method of increasing the weight in the 1-RM approach (particularly if it's combined with an adrenaline rush or a machismo-driven attempt to validate an unrealistic exhibition of strength) often leads the individual to use too much weight. The 1-RM approach to strength testing can also increase your blood pressure to a risky level. Lifters—particularly at the upper end of the trial and error 1-RM method—tend to hold their breath while performing the exercise, an action which increases their blood pressure beyond that which they normally encounter when lifting less (submaximal) resistance.

Another safety issue involved in 1-RM testing is the fact that if you attempt to lift too much, you may compromise the proper techniques for performing the exercise and injure yourself. For example, one of the most common problems which occurs with 1-RM testing is back injuries during the 1-RM bench press test. Using excessively high loads, individuals arch their backs during the lift, thereby placing undue stress on the lumbar spine. Finally, in a few isolated instances, individuals have actually lost control of the weight at some point in the 1-RM lift and injured themselves. Accordingly, if you decide to perform 1-RM testing, you must use a competent spotter to help you maintain control of the weight during the exercise, if necessary, and to serve as a valuable source of direct feedback regarding your adherence to the proper techniques for performing a particular exercise.

Given the fact that individuals have their own unique genetic potential for achieving (and demonstrating) muscular strength, comparing the strength of one person to another is of dubious value. A more logical approach would be to compare the results of your strength testing to your previous performances. Even accounting for the occasional glitch in testing results that can be attributed to emotional/mental factors, comparing your test results over time should provide you with a reasonable basis for measuring the relative progress of your training efforts.

In lieu of the inherent problems with assessing strength (e.g., genetic differences, safety limitations, etc.), what measures should you use to assess strength? Two of the better approaches are the strength-to-weight ratio and the one-rep predicted max from reps-to-fatigue.

The strength-to-weight ratio is a relative method of determining how much you lifted on a given exercise compared to the listed values. This approach uses your body weight and gender to categorize your performance on a scale ranging from excellent to poor. Tables 12-4 and 12-5 present the 1-RM/BW values for both the bench press and the leg press exercises, respectively. To use either table all you have to do is to divide how much you lifted by your body weight, and then compare the resultant dividend to the values listed in the table. For example, if you weigh 200 lbs. and you bench pressed 250 lbs., your 1-RM/BW ratio of 1.25 (250 divided by 200) would categorize your performance as "excellent."

The one-rep predicted max from reps-to-fatigue method is an approach which is based on the precept that a direct relationship exists between anaerobic endurance and strength. Given this relationship, it follows that you can determine your level of strength by assessing your level of anaerobic endurance (and vice versa). Unquestionably, the most positive aspect of this approach is the fact that measuring anaerobic endurance is a much safer process than directly determining your 1-RM because it involves lifting submaximal loads.

The critical issue is how to assess anaerobic endurance. Based upon research that shows that a near linear relationship exists between the number of reps you can perform before you reach a state of fatigue and the percentage of maximum load you can lift, Matt Brzycki, the health fitness coordinator and strength coach at Princeton University, developed an equation for predicting 1-RM when the number of reps-to-fatigue performed is less than 10 (refer to page 145). If the number of reps-to-fatigue is exactly 10, you should divide the weight you lifted by 0.75 to get your predicted 1-RM. Because Brzycki's equation has been found to be less reliable if the number of reps-to-fatigue exceeds 10, the reps-to-fatigue method for predicting 1-RM should not be used if the rep count exceeds 10. A user-friendly matrix for predicting 1-RM based on reps-to-fatigue with weights ranging from 45 to 310 pounds is presented in Table 12-6.

Equation for Predicting 1-RM Based on Reps-to-Fatigue

$$\text{Predicted 1-rm} = \frac{\text{Weight Lifted}}{1.0278 - .0278X}$$

where X = the number of reps
performed

BODY COMPOSITION

Body composition is defined as the ratio of fat to fat-free mass in your body. For the most part, fat-free mass is comprised of muscle, bone, water, and protein, while adipose tissue makes up the fat mass component of your body. Determining whether you have a ratio appropriate for good health is important, since excessive fat (obesity) has been shown to be a risk factor for a number of diseases, such as coronary heart disease, hypertension, and diabetes. Assessing body composition can be accomplished through a variety of laboratory (e.g., hydrostatic weighing, etc.) and non-laboratory (e.g., skinfold testing, U.S. Navy circumference measurements, waist-to-hip ratio, etc.) methods.

Hydrostatic weighing. The most widely accepted procedure in a laboratory setting for assessing body composition is hydrostatic weighing—commonly referred to as *underwater weighing.* Based on Archimede's Principle (which states that the weight of an object in water subtracted from its dry land weight gives the weight of the water displaced), underwater weighing involves determining whole body density by measuring how much you weigh when you are totally submerged in water. Your weight underwater and on land are then used in an equation which has been developed to predict body density. Such a calculation is possible because fat and lean tissue do not have the same level of density. Fat tissue is less dense. As a result, an individual with a high percentage of fat weighs less underwater than an individual with the same weight on land but with a lower percentage of body fat. Experts estimate that hydrostatic weighing will provide you with a calculation of your percent body fat that is within ± 2.5 percent of the "true" value. Despite its accuracy, hydrostatic weighing is not widely used because the technique is relatively inefficient time-wise, involves expensive equipment, and requires trained, experienced technicians to administer.

Skinfold techniques. Because underwater weighing is not a very feasible technique for most settings, several non-laboratory techniques have been developed which assess percent body fat with a reasonable degree of accuracy. Without question, the most popular of these approaches is skinfold testing. Skinfolds (perhaps more appropriately titled "fatfolds") are the amount of skin and fat just beneath the skin at any given location (site) on your body. By "pinching" everything but muscle at a site, a tester can measure the thickness of the pinch, which is made up mostly of fat. From an assessment standpoint, the value of this procedure stems from the fact that certain skinfold site "pinches" (e.g., triceps, chest, abdomen, thigh) can be used in specific equations to predict your level of percent body fat.

The usual procedure for measuring skinfolds involves simply grasping the skin and its underlying fat with the thumb and index finger into a double fold. With the other hand, the arms of the caliper are opened and gently closed over the skinfold which is being held by the opposite hand. The tips of the caliper arms are placed approximately one-half inch from the thumb and index finger. The caliper then grasps the skinfold for about 2-3 seconds. A value representing the relative "thickness" of the measured skinfold is then noted and recorded in millimeters. The caliper tips are subsequently released from the skinfold, and the person doing the testing lets go of the skinfold.

Several factors affect the degree of accuracy you can achieve in calculating percent body fat by measuring skinfold thickness. First, and foremost, is the experience of the tester. A large number of research studies have shown conclusively that the results obtained by an inexperienced tester will not be comparable (i.e., validity, reliability) to those measurements performed by an individual with extensive experience in performing such testing. The "experience inconsistency" stems from the fact that the failure to pinch appropriately will lead to either too much or too little of a skin- and fat-fold being measured on any given trial. Over time, practice enhances your ability to pinch just the right amount (i.e., according to published guidelines). Second, the tester should take three measurements of the same site and average them. Empirical evidence suggests that even the most experienced testers often will make small measurement errors each time they assess a skinfold thickness. By averaging several measurements (assuming some are over and some are underestimates of the true skinfold thickness), you increase the likelihood that you will obtain a more stable and accurate measurement of your percent body fat.

Several equations have been developed over the years that employ a variety of skinfold sites to estimate body density and predict percent body fat. These equations are gender- and age-specific and are designed to be used only with a similar population from which they were derived. Of equal importance, each equation is based on specific sites and requires that specified techniques for measuring the skinfolds at each site be employed.

Two of the most popular equations that have been successfully employed over the years (using Lange calipers) to assess body composition were developed by Jackson-Pollock for men, ages 18-61 years, and Jackson-Pollock-Ward for women, ages 18-55 years:

<u>Men</u>
- Body density = $1.1093800 - 0.0008267(x1) = 0.0000016(x1)2$
  $- 0.0002574(x2)$. x1 = sum of skinfolds. x2 = age in years.
  Sites: chest, abdomen, and thigh.

<u>Women</u>
- Body density = $1.089733 - 0.0009245(x1) = 0.0000025(x2)2$
  $- 0.0000979(x4)$. x1 = sum of skinfolds. x2 = age in years.
  Sites: triceps, suprailium, and abdomen.

The recommended techniques concerning how to properly place the skinfold calipers on the six distinct sites used in two aforementioned sample equations is as follows:

Chest: diagonal fold halfway between the anterior axillary line (frontal portion of the armpit) and nipple for men and one third the distance from the anterior axillary line to the nipple for women.

Triceps: vertical fold taken in the middle of the back of the upper arm, halfway between the tip of the shoulder and tip of the elbow, elbow extended and relaxed.

Subscapular: fold taken on a diagonal line coming from the vertebral border 1-2 cm from the inferior angle of the scapula.

Abdominal: vertical fold taken at approximately one inch to the right of the umbilicus (belly button).

Suprailium: diagonal fold taken above the crest of the ilium (hip bone). The fold should follow the natural diagonal line of the hip at this point.

Thigh: vertical fold taken on the front thigh, halfway between the hip and knee.

The U.S. Navy circumference method. The armed forces of the United States have identified a relatively accurate method for estimating percent body fat that almost anyone, with a minimum amount of training, can use. The U.S. Navy circumference method for estimating percent body fat is based on the fact that large circumferences at certain sites (e.g., waist, hips) are indicative of higher percent body fat and large circumferences at other sites (e.g., neck) are related to lower percent body fat. All the equipment that is required to perform this test is a weight scale and a cloth/fiberglass measuring tape (much like a tailor's tape that does not stretch when pulled).

Similar to skinfold measurements, circumference measures should also be taken at least three times, with the average used as the score. The tester should ensure that the tape stays in one plane and that the measurement is taken at the point of a slight tissue compression. The site selection must also be accurate; too high or too low on the waist, for example, could lead to a large measurement error. All measurements are recorded in inches.

The sites used in the equation to predict percent body fat for men are the waist and the neck. The waist measurement should be obtained parallel to the ground at the level of the umbilicus and should be taken only when the subject is in a natural relaxed state of exhalation. The waist measurements should be rounded down to the nearest one-half inch. The neck measurement should be taken just below the Adam's apple and perpendicular to the long axis of the neck, and rounded up to the nearest one-half inch. Most of the time, because this axis is not exactly vertical, the plane of the measurement will often not be parallel to the ground. You should be mindful that this measurement is often less than your neck size in a shirt.

For women, the U.S. Navy circumference method employs three sites: the abdomen (the narrowest portion of the waist, usually midway between the navel and the chest), the hips (the widest portion of the hips as viewed from the side), and the neck (the same as for men). Measurements taken at the hip and abdomen should be rounded down to the nearest one-half inch, and those taken at the neck should be rounded up to the nearest one-half inch.

The circumference values, along with the individual's height (to the nearest one-half inch) and weight (lbs.), are then substituted into the following equations—first to predict body density, then to predict percent body fat.

Men
- Body density = - .191[log10(waist - neck)] + .55 [log10(height)] + 1.032

Women
- Body density = - .350[log10(abdomen + hip + neck)] + .221[log10(height)] + 1.296

Men and Women
- Percent body fat = 495/body density - 450

The U.S. Navy circumference method offers several distinct advantages over the skinfold method. First, the method requires only a minimal level of skill by the tester to achieve reasonably accurate results. This feature has particular application in organizations (e.g., the military) where many members must be tested and only a few experienced testers (for skinfolding) would be available. Second, the equipment needed to perform the measurements costs relatively little compared to the $200 or so needed for a single set of skinfold calipers.

Waist-to-hip ratio. Over the past 15 years, many researchers have found that percent body fat is probably not as important for your long term health as where the fat is located on your body. Collectively, the fat deposited on your body is often termed "fat distribution" or fat patterning. Specifically, fat stored in your abdominal region, as opposed to your legs, hips, and arms, is considered more predictive of coronary heart disease (CHD). An individual who has this type of fat patterning is commonly referred to as an "apple", because the shape of an apple is wider at the top. Individuals classified as apples tend to have more fat on their chest and stomach areas than on their hips and legs. On the other hand, individuals who tend to have more fat stores below their waist are often referred to as "pears." Research has shown that "pears" are more likely to be at a relatively lower risk of CHD, even when they have comparable levels of body fat to "apples." Although the physiological reasons for the relationship between fat distribution and risk of heart disease exceed the scope of this chapter, the implications, from an assessment standpoint, are extremely important. Unfortunately, no accurate and feasible way exists to assess fat distribution in a typical exercise setting, because some type of x-ray (MRI, dual energy x-ray, etc.) is required.

One simple field test that has been developed for estimating your fat distribution is the waist-to-hip ratio (WHR) This ratio is simply the ratio of the narrowest portion of your waist (i.e., the circumference measured at the level of your bellybutton) to the widest portion of your hips (i.e., the circumference measured at the greatest protrusion of your buttocks). The larger the ratio, the higher your risk. In fact, some experts have established a criterion cut-off of 0.80 for women and 0.95 for men as being the maximal allowable WHR above which the risk for heart disease becomes significantly higher.

The WHR is a relatively easy field test that almost anyone can perform. It does, however, have some limitations. It should not be used with very lean subjects who might have not only a narrow waist, but narrow hips as well (leading to a high WHR with a corresponding, but erroneously assumed, higher risk of heart disease). Furthermore, some subjects might have an excessive level of abdominal fat but, because of very wide hips, have the WHR which masks their real fat distribution-related risk. Nevertheless, using the WHR can be very beneficial in providing you with a more realistic picture of your fat-related disease risk, than can relying merely on your assessed level of percent body fat.

FLEXIBILITY

Flexibility is generally defined as the ability of a skeletal joint to move fluidly through its full range of motion (ROM). Range of motion is highly specific to the joint and depends on the joint structure. Flexibility in one specific joint does not necessarily indicate flexibility in other joints. For example, triaxial joints (e.g., hip, shoulder) afford a greater degree of movement in more directions than either uniaxial (e.g., knee, elbow) or biaxial (e.g., wrist) joints. Accordingly, no general flexibility test exists for evaluating total body flexibility. Specific to each joint, your level of flexibility is affected by several factors, including age, gender, and the type and amount of physical activity in which you are involved.

Flexibility can be either static or dynamic. Static flexibility is a measure of the overall ROM at a specific joint; dynamic flexibility, on the other hand, is a measure of the amount of resistance to movement by the joint. Both types of flexibility play significant roles in physical activity. Despite the fact that assessing joint stiffness and resistance to movement (dynamic flexibility) may be more meaningful than absolute ROM data, relatively little research has been conducted to assess dynamic flexibility. Over the years, several techniques—both laboratory and field—have been developed to assess static flexibility. Traditionally, static flexibility is measured by determining ROM either directly or indirectly.

DIRECT METHODS FOR MEASURING STATIC FLEXIBILITY

Static flexibility can be measured directly through the use of a device specifically designed to measure ROM, such as a goniometer, an electrogoniometer, and a Leighton flexometer. Such tools are typically used in laboratory or clinical settings under very controlled conditions. A goniometer is a protractor-like instrument with two steel (or Plexiglas) arms that enable you to measure joint angles. The difference between the joint angles (in degrees) which are measured at the extremes of a movement is the ROM. An electrogoniometer is a device that allows you to assess ROM (joint angles) by means of electrical input. The Leighton flexometer is a device which consists of a weighted 360-degree dial and a weighted pointer. The ROM for a specific skeletal joint is measured in relation to the downward pull of gravity on the dial and the pointer. After you perform a movement, the pointer is locked in at the extreme ROM you achieved, which enables you to read the degree of arc through which the movement occurred directly from the dial.

INDIRECT METHODS FOR MEASURING STATIC FLEXIBILITY

Static flexibility can be assessed indirectly through linear measurements of the ROM. Among the examples of field tests which are commonly used for such purposes are: the sit-and-reach test, the modified sit-and-reach test, the shoulder rotation test, the ankle flexion test, the ankle extension test, the shoulder-and-wrist elevation test, and the trunk-and-neck extension test. Field tests are specific to the joints involved in the movement, should involve measuring to the nearest 1/4 inch how far you can either extend or flex during a specific movement, and usually require three trials or attempts—the best of which should be counted.

FUNCTIONAL FITNESS

Since the early 1970s, medical and exercise science experts have emphasized the importance of regular participation in aerobic exercise activities (e.g., walking, jogging, cycling, etc.) for developing a healthy heart and maintaining an optimal body weight. In recent years, however, the experts have become convinced that aerobic exercise alone is simply not enough. You can possess a heart and lungs which work efficiently and yet be too weak to perform certain activities of daily living, such as climbing stairs, cleaning house, or mowing your lawn. Unfortunately, with each passing year above age 30, you can expect to lose more strength. These losses will be significant if you do not engage in exercise specifically designed to enhance your level of muscular fitness. In other words, it is critical to your best interests that you develop and maintain an adequate level of functional fitness—which is defined as the ability to perform the tasks attendant to daily living (including leisure-time activities) without undue fatigue or risk of injury. In order to be functionally fit, you need to be both muscularly fit and aerobically fit.

How you structure an exercise program to enhance your level of functional fitness is somewhat subjective. At opposite ends of a time-efficiency continuum, your program can either include a specific workout to separately develop aerobic fitness and muscular fitness or feature an exercise regimen using one or more of the StairMaster Crossrobics® machines—modalities which enable you to simultaneously enhance your level of aerobic fitness and muscular fitness.

The point to remember is that a sound exercise program which focuses on functional fitness may reduce your risk for a sudden heart attack due to unaccustomed physical exertion that stresses both the skeletal muscles and the heart (e.g., carrying groceries up stairs or shoveling heavy snow). Equally important, an enhanced level of functional fitness will have a positive impact on the "quality" of your life.

Assessing your functional fitness level, however, is a much more difficult undertaking than simply defining it. The primary dilemma in this area arises from the fact that functional fitness is relative to each individual. Your ability to perform the activities of daily living (ADLs) in your life—at home, work, or play—without undue fatigue or injury is relatively specific to the level of challenges imposed by those tasks. What might be considered as a high level of functional fitness in one person's life might be a deficient level in someone else's life. Fortunately, it appears as if this entire area of concern will receive more attention in the future from the exercise science community, and that this increased level of emphasis on functional fitness will lead to valid, meaningful assessment measures for this critical component of life. ❑

Table 12-3. Standards for Evaluating Aerobic (Cardiovascular) Fitness

$\dot{V}O_{2\,max}$ (in METs)

AGE	LOW	FAIR	AVERAGE	ABOVE AVERAGE	HIGH	VERY HIGH	SUPERIOR
WOMEN							
20-29	<8.0	8.3-9.7	10.0-12.3	12.6-13.7	14.0-15.1	15.4-16.8	17.1+
30-39	<7.7	8.0-9.4	9.7-11.7	12.0-13.4	13.7-14.8	15.1-16.6	16.8+
40-49	<7.1	7.4-8.8	9.1-11.4	11.7-12.8	13.1-14.3	14.6-16.0	16.3+
50-59	<6.0	6.3-7.7	8.0-10.3	10.6-11.7	12.0-12.8	13.1-14.0	14.3+
60-69	<4.8	5.1-6.3	6.6-8.8	9.1-10.3	10.6-11.4	11.7-12.6	12.8+
MEN							
20-29	<10.8	11.1-12.3	12.6-14.6	14.8-16.0	16.3-17.7	18.0-19.7	20.0+
30-39	<9.7	10.0-11.1	11.4-13.4	13.7-14.6	14.8-16.3	16.6-18.3	18.6+
40-49	<8.6	8.8-10.0	10.3-12.3	12.6-13.4	13.7-15.1	15.4-17.1	17.4+
50-59	<7.1	7.4-8.8	9.1-11.1	11.4-12.3	12.6-13.7	14.0-15.7	16.0+
60-69	<6.0	6.3-7.4	7.7-10.0	10.3-11.1	11.4-12.6	12.8-14.0	14.3+

* To convert METs to ml/kg/min, simply multiply the values in Table 12-3. by 3.5.

Table 12-4. Standard Values for Bench Press Strength in 1-RM lb./lb. Body Weight

RATING	Age (in years)				
	20-29	30-39	40-49	50-59	60+
MEN					
Excellent	<1.26	>1.08	>0.97	>0.86	>0.78
Good	1.17-1.25	1.01-1.07	0.91-0.96	0.81-0.85	0.74-0.77
Average	0.97-1.16	0.86-1.00	0.78-0.90	0.70-0.80	0.64-0.73
Fair	0.88-0.96	0.79-0.85	0.72-0.77	0.65-0.69	0.60-0.63
Poor	<0.87	<0.78	<0.71	<0.64	<0.59
WOMEN					
Excellent	>0.78	>0.66	>0.61	>0.54	>0.55
Good	0.72-0.77	0.62-0.65	0.57-0.60	0.51-0.53	0.51-0.54
Average	0.59-0.71	0.53-0.61	0.48-0.56	0.43-0.50	0.41-0.50
Fair	0.53-0.58	0.49-0.52	0.44-0.47	0.40-0.42	0.37-0.40
Poor	<0.52	<0.48	<0.43	<0.39	<0.36

Note. Unpublished data from Institute for Aerobics Research (1985) as it appeared in *ACSM Guidelines for Exercise Testing and Prescription Resource Manual* (pp. 161-170) by Institute for Aerobic Research, 1988, Dallas: Author. Reprinted by permission.

Table 12-5. Standard Values for Bench Press Strength[a] in 1-RM lb./lb. Body Weight

RATING	Age (in years)				
	20-29	30-39	40-49	50-59	60+
MEN					
Excellent	<2.08	>1.88	>1.76	>1.66	>1.56
Good	2.00-2.07	1.80-1.87	1.70-1.75	1.60-1.65	1.50-1.55
Average	1.83-1.99	1.63-1.79	1.56-1.69	1.46-1.59	1.37-1.49
Fair	1.65-1.82	1.55-1.62	1.50-1.55	1.40-1.45	1.31-1.36
Poor	<1.64	<1.54	<1.49	<1.39	<1.30
WOMEN					
Excellent	>1.63	>1.42	>1.32	>1.26	>1.15
Good	1.54-1.62	1.35-1.41	1.26-1.31	1.13-1.25	1.08-1.14
Average	1.35-1.53	1.20-1.34	1.12-1.25	0.99-1.12	0.92-1.07
Fair	1.26-1.34	1.13-1.19	1.06-1.11	0.86-0.98	0.85-0.91
Poor	<1.25	<1.12	<1.05	<0.85	<0.84

Note. Unpublished data from Institute for Aerobics Research (1985) as it appeared in *ACSM Guidelines for Exercise Testing and Prescription Resource Manual* (pp. 161-170) by Institute for Aerobic Research, 1988, Dallas: Author. Reprinted by permission.

[a] Using upper plate of leg press machine.

Table 12-6. Predicted Max Based on Reps-to-Fatigue

WT	Repetitions									
	1	2	3	4	5	6	7	8	9	10
45	45	46	48	49	51	52	54	56	58	60
50	50	51	53	55	56	58	60	62	64	67
55	55	57	58	60	62	64	66	68	71	73
60	60	62	64	65	67	70	72	74	77	80
65	65	67	69	71	73	75	78	81	84	87
70	70	72	74	76	79	81	84	87	90	93
75	75	77	79	82	84	87	90	93	96	100
80	80	82	85	87	90	93	96	99	103	107
85	85	87	90	93	96	99	102	106	109	113
90	90	93	95	98	101	105	108	112	116	120
95	95	98	101	104	107	110	114	118	122	127
100	100	103	106	109	112	116	120	124	129	133
105	105	108	111	115	118	122	126	130	135	140
110	110	113	116	120	124	128	132	137	141	147
115	115	118	122	125	129	134	138	143	148	153
120	120	123	127	131	135	139	144	149	154	160
125	125	129	132	136	141	145	150	155	161	167
130	130	134	138	142	146	151	156	161	167	173
135	135	139	143	147	152	157	162	168	174	180
140	140	144	148	153	157	163	168	174	180	187
145	145	149	154	158	163	168	174	180	186	193
150	150	154	159	164	169	174	180	186	193	200
155	155	159	164	169	174	180	186	192	199	207
160	160	165	169	175	180	186	192	199	206	213
165	165	170	175	180	186	192	198	205	212	220
170	170	175	180	185	191	197	204	211	219	227
175	175	180	185	191	197	203	210	217	225	233

Table 12-6. Predicted Max Based on Reps-to-Fatigue

WT	Repetitions									
	1	2	3	4	5	6	7	8	9	10
180	180	185	191	196	202	209	216	223	231	240
185	185	190	196	202	208	215	222	230	238	247
190	190	195	201	207	214	221	228	236	244	253
195	195	201	206	213	219	226	234	242	251	260
200	200	206	212	218	225	232	240	248	257	267
205	205	211	217	224	231	238	246	254	264	273
210	210	216	222	229	236	244	252	261	270	280
215	215	221	228	235	242	250	258	267	276	287
220	220	226	233	240	247	255	264	273	283	293
225	225	231	238	245	253	261	270	279	289	300
230	230	237	244	251	259	267	276	286	296	307
235	235	242	249	256	264	273	282	292	302	313
240	240	247	254	262	270	279	288	298	309	320
245	245	252	259	267	276	285	294	304	315	327
250	250	257	265	273	281	290	300	310	321	333
255	255	262	270	278	287	296	306	317	328	340
260	260	267	275	284	292	302	312	323	334	347
265	265	273	281	289	298	308	318	329	341	353
270	270	278	286	295	304	314	324	335	347	360
275	275	283	291	300	309	319	330	341	354	367
280	280	288	296	305	315	325	336	348	360	373
285	285	293	302	311	321	331	342	354	366	380
290	290	298	307	316	326	337	348	360	373	387
295	295	303	312	322	332	343	354	366	379	393
300	300	309	318	327	337	348	360	372	386	400
305	305	314	323	333	343	354	366	379	392	407
310	310	319	328	338	349	360	372	385	399	413

BIBLIOGRAPHY •

1. American College of Sports Medicine. *Guidelines for Exercise Testing and Prescription,* 4th Ed. Philadelphia, PA: Lea and Febiger, 1991.
2. American Heart Association. *Exercise and Training of Apparently Healthy Individuals: A Handbook for Physicians.* Dallas, TX: American Heart Association, 1972.
3. Åstrand, I. "A method for prediction of aerobic work capacity for females and males of different ages." *Acta Physiol Scand* 49(Suppl.):S43-S60, 1960.
4. Åstrand, P.O., Rodahl, K. *Textbook of Work Physiology,* 3rd Ed. New York, NY: McGraw-Hill, 1986.
5. Ben-Ezra, V., Verstraete, R. "Stair climbing: An alternative exercise modality for firefighters." *J Occup Med* 30:103-105, 1988.
6. Brozek, J., Grande, F., Anderson, J., et al. "Densitometric analysis of body composition: Revision of some quantitative assumptions." *Ann NY Acad Sci* 110:113-140, 1963.
7. Brzycki, M. "Strength testing—Predicting a one-rep max from a reps-to-fatigue." *J Phys Ed Rec Dance* 64(1):88-90, 1993.
8. Cooper, K. "A means of assessing maximal oxygen uptake." *J Am Med Assoc* 203:201-204, 1968.
9. Carroll, K., Marshall, D., Sockler, J., et al. "An equation for predicting maximal oxygen consumption on the StairMaster." *Med Sci Sports Exerc* 22(2):S11, 1990.
10. Foster, C., Jackson, A.S., Pollock, M.L., et al. "Generalized equations for predicting functional capacity from treadmill performance." *Am Heart J* 107:1229-1234, 1984.
11. George, J., Vehr, P., Allsen, P., et al. "$VO_{2\,max}$ estimation from a submaximal 1-mile track jog for fit college-age individuals." *Med Sci Sports Exerc* 25(3):401-406, 1993.
12. Golding, L.S., Myers, C.F., Sinning, W.E. *The Y's Way to Physical Fitness, Revised.* Chicago, IL: National Board of YMCA, 1982.
13. Heyward, V.H. *Advanced Fitness Assessment & Exercise Prescription,* 2nd Ed. Champaign, IL: Human Kinetics Publishers, 1991.
14. Hodgdon, J. "Body composition in the military services: Standards and methods." In *Body Composition and Physical Performance, Applications for the Military Services.* Marriott, B. & Grumstrop-Scott, J. (Eds.). Washington, DC: National Academy Press, p. 65, 1992.
15. Holland, G.J., Weber, F., Heng, et al. "Maximal steptreadmill exercise and treadmill exercise by patients with coronary heart disease: A comparison." *J Cardiopul Rehabil* 8:58-68, 1988.
16. Jackson, A.S., Pollock, M.L. "Generalized equations for predicting body density of men." *Brit J Nutr* 40:497-504, 1978.
17. Jackson, A.S., Pollock, M.L. "Practical assessment of body composition." *Phys Sportsmed* 13(5):76-90, 1985.
18. Jackson, A.S., Pollock, M.L., Ward, A. "Generalized equations for predicting body density of women." *Med Sci Sports Exerc* 12:175-182, 1980.
19. Kline, G.M., Porci, J.P., Hintermeister, R., et al. "Estimation of $VO_{2\,max}$ from a one-mile track walk, gender, age, and body weight." *Med Sci Sports Exerc* 19(3):253-259, 1987.
20. Leighton, J. "Instrument and technique for measurement of range of joint motion." *Arch Phys Med Rehabil* 36:571-578, 1955.
21. McArdle, W.D., Katch, F.I., Pechar, G.S., et al. "Reliability and interrelationships between maximal oxygen intake, physical work capacity and step-test scores in college women." *Med Sci Sports* 4:182-186, 1972.
22. Nieman, D.C. *Fitness and Sports Medicine: An Introduction,* 2nd Ed. Palo Alto, CA: Bull Publishing Company, 1990.

23. Pollock, M.L., Foster, D., Schmidt, D., et al. "Comparative analysis of physiologic responses to three different maximal graded exercise test protocols in healthy women." *Am Heart J* 103:363-373, 1982.

24. Sharkey, B.J. *Physiology of Fitness*, 2nd Ed. Champaign, IL: Human Kinetics Publishers, Inc., 1984.

25. Siri, W.E. "Body composition from fluid spaces and density." In *Techniques for Measuring Body Composition*. Brozek, J., Henschel, A., (Eds.). Washington, DC: National Academy of Sciences, 1961.

26. Storer, T., Davis, J., and Caizzo, V. "Accurate prediction of $\dot{V}O_{2\,max}$ in cycle ergometry." *Med Sci Sports Exerc* 22(5):704-712, 1990.

27. Vanderburgh, P. "The 12-minute stationary cycle ergometer test: An efficacious $\dot{V}O_2$ peak prediction test for the injured." *J Sport Rehabil* 2(3):189-195, 1993.

28. Vanderburgh, P. "Fat distribution: Its physiological significance, health implications and its adaptation to exercise training." *Military Med* 157(4):189-192, 1992.

CHAPTER 13

• •

DEVELOPING A PERSONALIZED EXERCISE PROGRAM: PRESCRIPTION GUIDELINES

by

Gerald D. Thompson, M.S.
and
B. Don Franks, Ph.D.

• • •

"My present prescription for exercise is as follows: Daily —at least 60 minutes of physical activity, not necessarily vigorous, nor all at the same time. Weekly—at least two or three periods of 30 minutes of intermittent or sustained activity at a submaximal rate of work are necessary for maintaining good cardiovascular fitness."
Dr. Per-Olof Åstrand

*I*n general, the statement made by Dr. Åstrand concerning what constitutes a sufficient quantity of exercise for maintaining personal fitness is supported by the American College of Sports Medicine (ACSM) and prevailing exercise science research. His statement, however, needs some qualification and further quantification. An exercise prescription is a personalized program of recommended physical activity which is designed to enhance, maintain, or restore positive health and fitness. Specific guidelines for the intensity, duration, frequency, type, and progression of exercise are integral components of a sound exercise prescription.

An individual's health and fitness status, the exercise setting, the program goals, and the participant's goals are critical factors in the development of an exercise prescription. As a general rule, exercise prescriptions are either self-developed or designed by professionally trained personnel who are employed at health-fitness facilities. Regardless of what option is followed, the prescription must be based on the aforementioned factors. Health-Fitness facilities usually administer some type of Health Status Questionnaire (refer to Chapter 3) to gather information on those factors to decide which activities (as outlined by criteria established by the ACSM) will be most appropriate to include in an individual's initial exercise program. Finally, it should be noted that once an exercise program has actually begun, periodic evaluations of an individual's health and fitness status need to be conducted to assess the individual's adaptation to the exercise regime and whether or not adjustments in the program's protocol should be undertaken.

If you are engaging in a "self-administered" exercise program and are charged with conducting your own periodic assessments of your personal level of fitness, you need to ensure that your efforts are based on sound information and techniques. If, however, you are one of the more than ten million Americans who belong to a health-fitness facility, the professional staff at that facility—in all likelihood—will include periodic evaluations of your health status and fitness progress as part of their efforts to serve you. In fact, the ACSM—in its recently developed "Consumer Guidelines for Selecting a Health-Fitness Facility," recommends that if you are considering becoming a member of a health-fitness club, you examine the policies of that facility with regard to medical clearance and personal fitness assessment before you join. In general, a health-fitness facility should adhere to the following fundamental policies:

- Recommends routine medical checkups and health screening as part of its standard operating procedures.
- Recommends low-intensity exercise (40 to 60% of maximal heart rate reserve) initially, for all apparently healthy individuals who display no unusual physiological signs or symptoms.
- Requires medical clearance before moderate or high-intensity exercise participation for individuals with:
    - known health problems, two or more major coronary risk factors, or signs or symptoms indicative of potential health problems (individuals at higher risk) refer to Chapters 3 and 4, or
    - intentions of engaging in very strenuous activities (in athletic performance where the level of intensity is much higher than that needed for fitness gains).
- Recommends maximal graded exercise (stress) test (GXT), with physician's interpretation of ECG, prior to exercise participation for individuals with known cardiovascular disease, symptoms related to cardiovascular disease, significant risk factors for cardiovascular disease, and men over 40 years of age or women over 50 years of age.

The primary focus of this chapter is to provide an overview regarding factors that should be considered in developing fitness programs for apparently healthy adults. The apparently healthy population is generally characterized as being both symptom free and engaging in relatively routine physical activity. They can begin low intensity exercise programs without the need for exercise testing or medical examination as long as the exercise program progresses gradually and the individual is alert to the development of any unusual signs or symptoms. A simple, brief questionnaire called the Physical Activity Readiness Questionnaire (PAR-Q) has been found to be a valid screening instrument for both submaximal exercise testing and for beginning low-intensity and gently progressive (but not heavy or overly challenging) exercise programs (refer to Chapter 3). Moderate-intensity exercise (60 to 80% $VO_{2\,max}$) is sufficiently intense to represent a substantial challenge to an individual because it will elicit significant increases in specific physiologic responses (e.g., heart rate and respiration). At or above age 40 in men, or age 50 in women, it is desirable for individuals to have both a medical examination and a supervised maximal exercise test before beginning a vigorous exercise program (refer to Chapter 5 for a summary of the basic guidelines for exercise testing).

CARDIORESPIRATORY CONDITIONING

Based on the existing scientific evidence concerning exercise prescription for healthy adults and the need for such guidelines, the American College of Sports Medicine developed a position paper on exercise prescription which included the following recommendations concerning the quantity and quality of (exercise) training for developing and maintaining cardiorespiratory fitness and desirable body composition in a healthy adult.

1. <u>Frequency of training:</u> 3 to 5 days per week.

2. <u>Intensity:</u> 50% to 85% of maximum oxygen uptake ($VO_{2\,max}$), 50% to 85% of maximum heart rate reserve, or 60% to 90% of maximal heart rate. It should be noted that exercise of low and moderate intensity may provide important health benefits and may result in increased fitness in some persons (e.g., those who were previously sedentary and low fit).

3. <u>Duration of training:</u> 20 to 60 minutes of continuous aerobic activity. The actual length of time you should exercise aerobically is generally dependent on the relative intensity level of the activity. For example, activities involving a lower intensity should be conducted over a longer period of time. Your emphasis should be placed on the total work you perform. Total work can be estimated by the caloric expenditure associated with the activity—a subject which will be discussed later in this chapter.

4. <u>Mode of activity:</u> An appropriate modality for developing cardiorespiratory fitness is any activity that uses the large muscle groups, that can be maintained continuously, and is rhythmical and aerobic in nature (e.g., running, jogging, walking, machine-based stair climbing, swimming, skating, bicycling, rowing, cross-country skiing, and various endurance game activities). Note: At the beginning of an exercise program, activities such as walking, jogging, machine-based stair climbing, and cycling are most recommended.

5. <u>Rate of progression</u>: In most instances, the ability of the body to adapt to the stresses imposed upon it (sometimes referred to as the training effect) allows individuals to gradually increase the total work they do over time. In continuous exercise, increasing the work performed can be achieved by increasing the intensity of the exercise, the duration of the exercise bout, or by some combination of the two. The most significant conditioning effects are typically observed during the first six to eight weeks of an exercise program. An individual's exercise prescription is normally adjusted as these conditioning effects occur. The extent of the adjustment depends on the individual involved, additional feedback from assessment efforts, and/or the exercise performance of the individual during exercise sessions.

DEVELOPING AN APPROPRIATE EXERCISE PRESCRIPTION

It should be noted that desirable outcomes can be attained with exercise programs that vary considerably in terms of mode, frequency, duration, and intensity. In addition, it should be remembered that some individuals achieve a faster (or greater) rate of improvement than others.

For example, if you have been relatively sedentary for years, you should expect to progress more slowly. In this instance, you should begin exercising at a level that you can easily complete and should then gradually increase the amount of work that you perform during a workout. On the other hand, if you are an individual who has been somewhat active, you may progress more rapidly in your exercise programs than a sedentary individual whose slower progression is necessary primarily to reduce injury potential and to assure appropriate adaptation in previously unused muscles. Finally, depending upon how your body responds (and adapts) to the demands imposed upon it by your exercise program, you need to be both willing and able to modify your exercise prescription as appropriate.

WARM-UP AND COOL-DOWN PHASES

Warm-up and cool-down activities should be an essential part of all exercise programs. The purpose of the warm-up is to prepare your body, especially your cardiovascular and musculoskeletal systems, for the conditioning or stimulus phase of the exercise session. The cool-down phase assures that venous return to your heart is maintained in the face of significant amounts of blood going to previously working muscles. Light aerobic endurance activities, coupled with stretching activities, provide the recommended basis for both the warm-up and cool-down phases.

The length of the warm-up and cool-down periods depends on several factors, including the type of activity engaged in during the conditioning period, the level of intensity of those activities, as well as the age and fitness level of the participant. In general, the warm-up and cool-down phases last approximately five to ten minutes each. If the time you have available to work out is less than usual, it is recommended that you reduce the time allotted for the conditioning phase of your workout, while retaining sufficient time for the warm-up and cool-down phases.

CARDIORESPIRATORY ENDURANCE ACTIVITIES

The ACSM differentiates between several types of cardiorespiratory endurance activities. Activities like walking, jogging, machine-based stair climbing, or cycling (referred to as Group 1 activities) can be easily maintained at a constant level of intensity. The variability between subjects in terms of energy expenditure is relatively low in these types of activities. In Group 2 activities, such as swimming or cross-country skiing, the rate of energy expenditure is highly related to skill. Although the level of intensity involved in Group 2 activities tends to vary between individuals, a relatively constant level of intensity can be maintained within a given individual. Tennis, basketball, and racquetball (referred to as Group 3 activities) by their very nature are highly variable in intensity both between individuals and within a specific individual.

The type of activities (Group 1, 2, or 3) prescribed for you will be highly dependent upon the results of your health risk appraisal assessment and your current fitness level. For example, Group 3 activities are generally not prescribed for unfit, at risk, or diseased individuals, because such activities can vary a great deal in their intensity.

INTENSITY OF EXERCISE

Perhaps the most important component of an exercise prescription is the level of exercise intensity. The prescribed level of intensity must be sufficient to overload the cardiovascular system, but not so severe that it overtaxes the system. For the apparently healthy individual who wants to develop and maintain cardiorespiratory fitness, the American College of Sports Medicine recommends that the intensity level of the exercise needs to be between 50% to 85% of the person's maximum oxygen uptake capacity ($\dot{V}O_{2max}$). Exercise intensities between 60% to 80% of $\dot{V}O_{2max}$ are prescribed for most participants. It is generally believed, however, that the intensity threshold for a training effect is at the low end of this continuum for those who have been sedentary, and at the high end of the scale for those who are physically active.

CALCULATING EXERCISE INTENSITY

Exercise intensity can be prescribed in terms of heart rate (HR) by using specific heart rate values that are approximately equal to 60 to 80% of $\dot{V}O_{2max}$. One method involves monitoring HR at each stage of a maximal graded exercise test (GXT). The HR is plotted on a graph against the $\dot{V}O_2$ (or MET) equivalents of each stage of the test in order to define the slope of the heart rate response to exercise. From this relationship the exercise heart rate associated with a given percent of $\dot{V}O_{2max}$ can be obtained. While such a method is generally preferred, it does require a participant to complete a maximal GXT—with its associated logistical and safety considerations. Another method for assessing exercise intensity is based on the observation that 70 and 85% of maximal heart rate is equal to approximately 60 and 80% of functional capacity ($\dot{V}O_{2 max}$). For example:

> THR range = maximal HR x 0.70 and 0.85
> where:
> THR = training heart rate
> maximal HR = 220 - age (in years)

The third method for determining the exercise heart rate for training is to calculate the heart rate reserve (HRR). The HRR method of determining the training or target heart rate range, made popular by Karvonen, requires a few simple calculations:

> First, subtract resting HR from maximal HR to obtain HR reserve.
> Then, take 60% and 80% of the HR reserve.
> Then, add each value to resting HR to obtain the THR range.
>
> • THR range = [(maximal HR - resting HR) x 0.60 and 0.80] + resting HR[*]

Whenever possible, use an accurate measurement of maximal heart rate rather than a predicted or estimated one. Estimated maximal heart rates have the distinct disadvantage in that they are based on population averages, and, as a result, have a standard deviation of plus or minus 10-12 bpm.

Another method for prescribing and monitoring exercise intensity involves using ratings of perceived exertion (RPE—refer to Table 13-1). This method, developed by Swedish psychologist Gunnar Borg, uses a 15-point numerical scale ranging from 6 to 20 with the individual who is exercising providing a verbal description of how (relatively) difficult the exercise is based on categories assigned to every odd number. A perceived exertion rating of 12 to 13 has been shown to correspond to approximately 60% of $\dot{V}O_{2 max}$. A rating of 16 corresponds to approximately 80% to 85% of $\dot{V}O_{2 max}$. Therefore, an RPE range of 12 (somewhat hard) to 16 (hard) is recommended for most healthy adults.

Participants skilled at using RPE as an indicator of overall feeling of exertion can use it to specify an RPE level for conditioning. It can also be used in conjunction with a THR prescription. In addition, RPE can be used to modify an exercise prescription. RPE, for example, is often one of the first readily recognizable measures of (positive) changes in cardiorespiratory fitness.

---

[*] Resting HR is best determined while in a seated position immediately upon waking in the morning.

Table 13-1. The 15-point and 10-point Borg RPE scales.

Category (15-point) RPE Scale		Category/Ratio (10-point) RPE Scale	
6		0	Nothing at all
7	Very, very light	0.5	Very, very weak
8		1	Very weak
9	Very light	2	Weak
10		3	Moderate
11	Fairly light	4	Somewhat strong
12		5	Strong
13	Somewhat hard	6	
14		7	Very strong
15	Hard	8	
16		9	
17	Very hard	10	Very, very strong
18		*	Maximal
19	Very, very hard		
20			

From Noble, B.J., et al. *Med Sci Sports Exerc* 15:523-528, 1983.

DURATION OF THE EXERCISE SESSION

The duration of exercise refers to the amount of time (in minutes) that the proper intensity level should be maintained. Typically, a conditioning phase lasts for at least 20 to 30 minutes, which corresponds to the amount of time required for the improvement or maintenance of functional capacity. Individuals just beginning an exercise program should start with approximately 10-20 minutes of aerobic activity. On the other hand, individuals in average shape can exercise for a longer period of time (e.g., 20-30 minutes). Keep in mind that the optimum duration of an exercise session usually depends on the intensity level of the workout. More importantly, in order to achieve health and fitness benefits, exercise should be long enough to expend about 300 kcal.

FREQUENCY OF EXERCISE SESSION

Frequency of exercise refers to the number of exercise sessions per week. While some studies have been able to demonstrate improvements in cardiorespiratory fitness with an exercise frequency of less than three days per week, such improvements have tended to be minimal. It appears that the body responds best to three to five days per week of moderate-intensity aerobic exercise with sessions lasting 20-30 minutes. The traditional recommendation of a "work-one-day and rest-one-day" routine remains a valid approach if you want to improve your level of cardiorespiratory fitness. It should be pointed out that for previously sedentary individuals, the frequency level of their exercise program should initially be established at three days per week. More sessions would place them at undue risk for orthopedic injuries and expose them to an exercise environment which might have a negative effect on their level of exercise adherence. Individuals who desire to increase their frequency of training should gradually do so, depending on their age, initial and existing fitness status, and their personal needs, interests, and exercise objectives.

Mode Of Exercise

Activities should be selected on the basis of individual functional capacity, interest, time, personal goals, and objectives. A fitness program usually starts with activities quantifiable, such as walking, exercise cycling, or stair climbing, so that the proper exercise intensity which is appropriate for you can be determined and achieved. When you can exercise 3-4 days a week 30-40 minutes a day at that level, any activity utilizing large muscle groups can be incorporated into your exercise program.

Rate Of Progression

The recommended rate of progression in your exercise program depends on several interrelated factors, including your fitness status, health status, age, needs or goals, and support provided by friends and family. The American College of Sports Medicine defines three distinct stages of an exercise prescription.

1. Initial Conditioning Stage: This stage typically lasts 4-6 weeks, but may be longer depending on the participant's adaptation to the exercise program. ACSM suggests that you exercise at a level of intensity which is approximately 1 MET* lower than the one corresponding to an estimate of 40 to 85% (or lower than 50 to 90% of maximal heart rate) of your functional capacity in order to avoid undue muscle soreness, injury, discomfort, and discouragement.

2. Improvement Conditioning Stage: This stage lasts 12-20 weeks, and is the period during which progression is most rapid. The intensity level is increased to 50 to 85% of $VO_{2 max}$ (60 to 90% of maximal heart rate), while the duration of the exercise session is increased as frequently as every two to three weeks. The frequency and magnitude of increments are dictated by the rate at which you adapt to the conditioning program.

3. Maintenance Conditioning Stage: When the desired level of conditioning is attained, the maintenance stage begins—usually after the first six months of training. At this time, the emphasis is often refocused from an exercise program involving primarily fitness activities to one which includes a more diverse array of enjoyable (lifetime) activities.

---

* One MET is assumed to be equal to an oxygen uptake of 3.5 milliliters per kilogram of body weight per minute. It is a measure of energy output equal to the resting metabolic rate of an average individual.

PRESCRIPTION GUIDELINES

• • •

MUSCULOSKELETAL CONDITIONING

Musculoskeletal conditioning includes exercises for ensuring that you have an adequate level of flexibility, as well as for developing an appropriate level of muscular fitness. Flexibility was previously discussed in the sections on the warm-up and cool-down phases of an exercise bout. Achieving and maintaining an adequate range of motion should always be an objective of a comprehensive exercise prescription. Flexibility is important for several reasons, including the fact that it reduces an individual's potential for injury and improves an individual's ability to perform certain physical and sports-related tasks.

The warm-up phase of your exercise session should include some type of light warm-up activity to increase both your heart rate and your internal body temperature, which is then followed by flexibility exercises which are specifically designed to stretch the musculature around your body's major skeletal joints. Attempting to stretch a cold muscle can be dangerous to the soft tissues surrounding the muscle. No matter how controlled the movement, forcing a muscle through a full normal range of motion (and beyond) without appropriately warming it up is both unsafe and counterproductive.

A general exercise prescription for achieving and maintaining flexibility should adhere to the following guidelines:

- Frequency   - daily
- Intensity   - to a position of mild discomfort
- Duration   - 10-30 seconds for each stretch
- Repetitions   - 2-6 for each stretch
- Type   - static, with a major emphasis on the low-back and hamstrings area because of the high prevalence of low-back pain syndrome in our society.

Specific guidelines for developing muscular fitness are not nearly as universally accepted as are those for attaining flexibility. Considerable debate exists regarding what constitutes the most appropriate protocol for developing muscular strength and muscular endurance (collectively referred to as muscular fitness). What is generally accepted, however, is the fact that like any system of your body, your muscular system responds to the demands placed upon it. In the exercise arena, the particular form of physical activity that is designed to develop muscular fitness is referred to as resistance training. A growing awareness also exists that resistance training of at least a moderate intensity level, sufficient enough to develop and maintain lean body tissue, must be an integral part of a comprehensive (adult) fitness program.

According to the ACSM, one set of 8 to 12 repetitions of 8 to 10 exercises that train the major muscle groups at least two days per week is the recommended minimum amount of resistance training that should be performed to achieve a training effect. Considerable evidence also suggests that in order for your resistance training efforts to be as safe, effective, and efficient as possible, you should:

- Adhere as closely as possible to the specific techniques for performing a particular exercise.
- Exercise to the point of momentary muscular fatigue.
- Perform every exercise through a full range of motion.
- Exercise antagonist muscle groups.
- Perform the eccentric (lowering) portion of a lift in a controlled manner, as well as the concentric (raising phase).
- Include exercises in your training program for all of the major muscle groups of your body—not just a few selected muscle groups.
- Work out (if possible) with a training partner who could, as appropriate, provide you with feedback, support, and motivation.
- Never hold your breath while strength training, since holding your breath can raise your blood pressure to an unsafe level (refer to Valsalva maneuver in Appendix A).

ENVIRONMENTAL CONSIDERATIONS

Environmental factors exist, such as heat, humidity, altitude, and pollution, that can cause HR and perception of effort to increase during an exercise session. The RPE scale and heart rate are two of the primary indicators that you can use to adjust the intensity and duration of your exercise efforts in diverse environments. In extremely warm conditions, such as very humid and arid climates, the intensity level of your exercise bout should be somewhat restricted. Care should be taken to replace any fluids you lost during and after your exercise sessions. When exercising during extremely cold conditions, you should wear clothing that adequately protects your head (a major avenue of heat loss) and extremities (common sites for frostbite injuries). The intensity and the duration of exercise may also have to be modified (i.e., reduced) when you exercise at high altitudes and in areas with high levels of air pollution (for more information regarding exercise and environmental factors refer to chapter 19).

PROGRAM SUPERVISION

As a basic guideline, apparently healthy, asymptomatic individuals who want to engage in unsupervised exercise programs should have a functional capacity of at least 8 METs. Whatever your fitness level, it is recommended that, if you want to engage in an unsupervised exercise program, you should begin with low-intensity exercises, at or below 50% of your functional capacity (60% HR max) and then increase the intensity of your efforts gradually as your body adapts to the stress you've imposed upon it. You should be acutely aware of the signs or symptoms of exertional intolerance (e.g., dizziness, pallor, angina, dypsnea, etc.). It is also in your best interests to have a basic understanding of the fundamental prescription variables of the intensity (THR), duration, and frequency of exercise.

One of the major advantages of joining a health-fitness facility is the fact that they have trained professionals on site to provide you with exercise leadership and guidance. For high-risk or symptomatic individuals, such assistance is extraordinarily valuable. However, these programs are also useful for those individuals who would benefit from hands-on instruction regarding proper exercise technique. In addition, supervised programs can also offer valuable social support for those individuals having difficulty initiating and sustaining lifestyle behavioral changes.

A Prescription For Life

Exercise training can be a valuable tool in improving your relative health and functional status. In order to ensure that you fully receive all of the benefits of a sound exercise program, you need to first identify the existence (if any) of risk factors that may influence the design of your exercise program. Based upon a comprehensive analysis of your personal exercise needs and interests, you should then develop (or have developed for you) an individualized program of exercise that will meet your unique requirements. This program should closely adhere to the primary prescription variables for a sound exercise regimen. Periodically, the manner in which your body has adapted to these variables should be reevaluated. Whenever necessary, you should make adjustments in your personal exercise prescription as appropriate. In so doing, you will be giving yourself a prescription for life . . . a R_X for health and wellness. ❏

BIBLIOGRAPHY •••

1. American College of Sports Medicine. *Guidelines for Exercise Testing and Prescription*, 4th Ed. Philadelphia, PA: Lea & Febiger, 1991.
2. American College of Sports Medicine. "Position stand on the recommended quantity and quality of exercise for developing and maintaining cardiorespiratory and muscular fitness in healthy adults." *Med Sci Sports Exerc* 22:264-274, 1990.
3. Åstrand, P.O., Rodahl, K. *Textbook of Work Physiology*, 3rd Ed. New York, NY: McGraw-Hill, 1986.
4. Brooks, G.A., Fahey, T.D. *Exercise Physiology: Human Bioenergetics and Its Applications*. New York, NY: Macmillan Publishing Company, 1985.
5. Franklin, B.A., Gordon, S., Timmis, G.C. (Eds). *Exercise in Modern Medicine*. Baltimore, MD: Williams & Wilkins, 1989.
6. Gledhill, N. "Discussion: Assessment of Fitness." *Exercise, Fitness, and Health: A Consensus of Current Knowledge*. Bouchard, C., et al. (Ed). Champaign, IL: Human Kinetics Publishers, 1990.
7. Heyward. V.H. *Advanced Fitness Assessment & Exercise Prescription*, 2nd Ed. Champaign, IL: Human Kinetics Publishers, 1991.
8. Howley, E.T., Franks, B.D. *Health/Fitness Instructor's Handbook,* 2nd Ed. Champaign, IL: Human Kinetics Publishers, 1992.
9. Nieman, D.C. *Fitness and Sports Medicine: An Introduction*, 2nd Ed. Palo Alto, CA: Bull Publishing Company, 1990.
10. Noble, B.J., Borg, G.A., Jacobs, I., et al. "A category-ratio perceived exertion scale: Relationship to blood and muscle lactate and heart rate." *Med Sci Sports Exerc* 15:523-528, 1983.
11. Painter, P. "Exercise Programming." *Resource Manual for Guidelines for Exercise Testing and Prescription*. American College of Sports Medicine. Philadelphia, PA: Lea & Febiger, 1988.

CHAPTER 14

EXERCISE AND CARDIAC REHABILITATION

by

Donald B. Bergey, M.A.
and
Paul M. Ribisl, Ph.D.

• • •

*C*onsiderable research and empirical practice have shown that properly prescribed exercise training can be an effective part of a treatment program for patients with coronary artery disease (CAD). Previous chapters in this book have discussed the benefits and physiological basis of exercise training. The fundamental purpose of exercise training for CAD patients is threefold: *primary prevention* (i.e., enhancing positive health), *secondary prevention (i.e.,* slowing of the progression of the CAD process) and *rehabilitation* (i.e., restoring normal function). Prescribing exercise for cardiac patients (as well as for other special populations) should follow the basic prescription and training guidelines for healthy populations, with the exception of modifications arising from several specific principles which are unique to cardiac patients. This chapter examines the special principles of training which should be applied to CAD patients and offers suggestions regarding how to apply them to an individual training program designed for an individual with CAD.

THE TRAINING STIMULUS

An appropriate discussion of exercise training should initially focus on the size of the training stimulus required to cause a positive physiological adaptation to occur (i.e., an improvement in functional capacity). Most of the literature concerning exercise training suggests specific thresholds which must be exceeded in order to improve functional capacity. The recommended work loads include a range of 40 - 60% of maximal oxygen uptake, 50 - 70% of maximal heart rate response, or the expenditure of 300 kilocalories per exercise session. It is important to realize that the training stimulus for adaptation is based on the *overload principle*. Any work load that is greater (within limits) than that to which any given system is accustomed will produce an increase in the functional capacity of that system. The aforementioned thresholds are actually appropriate work loads for maintenance levels of training in presumably healthy individuals. When training extremely deconditioned, diseased individuals, it may be more appropriate to use lower than the standard or "usual" work loads, especially when designing the beginning or "initial" phase of the program.

DEVELOPING A SAFE EXERCISE PRESCRIPTION

Safety is the most important factor that must be addressed when you are developing an exercise prescription for cardiac patients. As you will see in the later discussion, several methods can be used to compute a training work load for CAD patients—each with its advantages and disadvantages. The unyielding guideline for developing an appropriate exercise prescription for an individual with CAD, however, is that the work load must be both safe and realistic for the patient. Making a safe exercise prescription is based on the concept of the level of the "symptom-limited end point." The purpose of a graded exercise (stress) test (GXT) is to evaluate an individual's ability to tolerate gradual increases in the intensity of exercise. The point at which the individual demonstrates an abnormal response pattern to the work load which precludes continuing the exercise is termed the "symptom-limited end point" (i.e., the maximum level of exercise before signs or symptoms of physiological intolerance occur).

Another important part of exercise training is identifying individuals whose participation in exercise programs may be contraindicated (i.e., not recommended) because of specific health/medical conditions they possess. The American College of Sports Medicine (ACSM) in its most recently published guidelines on exercise prescription, developed several criteria which can be used to identify those individuals for whom an exercise program may be contraindicated (refer to Table 14-1).

If you have cardiovascular disease, you should get permission from your physician before you begin an exercise program. Specifically, you should ask your physician if you have any of the contraindicative conditions specified by the ACSM.

Once you begin an exercise program, it is important to know when it is unsafe to continue to exercise. Neil F. Gordon, M.D. and Larry W. Gibbons, M.D., on the staff of the Cooper Clinic in Dallas, Texas, offer the following guidelines* concerning what actions you should take if you experience certain symptoms:

---

* Authors' Note: These guidelines have been modified from Gordon and Gibbons (1991), p.159.

Table 14-1. Contraindications for Entry into Inpatient and Outpatient Exercise Programs.

The following criteria may be used as contrindications for program entry:

1. Unstable angina (unpredictable or recurring chest pain)
2. Resting systolic blood pressure >200 mm Hg or resting diastolic blood pressure > 100 mm Hg.
3. Orthostatic hypotension (a drop in blood pressure $\geq$ 20 mm Hg when an individual stands after sitting or lying down)
4. Moderate to severe aortic stenosis (narrowing of the aorta)
5. Acute systemic (whole body) illness or fever
6. Uncontrolled dysrhythmias (abnormal heart rhythms of either the atria or the ventricles)
7. Uncontrolled sinus tachycardia (elevated resting heart rate—greater than 120 bpm)
8. Uncontrolled congestive heart failure
9. Complete (3^0 A-V) heart block
10. Active pericarditis (inflammation of the membrane covering the heart) or myocarditis (inflammation of the heart muscle)
11. Recent embolism (a traveling blood clot)
12. Thrombophlebitis (inflammation of a vein, often due to a blood clot)
13. Greater than 3 mm resting ST displacement (an ECG abnormality that is indicative of coronary insufficiency)
14. Uncontrolled diabetes
15. Orthopaedic problems that would prohibit exercise

Modified from the American College of Sports Medicine (1991).

- *Pain or discomfort in your chest, abdomen, back, neck, jaw, or arms.* You should never exercise to the point where you develop even a mild form of these symptoms of myocardial ischemia. Even a rating of 1+ ("light, barely noticeable") on the angina scale (refer to Table 14-2) is an indication you've overstepped the bounds of safe exercise. Upon experiencing these symptoms, slow down immediately and notify a rehabilitation staff member. If you're exercising alone and the discomfort doesn't subside within two or three minutes, follow our nitroglycerin guidelines outlined in the following statement. Remember, if ischemia continues for a prolonged period of time, you run the risk of sustaining permanent damage to your heart muscle.
- *If you are alone and you think that it is angina.* Slow down or stop what you are doing immediately. The symptoms should subside within a minute or two, in which case you needn't be unduly alarmed. If your symptoms continue, your physician may have prescribed nitroglycerin tablets (or an oral spray) for just such an occurrence. Take one tablet or dose as directed. If the discomfort is still present after another five minutes, take a second tablet. Again, wait for five minutes. If this doesn't work either, take a final nitroglycerin tablet and call your physician immediately.
- *Unaccustomed shortness of breath during exercise.* For example, if you've always been capable of walking three miles in forty-five minutes with no

breathlessness, then you should be alarmed if suddenly you can't any-more. Notify your doctor.

- *Dizziness or fainting.* During or immediately after exercise, if you get very dizzy and feel as if you are about to faint, it is usually best to lie down flat on your back with your head either level with your body or below your feet.
- *A nauseous sensation during or after exercise.* Treat the same as for dizziness or fainting.
- *An irregular pulse, particularly when it's been regular in past exercise sessions.* If you notice what appear to be either extra heartbeats or missed beats, you may be experiencing premature ventricular contractions (PVC). Once again, summon a staff member or tell your doctor.

Table 14-2. Angina Pain Scale.

1+ Light, barely noticeable
2+ Moderate, bothersome
3+ Severe, very uncomfortable
4+ Most severe pain ever experienced

Everyone who exercises or supervises an exercise program should be familiar with certain warning signs that may indicate that your cardiovascular system is not coping with or adapting to an exercise bout, and that a cardiovascular event may be impending. The ACSM (1991) in its guidelines recently identified specific criteria concerning when an exercise session should be terminated. If any of the following signs or symptoms are experienced, you should stop exercising and seek a medical consultation. Also, no further exercise should be undertaken until you have been seen by a physician. Your exercise session should be terminated if you experience any of the following:

- Excessive fatigue
- Failure of monitoring equipment
- Light-headedness, confusion, ataxia, pallor, cyanosis, dyspnea, nausea, or any peripheral circulatory insufficiency
- Onset of angina with exercise
- Symptomatic supraventricular tachycardia
- ST displacement (3 mm) horizontal or downsloping from rest
- Ventricular tachycardia (3 or more consecutive PVCs)
- Exercise-induced left bundle branch block
- Onset of second degree and/or third degree A-V block
- R-on-T PVCs (one)
- Frequent multifocal PVCs (30% of the complexes)
- Exercise hypotension (> 20 mm Hg drop in systolic blood pressure during exercise)
- Excessive blood pressure rise: systolic $\geq$ 220 or diastolic $\geq$ 110 mm Hg
- Inappropriate bradycardia (drop in heart rate greater than 10 bpm) with increase or no change in work load

Medications are the final consideration concerning how to ensure that your exercise prescription is safe. The safest approach in obtaining an exercise prescription is to consult an experienced or certified exercise physiologist or physician and undergo a GXT. If you are taking any of the class of cardiac medications called beta blockers or calcium channel blockers, you must have a GXT. It is important that you take your medication as you normally would if you are going to use the heart rate method to prescribe the intensity of your exercise program, since these medications alter the heart rate response to exercise. It is best if you can undergo your GXT at about the same time of day as you plan to exercise. The *beta blockers* are Propranolol (Inderal®), Nadolol (Corgard®), Metoprolol (Lopressor®), Atenolol (Tenormin®), Timolol (Blocadren®), Pindolol (Visken®), and Labetalol (Trandate® and Normodyne®). Sectral® and Tenoretic® are combination drugs that also contain a beta-blocker. The *calcium channel blockers* include Nifedipine (Procardia®), Diltiazem (Cardizem®), Verapamil (Calan® and Isoptin®), Bepridil (Vascor®), and Nicardipine HCL (Cardene®).

TYPE OF ACTIVITIES

One of the first decisions to be made concerning an exercise prescription is the type of activity to be used. To make this choice properly, the principle of specificity must be clearly understood. All physical activities can generally be classified into three basic types of exercise: *aerobic*, *flexibility*, and *resistance*. Aerobic exercise is specific to training the cardiovascular system. It is also the most beneficial type of exercise for making changes in body composition (fat reduction). *Flexibility* exercise is specific for improving the range of motion of the joints and muscles. *Resistance* exercise is specific to training the skeletal muscles for strength and endurance. An overall training program incorporates activities that include each of these types of exercise.

Aerobic exercise is an example of fitness training which involves activities that require your body to be physically moved. No activity is entirely aerobic. The extent to which an activity can be judged as an aerobic exercise depends on how much oxygen is used by the body—a factor which is related to how many of the muscles of the body are used. Fitness activities such as walking/jogging, cycling, swimming, cross country skiing, rowing, stair climbing*, dance, and rope skipping are examples of the most efficient types of aerobic activities because they can be conducted on a non-stop (continuous) basis. They enable you to achieve the most from your training in the least amount of time. Recently conducted research at St. Joseph's Hospital in Phoenix, Arizona, the University of Florida, and Arizona State University indicates that exercising on an independent-step action stair climbing machine may be particularly appropriate for CAD patients because of the fact that it offers weight bearing exercise without the usual accompanying orthopaedic trauma.

---

* Editors' Note: The recently introduced StairMaster® 4000CT® allows individuals to perform stair climbing exercise within an intensity range of 2.0-8.5 METs.

Most sport activities also involve an aerobic component. A few examples of the more popular athletic endeavors that often place a demand on your aerobic system are basketball, soccer, tennis, racquetball, and even golf (if you walk!). Several dimensions of sport activities diminish their value as aerobic conditioners. First, it is hard to control the intensity level in sports. In most instances, they are usually discontinuous. In addition, if the activities are team sports, you must depend to some degree on other people to get your exercise. Finally, the competitive aspect of sports also makes the intensity level difficult to control.

Flexibility exercise is an example of fitness training which involves activities that move a joint through a full range of movement. The most common type of activity that is used for range of motion is stretching.

Resistance exercise is an example of fitness training which involves activities that require the skeletal muscles to work against a resistance. The most common types of this exercise are weight training and calisthenics.

Most exercise scientists believe that the most important element of your exercise training program is the aerobic component. Accordingly, they conclude that the greatest portion of your workout should be devoted to an aerobic activity. As a general rule, the best aerobic activity is one that you enjoy and will engage in on a regular basis. All factors considered, the best aerobic activity which involves the largest number of people is walking. Range of motion activities involving the major joints in your body should be employed as part of the warm-up that precedes your aerobic activity (but should be applied gently before exercise). On the other hand, range of motion training, which is intended to improve your level of flexibility, should be performed after you engage in aerobic activity (because a warmed muscle can be stretched more safely and effectively). Resistance training should be employed to develop a higher level of muscular fitness, which, in turn, should help alleviate some of the demands on your cardiovascular system that occur with normal, everyday activities.

TRAINING VARIABLES

Several fundamental training variables can be applied to all types of exercise training, including: intensity, duration, frequency, starting level, progression, and warm-up, cool-down. *Intensity* defines how hard the exercise should be performed. *Duration* defines how long the exercise should be performed. *Frequency* defines how often the exercise should be performed. The *starting level* defines at what training level an exercise program should be initiated. *Progression* defines how to gradually adjust your training program as you become more fit. *Warm-up* and *cool-down* define how to properly prepare the body for exercise and how to enable the body to properly recover from the exercise bout, respectively.

INTENSITY

The intensity level of the aerobic activity is the most critical part of an exercise prescription for a CAD patient. In order to identify a proper intensity level, a GXT should be administered at approximately the same time of day as the exercise program will be conducted. In the time period immediately after an event (heart attack, open heart surgery, or angioplasty) and before a GXT can be administered, all physical activity can be monitored by using a heart rate upper limit that is equal to the resting heart rate plus 20 beats. This time frame occurs while the individual is still involved in a hospital-based rehab program (Phase I and II or inpatient and outpatient programs). As soon as a GXT is administered, even if it is a "low level" or "discharge" GXT (an exercise stress test which is used only for prognostic purposes), the subsequent exercise level can be set using the GXT results.

The primary focal point in establishing a proper intensity level for the exercise program of a CAD patient involves the concept of the symptom-limited end point. This end point identifies the maximum level of safe exercise that can be performed. This parameter is determined by establishing the level of exercise at which an abnormal response is elicited during the performance of the GXT. If no abnormal responses are seen, then the symptom-limited end point is volitional fatigue—or the highest attainable level of exercise. Once this end point is determined, then the intensity level of the exercise session should be prescribed at a level below this end point. Several methods of prescribing intensity exist—each of which has advantages and disadvantages associated with it. Regardless of which method is used, the concept of the symptom-limited end point is an underlying principle that must be followed.

The simplest method is to use the level of the end point as the maximum level of exercise and allow any training below it. This method has two serious problems, however. By allowing an individual to exercise to the point of an abnormal response, it increases the risk of exceeding this end point, thus entering the "danger zone." Also, by not setting a lower limit, the individual may not be exercising "hard enough" to stimulate a positive training adaptation. A more prudent approach is to adopt a training intensity level that falls within two subjective range limits relative to the end point. This approach enables you to establish a lower limit of training and also to set an upper limit that has a built-in "buffer zone" between it and the end point. Three commonly used methods of setting the intensity level based on the symptom-limited end point are:

1. **Oxygen uptake (50-85% of the symptom-limited end point).** The most direct method to set the intensity level is to use the amount of oxygen utilized by the body in an aerobic activity. The measurement most easily used for this method is the MET level. A MET is the metabolic equivalent or amount of oxygen used by your body at rest. Thus, five METs would equal five times the amount of oxygen used at rest. This method is relatively easy to apply. The intensity level is set to equal a range using 50% of the symptom-limited end point as the lower limit of the exercise prescription and 85% of the symptom-limited end point as the upper limit (e.g., an individual with a 10-MET capacity would exercise between 5 and 8.5 METs).

Using METs to establish the intensity level of an exercise program is the most direct method because it uses the rate of oxygen consumption to prescribe the exercise level, which most accurately reflects the intensity of an aerobic activity. Unfortunately, this method has some clear disadvantages that must be understood if it is to be used properly. If the MET level is *estimated* from the work load on the treadmill (or any other ergometer), as opposed to actually *measuring* the work load, the prescription level may be inaccurate because of individual variations in oxygen uptake. (Note: In our laboratory we have found rather large variations in the measured MET levels of our cardiac patients compared to the estimated MET levels.) The major problem with this method is encountered when applying the MET level to a specific bout of exercise. If the aerobic exercise is going to be carried out on an ergometer (treadmill, cycle, arm, or etc.), the MET level becomes very difficult to define. You simply cannot tell someone to walk at six METs, for example. Also, extreme conditions of the environment (heat, cold, and humidity) can change the way the cardiovascular system responds to a given MET level. As a result, the cardiovascular system may be working harder at the same MET level.

2. **Heart rate response (50-85% of symptom-limited end point using the HR-Reserve method).** The heart rate response is an indirect method of applying the exercise prescription because your heart rate does not accurately reflect the work of your cardiovascular system in all activities. As a result, caution must be taken when using heart rate to determine exercise intensity for non-aerobic activities or activities that do not have a large aerobic component. When heart rate is used with aerobic activities, however, it is probably the best method, because it is the easiest to apply and will reflect the effect of the environment on the cardiovascular system more accurately. Two methods are commonly used for computing training heart rate: the percent of heart rate-maximum (% HR-max) and the heart rate reserve method (HR-Reserve). The HR-Reserve method is also known as the Karvonen method. The % HR-max method is applied by simply computing a given percent of a set heart rate-maximum (e.g., the symptom-limited end point). The HR-Reserve method uses the following formula:

> **THR = [(SLHR - RHR) X (CI/100)] + RHR**
>   where:
>   THR = Training heart rate
>   SLHR = Symptom limited end point heart rate
>   RHR = Resting heart rate
>   CI = Conditioning intensity

The HR-Reserve method has two features which make it particularly appropriate for use with cardiac patients:

- Heart rates computed by this formula very closely approximate heart rates computed by using the relationship to oxygen uptake.
- If the resting heart rate is not used to compute the training heart rate, it is possible that the training heart rate will be actually lower than the resting heart rate for some patients.

3. **The Borg Scale or RPE (Rating of Perceived Exertion) (11-14 on the 15-point scale or 3-5 on the 10-point scale).** The RPE scales developed by Swedish psychologist, Gunnar Borg, enable individuals to monitor the intensity level of an exercise bout by rating how hard they perceive themselves to be exercising (refer to Table 14-1).

Caution should be used if applying RPE levels with patients just beginning an exercise program, especially if the individuals have not engaged in exercise training for a significant period of time. The RPE scale is appropriate for use after patients have exercised for some time and if they change the dosage of a beta blocker or calcium channel blocker medication. While the change in dosage will affect their heart rate response, it will not affect their interpretation of the RPE scale.

Both the Heart Rate Reserve and the RPE scale should be explained to the patient. Patients can be safely monitored in an outpatient program through either self monitoring of their heart rate or through the use of a HR monitoring technique which employs a tool specifically designed to measure HR (e.g., PhysioControl Lifepak paddles).

Duration (30 ≥ minutes/day)

The duration of an activity, which should be at least 30 minutes, applies directly to the stimulus phase of the program and is exclusive of the time spent in warm-up and cool-down. This time period can be used intermittently (especially by extremely deconditioned individuals, or those just beginning an exercise program) or split up among two or three sessions in a single day.

Duration is best quantified in terms of time, as opposed to distance. The only appropriate method for equating training routines using different activities is to compare intensity as a work rate and duration as time. Distance will not equate among different activities. Jogging three miles, for example, does not compare with swimming three miles or cycling three miles. Training at a given heart rate for a given period of time will produce approximately the same cardiovascular training stimulus, even if you're performing a different type of aerobic activity.

Frequency (3 or 4 days/week)

The frequency of training defines how many times or days per week that a given work bout should be performed. An important principle of frequency that should be understood involves the necessity for alternating easy and hard training days/sessions. This guideline suggests that an individual should not engage in "hard" training sessions for two or more consecutive days. A hard training session may be defined as one involving either high intensity or long duration. It should also be understood that "easy" and "hard" are relative terms and must be judged according to the individual. An "easy" day for a *beginning* or *low functional capacity* patient might be considered to be a day of light or no exercise, or if weight bearing exercise is the usual training, a session using a non-weight bearing exercise.

While research has found that two days per week of exercise training are required to *maintain* functional capacity, three days and possibly four days of training per week are probably needed to *improve* functional capacity. Depending on whether your exercise program is designed for maintenance or improvement, the aforementioned are the *optimal* training frequencies. Five to seven days per week can be used by patients if they are engaging in very low intensity and very low duration sessions, or by patients who have very high functional capacity and have been training for a long period of time. In the latter case, caution must be observed because of the high incidence of orthopaedic injuries that often occurs in individuals who exercise on a high frequency basis.

STARTING LEVEL (1 - 6 WEEKS)

Setting the initial work bout in an exercise program is a very important part of the exercise prescription. If the first training session that a patient performs is too difficult, the experience can be very discouraging and even dangerous. If the first session is too easy, the patient might not perceive any benefit from the program. As a result, establishing a work load that is between these two extremes is the ideal approach. Because setting a work load is always an "educated guess," it is better to err on the side of conservatism. As a basic rule of thumb, it is better to establish an exercise level that will allow a patient to succeed, rather than fail. This is where the "art" of exercise prescription comes in. The starting level should last from one to six weeks. How to set the initial level and how long it should last depends on a number of factors, including: age, exercise history, body weight, and the functional capacity of the patient. The basic rule is that the older, the less active, the heavier, and the more unfit the individual, the lower the starting level. Probably the most important fact to know about patients is how much exercise they have been doing before starting in your program. This information enables you to set an exercise level that is consistent with what the patient has already been doing. The following discussion relates how the training principles can be manipulated to set a proper starting level.

- *Type of Activity*. Consider using weight bearing activities with beginning patients, especially if the patient is a larger than normal individual (large because of fat tissue or muscle tissue). Weight bearing activities (e.g., running, walking) generally cause more stress on the joints and muscles than non-weight bearing activities.*

---

* Editors' Note: The StairMaster® 4000PT® and the StairMaster® 4000CT® offer a means for providing weight-bearing exercise with little or no orthopaedic stress.

- *Intensity.* Do not be afraid of using lower than the normal or traditional levels of intensity (50%) to start an exercise program for a patient. Remember that the training stimulus depends on the overload principle, and a 20% intensity may represent an overload for some patients.

- *Duration.* Consider using intermittent programs of walking/rest for beginning patients. If your client has the flexibility to exercise at different times of the day, another good plan is to split up work bouts into two or three sessions a day. For example, a 30-minute work bout can be split into a 15-minute session in the morning and a 15-minute session in the afternoon. Or a 30-minute work bout can be split into a 10-minute session in the morning, a 10-minute session at noon, and a 10-minute session in the late afternoon.

- *Frequency.* Remember the principle of alternating easy and hard training days. (Note: An easy day for a beginner may mean a day off.)

SLOW PROGRESSION (UP TO 6 MONTHS)

A sensible progression of the exercise prescription should be controlled by the training levels that move a patient from the starting level to the maintenance level. A safe rate of progression incorporates small increases in work loads that are adopted in a time schedule that enables positive physiological adaptations to take place. The period of time necessary to develop desirable baseline (starting) levels of fitness can take up to six months, depending on the goals of the individual. How fast a patient progresses should generally adhere to the same guidelines for setting the starting level, with the critical issue being how long to spend at each level. The general rule is that your body takes two weeks of training to adapt to a new work load. An example of a walking progression for a cardiac patient is presented in Table 14-3. The number of sessions required at each level can be adjusted both initially and throughout the training regimen according to the health/fitness status of, and the relative rate of adaptation by, the patient.

Table 14-3. Sample Walking Progression Program.

NAME_____ DATE STARTED _____

# of Sessions	Walking Routine	Dates
_____	Walk 5 min./Rest 3-5 min. (Repeat x 2)	_____
_____	Walk 5 min./Rest 3-5 min. (Repeat x 3)	_____
_____	Walk 5 min./Rest 3-5 min. (Repeat x 4)	_____
_____	Walk 10 min./Rest 3-5 min. (Repeat x 2)	_____
_____	Walk 10 min./Rest 3-5 min. (Repeat x 3)	_____
_____	Walk 15 min./Rest 3-5 min. (Repeat x 2)	_____
_____	Walk 20 min./Rest 3-5 min./Walk 15 min.	_____
_____	Walk 25 min./Rest 3-5 min./Walk 10 min.	_____
_____	Walk 30 min./Rest 3-5 min./Walk 5 min.	_____
_____	Walk 35 min./Rest 3-5 min.	_____
_____	Walk 40 min. (Maintenance)	_____

Warm-up (10 - 15 minutes)

The work bout or stimulus phase should be preceded by an adequate *warm-up* session. The purpose of the warm-up is to ensure that the cardiovascular system is prepared to function safely at an elevated level and that the joints and muscles are prepared for the exercise bout without undue risk of injury. Accordingly, a warm-up session should consist of two parts.

The first part of the warm-up period should raise your body core temperature. The best way to accomplish this is with the same activity that is going to be used in the stimulus phase, but performed at a lower level of intensity. Research has shown that even normal, healthy cardiovascular systems can demonstrate ischemic responses in reaction to abrupt and extreme increases in exercise intensity. This issue becomes an even more important safety factor when training cardiac patients. This part should last from five to ten minutes. The second part of the warm-up phase should include some very gentle range of motion activities such as light, static stretching. Your body temperature needs to be elevated in order to allow for safer and more productive stretching. The older the individual is and the earlier in the day the activities are being performed, the more time should be devoted to the warm-up and stretching.

Cool-down (10 - 25 minutes)

A *cool-down* session should follow the *stimulus* phase of the exercise bout. A cool-down phase should consist of the same two parts as the warm-up period. Similar to the warm-up, the first part of a cool-down should involve approximately five to ten minutes of the same aerobic activity performed at a lower level of intensity. This approach to cooling down is designed to permit your cardiovascular system to return to its resting functional status without compromising adequate circulation to your vital organs (heart and brain). The second part of a cool-down session involves performing additional repetitions of range of motion activities. Such exercise has several potential benefits. For example, some evidence exists to support the contention that post-activity stretching decreases the muscle soreness that is common in individuals who are starting an exercise program. Furthermore, because the muscles and joints are sufficiently warmed, it is also an ideal time to utilize a more vigorous stretching routine in order to train for increasing flexibility.

RESISTANCE TRAINING

The activities of everyday life require that you perform resistance exercises. For example, whenever you move your body or an object through space, you are doing a resistance exercise. Traditionally, heavy resistance exercise was perceived by members of the exercise science and medical communities to be more of a "strain" than a training stimulus on the cardiovascular system. As a result, for a number of years, resistance work was seldom prescribed for cardiac patients. In recent years, however, sufficient research has demonstrated conclusively that training the skeletal muscles to perform resistance exercise can, in fact, reduce the "strain" on the cardiovascular system.

The American College of Sports Medicine has adopted a position in support of the value of sound resistance training for CAD patients. The ACSM (1991) guidelines suggest that the following exclusion criteria for resistance training be used to identify individuals for whom resistance training would not be appropriate:

• Abnormal hemodynamic responses or ischemic changes on the electrocardiogram during graded exercise.
• Poor left ventricular function.
• Peak exercise capacity < 6 METs.
• Uncontrolled hypertension or dysrhythmias.

Resistance training to develop muscular fitness should adhere to the same basic training principles as for cardiovascular fitness. The application of these principles to resistance activities is different, however, than for aerobic activities.

Intensity. The intensity of a resistance activity is measured by the resistance against which the muscle must move. Heavy resistances (⁻ 60% of the maximum amount of weight that can be lifted one time) should be avoided by cardiac patients.

Duration. The duration of a resistance activity is measured by the number of times that the object is lifted. This number is referred to as the repetitions (REPs) performed. As with aerobic activity, there is an inverse relationship between intensity (weight) and duration (repetitions). The traditional DeLorme theory of resistance training theorizes that the higher the weight and the lower the repetitions, the more the training will increase muscular strength. By the same token, the lower the weight and the higher the repetitions, the more the training will increase muscular endurance.* The most commonly followed guideline for cardiac patients is to perform 10 to 15 REPs. Two or three sets (i.e., groups of repetitions of an exercise movement performed consecutively, without rest, until a given number, or momentary exhaustion, is reached) of each routine are also normally recommended.

Frequency. If more intense strength training (using heavier weights) is being performed, then the training should be done only every second or third day. At lower levels of relative resistance, the issue of adequate time to recover is not as critical.

Starting level. A critical element in developing a safe, sensible resistance training program for cardiac patients involves determining what initial level of resistance should be used for each exercise. Initial weights should not be more

---

* Editors' Note: The ACSM (1991) recommends that an effective protocol for developing either muscular strength or muscular endurance is to perform a single set of 8-12 repetitions of each exercise.

than 40 to 50% of the one-repetition maximal level (1-RM) of a patient. While 1-RM *testing* has been shown to be a relatively safe technique for most CAD patients, a more useful and prudent way is the "Titration" method. This method involves having patients start with 10 REPs with a lighter more comfortable weight, and then progressing to 15 REPs each training session. At their next workout, they raise the resistance level for a specific exercise to the next highest weight for 10 REPs of an initial set. During the session, they again progress to being able to perform one set of 15 REPs. This process continues until the patient identifies the level of resistance that is appropriate to the individual's training objectives.

Slow progression. The individual can progress to the next highest level of resistance for a particular exercise when 15 REPs of a weight can be performed for two or three sets without significant strain. The initial number of repetitions that should be performed at the new level of resistance is usually ten. If the individual can't perform at least ten, the amount of increase was too high or undertaken too soon.

Safety is the most crucial issue attendant to resistance training for cardiac patients. Specific guidelines for the safe and effective application of resistance training for cardiac patients have been developed by the American Association of Cardiovascular and Pulmonary Rehabilitation (1991), including the following:

- To prevent soreness and injury, initially choose a weight that will allow an individual to comfortably perform 10 to 12 REPs of an exercise. In general, this level of resistance will correspond to a level which is approximately 40 to 60 percent of the maximum weight load that can be lifted in one REP. High-risk adults and low-risk cardiac patients should select an initial weight load that can be lifted for 12 to 15 REPs.
- Generally, two to three sets of each exercise are recommended.
- Don't strain! Ratings of perceived exertion (6-20 scale) should not exceed "fairly light" (11) to "somewhat hard" (13) during lifting.
- Avoid breath holding. Breathe normally at all times.
- Increase the amount of resistance lifted by 2.5 to 10 pounds when 10 to 12 repetitions can be comfortably accomplished; for high-risk adults and cardiac patients, the weight should be increased only after the individual can easily manage 12 to 15 repetitions of an exercise.
- Raise the weight to a count of two, and lower the weight gradually to a count of four; emphasize complete extension of the limbs when lifting.
- Include exercises for all of the major muscle groups of the body.
- Organize the resistance training program so that muscles are generally exercised in a largest-to-smallest order two to three times per week.
- Avoid excessive hand gripping when possible, since this may evoke an excessive blood pressure response to lifting.
- Stop exercising in the event of any contraindicative warning signs or symptoms, especially dizziness, abnormal heart rhythm, unusual shortness of breath, and/or chest pain.
- Don't rest for an extended period of time between either the exercises or the sets of exercises.

• Whenever possible, all patients should be monitored and their responses recorded (heart rate, symptoms, etc.) to the resistance exercise following each set. ❏

BIBLIOGRAPHY •

1. American Association of Cardiovascular and Pulmonary Rehabilitation. *Guidelines for Cardiac Rehabilitation Programs*. Champaign, IL: Human Kinetics Publishers, 1991.
2. American College of Sports Medicine. *Guidelines For Exercise Testing and Prescription*, 4th Ed. Philadelphia, PA: Lea & Febiger, 1991.
3. Brannon, F.J., Geyer, M.J., Foley, M.W. *Cardiac Rehabilitation*. Philadelphia, PA: F. A. Davis Company, 1988.
4. Fardy, P.S., Yanowitz, F.G., Wilson, P.K. *Cardiac Rehabilitation, Adult Fitness, and Exercise Testing*, 2nd Ed. Philadelphia, PA: Lea & Febiger, 1988.
5. Gordon, N.F., Gibbons, L.W. *The Cooper Clinic Cardiac Rehabilitation Program*. New York, NY: Simon and Schuster, 1990.
6. Hall, L.K., Meyer, G.C. (Eds). *Cardiac Rehabilitation: Exercise testing and prescription*, Vol. II. Champaign, IL: Human Kinetics Publishers, 1988.
7. Hall, L.K., Meyer, G.C., Hellerstein, H.K. (Eds). *Cardiac Rehabilitation: Exercise testing and prescription*. Champaign, IL: Human Kinetics Publishers, 1984.
8. McKelvie, R.S., McCartney, N. "Weightlifting training in cardiac patients: Considerations." *Sports Med* 10(6):355-364, 1990.
9. Wilson, P. K. "Cardiac rehabilitation: Then and now." *Phys Sportsmed* 16(9):75-84, 1988.

CHAPTER 15

• •

EXERCISE
AND AGING

by

Walter M. Bortz, II, M.D., Cedric X. Bryant, Ph.D.,
James A. Peterson, Ph.D., and Dennis L. Colacino, Ph.D.

• • •

*T*he emergence of aging as a legitimate area of scientific inquiry has led to immense gains in the body of knowledge concerning the biological markers of life. The recognition that life is not a set of instantaneous events each judged at a specific moment in time, but rather a continuous series of interconnecting and developmental processes is an insight that has tremendous implications. The resulting explosion in knowledge is a direct byproduct of demographic change. When there were few people in the world who survived past age 60, little urgency existed to inquire as to the basic dynamics of aging. Now with hundreds of millions reaching and, in many cases, surpassing their seventh decade of life, the questions inherent to aging become pressingly significant.

BIOMARKERS OF AGING

Until the current era, the attempts to analyze the process of aging involved virtually no rigor. As a result, almost all the material in the older textbooks on aging is inaccurate—a byproduct of an inadvertent admixture of time-driven and non time-driven events which occur in older persons. Many of the supposed central decrements seen in old people, such as decreased metabolic rate, decreased lean body mass, and increased body fat, are artifacts, which are not due to aging, but to disuse. In simple terms, the supposed biomarkers of aging aren't.

Tuberculosis used to be considered a biomarker of aging since it was seen so frequently in old people. More recently arteriosclerosis was also felt to be a direct consequence of aging. The French pathologist Cazalis observed, "A man is as old as his arteries." Arteriosclerosis, however, is not an inevitable byproduct of aging for any number of reasons. First, arteriosclerosis sometimes afflicts young people. For example, many of our soldiers killed in Korea and Vietnam already had cholesterol in their arteries. Second, some old people don't get it; and third, it has been shown to be reversible, which should not be the case if the condition were truly due to the passage of time.

In contemporary society, perhaps the major act of mislabeling, as it relates to the process of aging, is Alzheimer's disease, which, it is important to keep in mind, is a disease—not a biomarker of aging. This confusion leads to several distorted expectations that aging inevitably brings consecutive decline, which is not the case. Yet, the widespread impression that Alzheimer's is somehow an irreversible part of growing older gives credence to the starkly negative image of aging held by many.

Overall ignorance about the human aging process has been so pervasive that even accurate information about the extent of the human life span has only recently become common knowledge in the medical and scientific communities. Previously, estimations of the human life span were obscured by extravagant reports of longevity in many ancient writings, and by the more common shortfall of life span caused by the precocious deaths of virtually everyone. It is certainly true that while there have always been old people, only a very few of such individuals existed until now. Similarly, in the wild, few animals grow old, due to nutritional scarcity, accident, and predation.

The times are changing, however. It is estimated that more people over the age of 65 are alive in the world today than in all previously recorded history. And this trend is just getting started. The world will never be young again. Life in a very real sense is a self-fulfilling prophecy. When all of your ancestors were dead by the age of 50, it was hard to project an old age for yourself.

LIFE SPAN

It is now generally acknowledged that the maximum human life span is 120 years, a time period which encompasses slightly more than one million hours. Considerable evidence exists to support this figure. This projection does not, of course, mean that everyone will or can live to 120, rather this estimate is the right-sided extreme of a bell-shaped curve. Manton has developed data which indicate that based on current health knowledge, if individuals were inclined to adopt a lifestyle of appropriate design, their mean life expectancy would be 100 years. A century of life is the fundamental goal for which people should strive. Such aspiration does not depend on technological advance or genetic improvement. In reality, it simply requires that people react intelligently to what is already known.

Having established for the first time in human history the natural duration of the human life is a momentous accomplishment. Such an act allows for all sorts of new analytic efforts in many domains—educational, political, psychological, financial, and personal. More importantly, it reinforces the fact that new planning, new structures, and new priorities are called for to adequately deal with the "new" realities of the process of aging.

A New Model for Medicine *

Among the essential tasks which must be undertaken as a result of the insights gained concerning human aging is a reformulation of the framework of medical science. Until now medical education has been structured along classical lines: anatomy, physiology, bacteriology, and then later on the clinical sciences. Medical textbooks and journals similarly reflect fractionated views of the whole of the human condition. The entire realm of specialization has been created by an apparent desire to know more about less and less. Such a dissection of the human life to its smallest parts has the inevitable result of the diminishment of the role of time in the greater order of things. Medical research focuses on instantaneous events and conditions. Regrettably, the obtaining of grant support does not deal gently with proposals which require decades to answer.

Pediatrics was the first domain of medicine which recognized a time dimension in biologic events. In the medical community, appropriate attention was drawn to the conditions found in children who were subsequently recognized as not being merely little adults, but rather as individuals with unique characteristics. Because pediatrics involves several inherent and unique processes of development, time eventually became an integral factor in the framework of pediatric practice. Adult medicine, on the other hand, has been dominated by the Disease Model. In this approach, pathology is characterized by episodic adverse encounters between some environmental agent and the host patient with the resultant outcome of illness. Medicine's appropriate response to each challenge is to identify the offending agents and their consequences, and somehow drug them or cut them out. Antibiotics and modern surgery are the logical and significant byproducts of adhering to the Disease Model. The participation of time in the Disease Model, however, is undeveloped. Most illness is conceived of as a time and situation insensitive event, for which a proximate cure exists. For practitioners of this approach, fee-for-service payment was the appropriate economic structure for such encounters. While such a model may offer a limited (but relatively effective) way of dealing with most infections and injuries and some malignancies, such an approach to medicine is wholly inadequate for preventing problems. We don't cure the conditions which afflict us today. We don't cure heart attacks, strokes, emphysema, diabetes, arthritis. We palliate. We treat symptoms, but cure is not possible. In short, Humpty Dumpty cannot be made whole again . . . under the Disease Model scheme.

Recognizing the serious shortcomings of the Disease Model leads to the development of a new model for considering aging which emphasizes two features, which previously had largely been overlooked—functionality and preven-

---

* Editors' note: Readers wishing to obtain more detailed information regarding Dr. Bortz' visionary concept of "the new model for medicine" should contact Dr. Bortz directly (refer to page vi).

tion. As people live longer and, in the process, develop chronic conditions, it becomes clear that the length of life is only part of the story. Quality of life is of at least as great a significance. Quality adjusted life years (QALYs) are an attempt to recognize that not all life is of equal value. Obviously, a lifetime spent in pain, crippled, or otherwise dysfunctional has a lower intrinsic value than a lifetime of high vitality. Katz et al. coined the term "active life expectancy," in which a statistical approach was developed in an attempt to determine the quality of future life. An integral part of Katz's approach was the identification of the activities of daily living (ADLs)

ACTIVITIES OF DAILY LIVING (ADL)
- Feeding
- Transferring
- Continency
- Dressing
- Toileting
- Bathing

and instrumental activities of daily living (IADLs).

INSTRUMENTAL ACTIVITIES OF DAILY LIVING (IADL)
- Transport
- Housework
- Shopping
- Finance
- Cooking

which were both measurable and quantifiable factors purported by Katz to reflect an individual's level of functionality, particularly in late life. Implicit in Katz's efforts is the concept that medical science should be redirecting its efforts from the mere preservation of life, no matter what its quality, to the extension of an active, fully functional, life. Further work in this area involves outcomes technology, as described initially by Stewart and Ware. This approach to dealing with life addresses not only the functionality of life, but also the subjective participation of the patient in his or her illness pattern.

The second implication of the New Model for Medicine is an emphasis on the prevention of illness. Such a switch from curing disease to promoting health presents a considerable change in focus for the medical community. The intimate participation of time in this reconceptualization is paramount. Health behaviors become not just a dry subject, often quite boring to medical students, but the very essence of medical science. McGinnis, Assistant Secretary of Health, estimates that 60%-70% of prescriptions and visits to doctors' offices, hospitals, and morgues are resultants of misapplied behavior, which over time yields adverse survival conditions. Hospital admissions are highly age-dependent. Fuchs estimates that people over 65 consume 40% of the health care dollar, a figure which will only go higher as America ages further. At this rate, most of medicine will soon be geriatrics.

The new model of medicine emphasizing that fact includes geriatrics in not only all of the other domains of medicine, but also, in the absolutely critical dimension of time. Such a recognition of time in the greater scheme of things brings medicine more in line with the physical sciences, which have had their own lack of appreciation for the role of time until recently. Common sense dictates that it is impossible to have any adequate sense of the whole without knowing what the last part of the particular item looks like. A ball game, a play, or a novel, for example, would all lack any sense of their course if interrupted part way through. So, too, it is with the human life. When we are able, as we now are for the first time, to know what the last of life is all about (relatively uncontaminated by other elements), then, and only then, can a scheme be formulated for medical sciences that makes sense. Such a scheme must have not only practical treatment and prevention strategies inherent in it, but also have derivative social and political implications to support it.

EFFECTS OF TIME

The cardiovascular system undergoes several changes as a person ages. These changes, coupled with alterations occurring in both the pulmonary and muscular systems, are responsible for a steady decline in maximal oxygen uptake ($\dot{V}O_{2\,max}$) as a person ages (refer to Figure 15-1). Some of the more prominent changes which occur include:

- A decrease in cardiac muscle size and heart volume, which decreases the heart's ability to pump blood.
- A decrease in the sympathetic nerve activity to the heart which results in a lower attainable maximal heart rate and a reduced strength of heart contraction.
- A decrease in the elasticity of the major blood vessels which results in elevated blood pressure (at rest and during activity).

Aging also produces some major changes in the pulmonary system. A decline in the structural integrity of the alveoli (the functional unit of the lung) reduces the surface area for gas exchange and thereby limits the diffusion capacity for oxygen to the blood. The elasticity of lung tissue and the strength of respiratory muscles decrease and rib cage stiffness increases with aging. The combined effect is an increase in the energy cost of breathing.

The musculoskeletal system undergoes numerous changes as individuals age. A progressive, steady decline in muscle mass and strength (especially of the lower extremities) occurs with age, leading to deficiencies in gait and balance, loss of functional mobility, increased risk of falling and ultimately a loss of independence. Muscle mitochondrial and enzymatic changes, which reduce muscle respiratory capacity (the muscle's ability to extract oxygen from the blood), occur as a result of aging. Aging is associated with a decrease in bone mineral content and mass (this occurs in both sexes), increasing the older person's risk for osteoporosis and bone fractures. With age, increased stiffness of connective tissue results in a loss of joint flexibility and mobility.

The aforementioned is but a brief overview of some of the various physiologic changes that occur with aging. While the fact that most bodily systems experience some form of decline in functioning presents a somewhat dismal picture, there is good news. A significant portion (some estimates have been as high as 50%) of the physiologic decline typically seen with aging can be attributed to disuse atrophy resulting from physical inactivity. In the words of Hippocrates, the father of medicine, "All parts of the body which have function, if used in moderation and exercised in labors in which each is accustomed, become thereby healthy, well developed, and age more slowly; but if unused and left idle, they become liable to disease, defective in growth, and age quickly."

Figure 15-1. Aging is accompanied by a decrease in cardiorespiratory and musculosketetal function. Many of these changes also occur during the transition from a trained to an untrained state. *Modified from Nieman, D.C. (1990).*

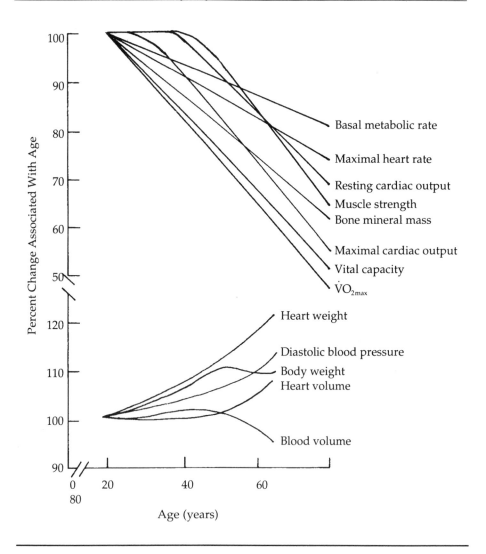

EXERCISE AND AGING

• • •

Effects of Exercise

A critical question concerning the aging process involves whether exercise can slow down the biological changes that occur over the course of an individual's lifetime. The answer appears to be a resounding "yes," although the extent to which exercising on a regular basis can affect the response of certain bodily systems to aging is generally unknown. At the least, a physically active lifestyle can positively affect age-associated declines that in large part may be attributed to the fact that most people become less active as they age.

Cardiorespiratory Adaptations

Numerous investigative efforts have shown that elderly individuals who exercise can achieve a demonstrable cardiorespiratory training effect. For example, even though $\dot{V}O_{2\,max}$ declines in everyone as we get older, physically active individuals are able to slow their average rate of decline in $\dot{V}O_{2\,max}$ to a level approximately half that of their sedentary counterparts. This means that an active 65-year-old person can be as aerobically fit as a 45-year-old sedentary person. In addition, older individuals who remain physically active do not experience the typical rise in blood pressure that occurs with aging.

Musculoskeletal Adaptations

Several recent studies support the belief that strength training can forestall the rate of deterioration of the musculoskeletal system in older persons. In these studies, individuals who engaged in a resistance training program maintained their strength. In fact, strength levels actually increased dramatically. In comparison, inactive individuals typically show a 20-30 percent loss in strength by age 65. Participants in the experimental training in these studies also incurred an increase in muscle mass, in contrast to the decrease in their inactive counterparts that traditionally occurs. Finally, proper strength training has been documented to maintain or increase joint flexibility, since it involves having an individual exercise through a full range of motion.

Body Composition Adaptations

Exercise can reduce the accumulation of body fat that accompanies aging and can slow, if not reverse, the substantial loss of fat-free mass that usually goes hand-in-hand with the increase in body fat. Older people can maintain the level of body fat they had in their youth if they remain consistently physically active and maintain an appropriate diet throughout their lives. Researchers suggest that proper strength training can attenuate the loss of lean muscle mass levels that often accompanies aging.

Lifestyle Changes

Exercise on a regular basis can have a positive effect on the overall quality of life in older adults in many ways, including:

- Regular exercise can provide older individuals with the functional capacity (attendant to having minimal levels of fitness in each of the primary components of physical fitness) necessary to perform basic living tasks, such as shopping, ambulation, personal care, and cooking meals.
- Physical activity can help an older person adapt to the changing social roles that sometimes accompany advancing age. For example, an activity program may replace work in the life of the individual.
- Social interaction can be promoted through exercise programs. Physical activity can help in adjusting to a traumatic event—e.g., retirement, the death of a loved one—by providing an avenue for social interaction and combating feelings of depression.
- Regular exercise can assist individuals in adjusting to retirement. Exercise, for example, can provide a relatively inexpensive activity for those on a reduced income. In addition, maintaining physical fitness enables older persons to remain independent, thereby incurring fewer of the costs for assistance that arise if they need home management and personal care.
- Old age frequently requires that older people must scale down their housing or move into an apartment or retirement community. Since many retirement communities do not take people who are physically dependent, maintaining physical fitness enables individuals to have more diverse options in their possible physical living arrangements. In several multi-level retirement communities, for example, the average cost for assisted living (e.g., help in making the bed, meals, home finances) is estimated to be more than double the monthly average cost required to live independently.

DEVELOPING AN EXERCISE PROGRAM

The first step is to ensure that the individual is medically safe to exercise. This involves seeing a physician and undergoing a physical examination and evaluation before an exercise program is initiated. The extent of the evaluation depends on the individual's age and health status. Men over age 40, women over age 50, and all individuals at high risk (e.g., having one or more of the following risk factors—smoking, hypertension, high blood cholesterol, obesity, stress, family history of medical problems, diabetes) are strongly encouraged to undergo a physician-supervised, graded exercise test.

The next step is to develop a sound exercise program based on scientifically documented information. A sound exercise prescription enables an individual to achieve as much as possible (effectiveness), as quickly as possible (efficiency), and most importantly, without undue risk of injury. If an exercise regimen is to be relatively risk-free for older individuals, it must be tailored to their age, gender, and current level of fitness.

A safety-oriented exercise program also involves starting at a level of intensity appropriate for the individual and then progressing gradually. The temptation to do too much too soon should be avoided. Moderation is essential. A major cause of musculoskeletal injuries is overuse—placing demands on the individual's body that the body simply is not capable of handling. A sound exercise program always includes provisions for stretching the major joints of the body before and after exercising. It also ensures that the individual get proper rest along with exercise. Rest enables individuals to recover from the demands of exercise placed on their bodies.

The final step is for individuals to listen to their bodies. They must respond accordingly to specific warning signals of exertional intolerance. These warning signs are grouped into three general categories according to their severity.

Category I: If individuals experience any of the following symptoms, they should stop exercising immediately and consult a physician before resuming exercise:

- Abnormal heart rhythm (irregular pulse; fluttering, pumping or palpitations in the chest or throat; a sudden burst of rapid heart beats or a very sudden slowing of the pulse).
- Pain or pressure in the arm or throat or in the middle of the chest (either during or after exercising).
- Acute heat or overuse-related signals (dizziness; light-headedness; sudden loss of coordination; mental disorientation; profuse sweating; glassy stare; unnatural pallor; blueness; fainting).

Category II: If an individual experiences any of the following symptoms and the suggested (listed) remedy doesn't work for the individual, the person should see a physician before exercising again:

- Persistent rapid heart rate (remedy—keep the heart rate at the lower end of the individual's aerobic training zone for several minutes at the start of the exercise session and then increase it very slowly as the individual continues to exercise).
- Flare-up of musculoskeletal conditions, such as osteoarthritis (remedy—stop exercising until the condition subsides; individuals should take their normal medicine for their condition).

Category III: The following warning signs can usually be handled without consulting a physician:

- Vomiting or nausea after exercising (remedy—reduce the intensity level of the present and future exercise bouts; take a more gradual cooling-down period after exercising).
- Extreme breathlessness that lasts more than ten minutes after the individual has stopped exercising (remedy—individuals should never exercise to the point where they're too breathless to talk while they're exercising).
- Prolonged fatigue or insomnia (remedy—exercise at the lower end

of the aerobic training zone for the next several exercise bouts, and then begin to gradually increase the exercise intensity level).

- Side-stitch (remedy—sit, lean forward, and attempt to push the abdominal organs against the diaphragm).

PRESCRIBING AEROBIC EXERCISE

The general principles of exercise prescription (refer to chapter 13) apply to individuals of all ages. However, the wide range of health and fitness levels observed among older adults make prescribing exercise for them more difficult. Great care must be taken in establishing the type, intensity, duration, and frequency of exercise.

TYPE

Selecting a mode of exercise for developing aerobic fitness can involve several factors. For most older persons (particularly those who have been sedentary), the exercise modality should be one that does not impose significant orthopaedic stress on the aged musculoskeletal system. Research has also shown that the activity should be something that is accessible, convenient, and enjoyable to the participant—all factors directly related to exercise adherence. Among the more popular methods of exercising that older adults use to develop aerobic fitness are the following:

Walking. Walking is an excellent form of exercise for young and old alike. It is beneficial for older adults for several reasons: it doesn't require learning a new skill; it can be done almost anywhere, indoors or outdoors; it doesn't require special clothing or equipment, except for a good pair of walking shoes; and, finally, if performed on a treadmill, it can be an activity in which preselected physiological and performance measures can be monitored by the person or an exercise specialist. The primary disadvantage of walking is the fact that a certain amount of orthopaedic stress is imposed on the skeletal joints of the user.

Stair Climbing. Recently, researchers at the University of Florida have shown that not only do older adults incur substantial improvement in both cardiorespiratory endurance and lower extremity musculoskeletal fitness as a result of exercising on independent step-action stair climbing machines, they also appear to greatly enjoy this form of exercise. Unlike the traditional forms of weight-bearing activities (e.g., walking, running, exercising on a treadmill), considerable evidence suggests that exercising on an independent step-action stair climbing machine does not impose injurious orthopaedic stress on the joints. Given the fact that lower-body musculoskeletal fitness is critical to the maintenance of functional mobility in the elderly, an orthopaedically safe weight-bearing exercise modality, such as an independent step-action stair climbing machine, can offer invaluable benefits to the exerciser. The primary downside of stair climbing is that an orthopaedically safe independent step-action stair climbing machine is relatively expensive.

Water Exercise. Swimming and water aerobic exercise (aquatic) classes offer certain advantages for older adults. The benefit most frequently cited is the fact that water-based activities have lower musculoskeletal injury rates and greater joint range of motion than most traditional weight-bearing activities. In addition, exercising in water offers the opportunity to engage in both upper and lower body muscular resistance exercise. The most obvious downside of water-based activities involves the need for access to a pool and the fact that an individual may not feel comfortable around water. Also, aquatic exercise classes do not promote positive bone adaptations since water-based activities are not weight bearing.

Stationary Cycling. Stationary cycling is a particularly safe modality for older adults. The weather is not a factor indoors. No substantial concern exists concerning the possibility of an older adult falling off the cycle. If adapting to the seat is a problem, equipping the cycle with an extra large seat tends to minimize the discomfort for people unaccustomed to a bicycle seat. If excessive fatigue in the user's thigh muscles is a problem (given the role of the quadriceps in exercise cycling), gradually increasing the exercise duration while reducing or holding intensity (i.e., pedal resistance) constant may minimize the problem of using a stationary cycle that employs wind resistance (e.g., the StairMaster® Spinnaker™ 3000 CE™ cycle ergometer). Stationary cycling has at least two significant shortcomings. First, an exercise cycle is needed. A quality exercise cycle can either be purchased or be part of the equipment offering of a health-fitness facility. Either option may be relatively expensive. Second, and more importantly, as a non-weight bearing activity, exercise cycling does not offer the beneficial effects on bone mass that weight-bearing activity does. The aerobic portion of the cycling exercise session may be broken into 10-minute segments and interspersed with 10-minute bouts of other forms of aerobic exercise, such as walking, simulated stair climbing, etc.

Aerobic Dance. Aerobic dance has several significant advantages and disadvantages for the older population. A list of the advantages includes: aerobic dance sessions are structured, yet social, events; aerobic dance can improve body awareness and can approximate everyday motions such as bending and reaching; aerobic dance exercise provides an opportunity to work on posture, gait and balance; and, finally, aerobic dance enables exercises involving coordination and flexibility to be integrated effectively with aerobic fitness activities. Among the more important possible disadvantages of this form of exercise are the following: an aerobic dance class must be comprised of persons with similar capabilities (to ensure safety); the risk of acute or chronic injuries is high; and the fitness benefits from class to class are not as predictable as from more structured forms of aerobic exercise (e.g., cycling, stair climbing, etc.) Finally, aerobic dance is more dependent than other forms of aerobic exercise on the skills of the exercise leader for direction, safety, motivation, and ultimate effectiveness.

INTENSITY

Perhaps the most important and, at the same time, potentially the most problematic training variable is exercise intensity. Exercise intensity must be sufficient to stress (overload) the cardiovascular, pulmonary, and musculoskeletal systems without overtasking them. In general, the intensity of exercise coincides with the training heart rate. Training heart rate (THR) is often determined by taking a straight percentage of age-predicted maximal heart rate (i.e., 220 minus age). This method of defining exercise intensity can, however, be very misleading in older individuals. High variability exists for maximal heart rates in persons over 55 years of age (maximal heart rates can range from as low as 100 bpm to as high as 190 bpm). Training heart rates calculated on the basis of age-predicted maximal heart rates can either underestimate or overestimate the exercise intensity. Thus, it is always better to use an accurate measurement of maximal heart rate (MHR) rather than age-predicted MHR.

The heart rate reserve method (Karvonen) is recommended for establishing THR in older individuals. Since MHR decreases and resting heart rate (RHR) increases with age, it would be possible to compute a THR that is lower than RHR, if the RHR is not used in the computation of the THR. The Karvonen method calculates the THR by using a percentage of the heart rate reserve as presented in chapter 11, (the difference between the maximum and resting heart rates).

The recommended level of exercise intensity for an older adult is 50-70% of maximal heart rate reserve (this also closely approximates a similar percentage of maximal oxygen uptake). Since many older persons suffer from a variety of medical conditions, a conservative approach to prescribing aerobic exercise is usually warranted. Individuals with a relatively low level of functional capacity should initially engage in aerobic exercise at an intensity range of 50-60% of maximal HRR, which can then be very gradually increased over a period of two to three months. For individuals with a normal level of functional capacity, an intensity range of 60-70 of maximal HRR is appropriate. When setting exercise intensity for older individuals, the general rule is "start low and go slow."

DURATION

Exercise duration and intensity go hand in hand. An increase in one often requires a decrease in the other. The prescription for duration is usually expressed in terms of time, distance, or calories. All three are interrelated. Most people prefer, however, to use time as their indicator of duration because of its comparative simplicity of use. Other than a watch or access to a clock, nothing is required except the ability to tell time.

The ACSM guideline (aimed at primarily healthy younger to middle-age adults) for duration recommends that an aerobic exercise workout take between 20 and 60 minutes. The goal of most older adults should be 20 to 30 minutes of sustained activity. Less than 20 minutes is often sufficient to provide for a significant training effect for many sedentary older people. During the initial stages of an exercise program, some older adults may have difficulty sustaining aerobic exercise for more than 10 minutes. For such individuals one viable option may be to perform the exercise in several 10-minute bouts throughout the day. If the exercise session is segmented, the individual should be encouraged to perform it at regularly scheduled times, so as to enhance compliance and adherence. For individuals with a low functional capacity (2-3 METs*), it may actually be preferable to schedule frequent 10-minute bouts of exercise throughout the day. Older persons who have a capacity of 3-5 METs may benefit from an exercise prescription involving two, ten-minute (at the minimum) bouts of aerobic sessions. To avoid injury and ensure safety, older individuals should raise the difficulty level of their workouts primarily through increases in exercise duration.

FREQUENCY

Researchers have found that an individual needs to exercise aerobically 3-5 days a week in order to achieve the intended training effect. Exercising less than twice a week has been found to produce little or no meaningful training response. By the same token, exercising more than five days a week results in little or no further improvement in an individual's maximum oxygen uptake level. In fact, the amount of positive change in a person's aerobic fitness level begins to plateau when the individual exercises more than three to four days per week. During the initial stages of weight-bearing aerobic exercise, exercising on alternate days is recommended to gradually give the individual's body an opportunity to adapt to the stresses being imposed upon it (thereby reducing the likelihood of an "overuse" injury). For persons who want to exercise aerobically on a daily basis, alternating between weight bearing (e.g., walking or stair climbing) and non-weight bearing (e.g., exercise cycling) is advised.

PRESCRIBING RESISTANCE TRAINING

The effects of resistance training and various strength training protocols have been relatively well-defined for younger populations. Recently published research findings suggest that muscular fitness (muscular strength and muscular endurance) offers considerable benefits to older adults. For example, it appears that strength training may enable elderly individuals (particularly women) to be able to perform their daily living tasks with greater ease, as well as leading to a heightened sense of self-confidence and self-worth. A certain level of muscular fitness is critical for individuals to retain their independence. Individuals obviously want and need to perform certain daily tasks for themselves. It is believed that strength training provides significant skeletal benefits for men and women of all ages. While the thought of "pumping up" to older adults might seem somewhat strange, it appears to be an inescapable fact that an appropriate level of muscular fitness is integral to ensuring that individuals are able to spend their latter years in a self-functioning, dignified manner.

Although the ability of older adults to realize significant strength gains has been documented, the specifics of resistance training protocols for older adults

---

* One MET is assumed to be equal to an oxygen uptake of 3.5 millimeters per kilogram of body weight per minute. It is a measure of energy output equal to the resting metabolic rate of an average individual.

have not been adequately addressed. For example, considerable research has shown that achieving a training effect for muscular fitness does not have to involve extended periods of time in the weight room, lifting massive amounts of free weights. On the contrary, calisthenics using body weight to stimulate an overload of the muscle, weighted and non-weighted stair climbing, and weight machines have all been found to produce substantial increases in muscular fitness.

Similar to aerobic fitness, the ACSM has developed recommendations concerning what constitutes an appropriate resistance training protocol. An ever-increasing number of experts are recommending that older adults participate in resistance training programs for the purposes of developing musculoskeletal fitness, improving body composition, and enhancing functional capacity.

INTENSITY

The ACSM recommends that, at the minimum, an individual should perform one set of 8 to 10 exercises that train the major muscle groups. Each set should involve 8 to 12 repetitions that elicit a perceived exertion rating of 12-13* (somewhat hard). The selection of exercises should ensure that all of the major muscle groups in the body are included in the training session. Depending on an individual's personal philosophy, additional sets could be performed. Recent research conducted at the University of Florida by Pollock et al. and previous investigations at the United States Military Academy suggest that additional sets may have limited value at best.

FREQUENCY

The ACSM recommends that resistance training be performed at least twice a week, with at least 48 hours of rest between workouts. Research indicates that as an individual becomes older, the need for sufficient time to recover from the resistance stress imposed upon the body increases.

DURATION

The ACSM suggests that resistance training sessions lasting longer than sixty minutes may have a detrimental effect on an individual's level of exercise adherence. Adherence to the guidelines of the ACSM would permit individuals to complete total body strength training sessions within 20-25 minutes.

Regardless of which specific protocol is adopted, several common sense guidelines pertaining to resistance training for older adults should be followed:

- Focus the major goal of the resistance training program on developing sufficient muscle fitness to enhance an individual's ability to live a physically independent lifestyle.

---

* Refer to Chapter 13 for more information regarding rating of perceived exertion.

- Have the first several resistance training sessions closely supervised and monitored by trained personnel who are sensitive to the special needs and capabilities of the elderly.
- Start out (the first eight weeks) with very minimal levels of resistance to allow for adaptations of the connective tissue elements.
- Teach the older participant the proper training techniques for all of the exercises to be used in the program.
- Instruct older participants to maintain their normal breathing patterns while exercising, since breath holding (i.e., performance of a Valsalva maneuver—see Appendix A) can induce excessive blood pressure elevations.
- As a training effect occurs, achieve an overload initially by increasing the number of repetitions, and then by increasing the absolute amount of resistance lifted.
- Never use a resistance that is so heavy that the exerciser cannot perform at least eight repetitions per set. Heavy resistances can be potentially dangerous and damaging to the skeletal and joint structures of an older individual.
- Stress that all exercises should be performed in a manner in which the speed is controlled. In order to prevent orthopaedic trauma to the joint structures, no ballistic (fast and jerky) movements should be allowed while exercising. Weights should be lifted and lowered in a slow, controlled manner.
- Perform the exercises in a range of motion that is within a "pain free arc" (i.e., the maximum range of motion which does not elicit pain or discomfort). As positive adaptations occur, individuals should gradually increase their exercise range of motion in order to improve their flexibility.
- Perform multi-joint exercises (as opposed to single-joint exercises) since they tend to help individuals develop functional muscular fitness.
- Given a choice, use machines to resistance train, as opposed to free weights. The primary advantages of machines are that they tend to require less skill to use, they protect the back by stabilizing the user's body position, and they allow the user to start with lower resistances, to increase by smaller increments (this is not true for all strength training machines), and to more easily control the exercise range of motion.
- Don't overtrain. Two strength training sessions per week are the minimum number required to produce positive physiological adaptations. Depending on the circumstances, more sessions may neither be desirable nor productive.
- Never permit arthritic participants to participate in strength training exercises during active periods of pain or inflammation, since exercise could exacerbate their condition.
- Engage in a year-round resistance training program on a regular basis, since it has been shown that the cessation of resistance training can result in a rapid significant loss of strength. When returning

from a lay-off, individuals should start with resistances that are equivalent to or less than 50% of the intensity at which they had been training before, and then gradually increase the resistance.

Prescribing Flexibility Exercises

An adequate range of motion in all of the joints of the body is important to maintaining an acceptable level of musculoskeletal function. Unfortunately, efforts to identify the most effective protocol for developing flexibility (defined as the ability of the muscle, tendon, and soft tissue to yield to stretch force—a factor which, in turn, determines how much motion a skeletal joint can actually achieve) have been somewhat limited, particularly in comparison to the other basic components of physical fitness. What is almost universally accepted, but not documented, is the fact that maintaining adequate levels of flexibility will enhance an individual's functional capabilities (e.g., bending and twisting) and reduce injury potential (e.g., risk of muscle strains and low back problems)— particularly for the aged. A well-rounded program of stretching has been shown to counteract the usual decline or improve flexibility in the elderly. Not surprisingly, it is critical that a sound stretching program be included as part of each exercise session for older adults.

Intensity

The ACSM recommends exercises involving a slow dynamic movement, followed by a static stretch that is sustained for 10 to 30 seconds. Exercises should be prescribed for every major joint (hip, back, shoulder, knee, upper trunk, and neck regions) in the body. Three to five repetitions of each exercise should be performed. The degree of stretch achieved should not be to the point of significant pain.

Frequency

The ACSM recommends that stretching exercises should be performed at least three times a week. In reality, stretching exercises should be included as an integral part of the warm-up and cool-down exercises that are performed prior to and at the conclusion of all workouts. Individuals can, however, choose to devote an entire exercise session to flexibility. This can be particularly appropriate for deconditioned older adults who are beginning an exercise program.

Duration

The stretching phase of an individual's exercise session should involve approximately 15 to 30 minutes collectively each workout. Several common sense guidelines pertaining to stretching by older adults should be followed:

- Always precede stretching exercises with some type of warm-up activity to increase heart rate and internal body temperature. It is safer and more productive to stretch a warm muscle.

- Stretch smoothly and never bounce. When individuals bounce while stretching, they cause the muscles to tighten to protect themselves— this actually inhibits effective muscle stretching. Moreover, ballistic (i.e., bouncing) movements can cause the very sort of muscle tears that stretching is designed to prevent.
- Do not stretch a joint beyond its range of motion. Tissue has a failure point and wide variations in range of motion exist between individuals.
- Gradually ease into a stretch, and hold it only as long as it feels comfortable. If individuals stretch to the point of feeling extreme pain, they increase their likelihood of being injured.

Balance Training

A great proportion, possibly up to 50% of older persons, report some difficulty with maintaining balance. Falls are the most evident byproduct. Poor balance is mostly multifactorial, involving visual, vestibular, peripheral neural, and muscular components. Increasing research is being devoted to the mechanisms behind poor balance and the countermeasures which can be used to offset them. Starting at approximately 70 years of age, individuals should be encouraged to include a balance training program into their regular exercise regimen. Several different types of exercise activities can be used to develop better balance. Perhaps the simplest technique to learn (the flamingo exercise) involves standing on one leg, then alternating to the other leg. The one-legged stance position should be maintained for 30 seconds on each leg for a total duration of five minutes. The ultimate goal is to be able to do this with your eyes closed. If this is not possible, keep your eyes open. If you still have difficulty performing the flamingo, hold onto the back of a chair with one finger, one hand, or both hands, depending on your degree of unsteadiness, eventually progressing to being able to stand on one leg with your eyes closed. Another basic balance exercise involves walking heel to two in a straight line forward and backward. Yet another balance exercise involves writing the alphabet with the foot of one leg while balancing on the opposite leg. One final exercise for developing balance involves standing near a wall and practicing leaning toward it in each direction. Any or all of these balance techniques have been shown to result in up to a 50% improvement in balance among older people.

Living Smart

Depending on an individual's point of reference, reflecting on the aging process may present a rather dismal picture. In fact, a generation ago much confusion and fatalism existed regarding aging. Old age was viewed as the time of inevitable and irretrievable decline. By no means, however, is the future as bleak as it might first appear. With respect to the effects of the aging process, to a great extent, individuals can control their own destiny. Regular exercise can and does slow down many of the debilitating effects of advancing years. The master guideline with regard to exercise and aging is that it is never too late to start. It is not "you're too old to exercise," it is "you're too old not to exercise." Irrefutable evidence exists to support the fact that mixing strict adherence to sound exercise principles with a personal commitment to common sense and patience could well serve as an appropriate recipe for improving and sustaining an independent lifestyle for the elderly. In other words, "living smart" is the fundamental priority for "living well" . . . at any age. ❑

BIBLIOGRAPHY •

1. American Dietetic Association Reports. "Nutrition, aging, and the continuum of health care." Technical support paper. *J Am Diet Assoc* 87:345-347, 1987.
2. Berger, B.G. "The role of physical activity in the life quality of older adults." In Spirduso, W.W., Eckert, H.M. (Eds), *The Academy Papers: Physical Activity and Aging.* Champaign, IL: Human Kinetics Publishers, 1989.
3. Bortz, W.M. *We Live Too Short and Die Too Long.* New York, NY: Bantam Books, 1991.
4. Bortz, W.M. "Disuse and aging." *JAMA* 248:1203-1208, 1982.
5. Bortz, W.M. "Effect of exercise on aging—effect of aging on exercise." *J Am Geriatr Soc* 28:49-51, 1980.
6. Brody, J.A., Brock, D.B., Williams, T.F. "Trends in the health of the elderly population." *Annu Rev Public Health* 8:211-234, 1987.
7. Dalsky, G.P., Stocke, K.S., Ehsani, A.A., et al. "Weight-bearing exercise training and lumbar bone mineral content in postmenopausal women." *Ann Intern Med* 108:824-828, 1988.
8. Evans W., Rosenberg, I. *Biomarkers.* New York, NY: Simon & Schuster, 1991.
9. Fiatarone, M.A., Marks, E.C., Ryan, N.D., et al. "High-intensity strength training in nonagenerians: Effects on skeletal muscle." *JAMA* 263:3029-3034, 1990.
10. Fowles, D.G. *A profile of older Americans.* Program Resources Department, American Association of Retired Persons. Administration on aging, U.S. Department of Health and Human Services, 1985.
11. Frontera, W.R., Meridith, C.N., O'Reilly, K.P., et al. "Strength conditioning in older men: Skeletal muscle hypertrophy and improved function." *J Appl Physiol* 64:1038-1044, 1988.
12. Jenkins, R., Goldfarb, A. "Introduction: Oxidants, stress, aging exercise. *Med Sci Sports Exerc* 25:210-212, 1993.
13. Kasch, F.W., Boyer, J.L., Van Camp, S.P., Verity, L.S., Wallace, J.P. "The effect of physical activity and inactivity on aerobic power in older men (a longitudinal study)." *Phys Sportsmed* 18(4):73-83, 1990.
14. Katz, S., Branch, L., Branson, J., et al. "Active life expectancy." *N Engl J Med* 309:1218-1223, 1983.
15. Katz, S., Ford, A., Moskowitz, R., et al. "Studies of illness in old age and the index of ADL: A standardized measure of biologic and psychologic function." *JAMA* 185:94-100, 1983.
16. Kisner, C., Colby, L.A. *Therapeutic Exercise.* Philadelphia, PA: F. A. Davis Company, 1990.
17. Larson, E.B., Bruce, R.A. "Health benefits of exercise in an aging society." *Arch Intern Med* 147:353-356, 1987.
18. Lewis, C.B. (Ed). "Exercise and Aging." *Topics in Geriatr Rehabil* 1:1, 1985.

19. Manton, K., Stallard, E. "Projecting the future size and health status of the U.S. elderly population." *Int J Forecasting* 8:433-458, 1992.
20. McGinnis, J. "Investing in health: The role of disease prevention." *In Emerging Issues in Biomedical Policy: An Annual Review*, Vol. 1. Blank, R., Bonnicksen, A., (Eds.) New York, NY: Columbia University Press, 1992.
21. Morey, M.C., Cowper, P.A., Feussner, J.R., et al. "Evaluation of a supervised exercise program in a geriatric population." *J Am Geriatr Soc* 37:348-354, 1989.
22. National Center for Health Statistics. "Health, United States, 1988." DHHS Pub. No. (PHS) 89-1232. Public Health Service. Washington. U.S. Government Printing Office, March 1989.
23. Nieman, D.C. *Fitness and Sports Medicine: An Introduction.* Palo Alto, CA: Bull Publishing Company, 1990.
24. Shephard, R.J. "The scientific basis of exercise prescribing for the very old." *J Am Geriatr Soc* 38:62-70, 1990.
25. Smith, E.L., Gilligan, C. "Physical activity prescription for the older adult." *Phys Sportsmed* 11:91-101, 1983.
26. Souminen, H., Heikkinen, E., Parkitti, T. "Effect of eight weeks' physical training on muscle and connective tissue of M vastus lateralis in 69-year-old men and women." *J Gerontol* 32:33-37, 1977.
27. Spirduso, W.W., Eckhert, H. (Eds). *Physical Activity and Aging.* Champaign, IL: Human Kinetics Publishers, Inc., 1989.
28. Stanford, B.A. "Exercise and the elderly." *Exerc Sport Sci Rev* 16:341-379, 1988.
29. Stewart, A., Ware, J. *Measuring Function and Well Being: The Medical Outcome Study Approach.* Durham, NC: Duke University Press, 1992.
30. Work, J.A. "Strength training: A bridge to independence for the elderly." *Phys Sportsmed* 17:134-140, 1989.

CHAPTER 16

EXERCISE AND NUTRITION

by

Karol J. Fink, M.S.
and
Bonnie Worthington-Roberts, Ph.D.

• • •

Nutrition can play a substantial role in almost every aspect of your life. Since inadequate nutrition can have a negative effect on your ability to engage in most of the tasks attendant to daily living, good nutrition is absolutely essential. Good nutrition involves providing your body with the required nutrients in appropriate amounts. Each distinct nutrient performs special functions that other nutrients cannot. Synergistically, the nutrients depend upon each other to provide the energy your body needs. Accordingly, obtaining all of the essential nutrients from food each day is especially important for you to be able to participate in physical activity programs.

The essential nutrients are grouped into two main categories—each with three separate entities. The nutrients without calories are water, vitamins and minerals; while the caloric nutrients are carbohydrates, protein and fat. The nutrients with calories supply the energy you require to perform your daily living activities. As such, they are particularly important during exercise. Although the non-caloric nutrients do not directly provide energy, they have an essential role because they participate in energy-producing reactions. Without their presence, your body could not produce energy.

How To Obtain Adequate Amounts Of Each Nutrient

Proper nutrition is an extremely important component of a sound training regime. When mapping out a workout schedule for the week, nutrition should be included. While sound nutritional practices will not convert a mediocre athlete into an Olympian, they will provide the requisite nutritional ingredients for enabling individuals to enhance their capability to perform at their (genetically determined) best.

News articles, friends, restaurants, physicians, dietitians, coaches, and trainers often refer to the terms "proper," "good," and "balanced" nutrition. Despite such a focus on nutrition, understanding what the words "proper," "good," or "balanced" nutrition really mean and how to attain proper nutrition is a frequently confusing undertaking.

A simple way to ensure that your body's nutrient needs are being met is to understand and adhere to the Four Food Group model, which was developed to aid the American public in attaining proper nutrition. Most American elementary schools use the Four Food Group model for educating students about nutrition. As a result, it is quite likely that most athletes and exercisers have had some exposure to the concept. The major benefit of the Four Food Group model is that it can be easily understood and integrated into the daily dietary habits of most people.

The four groups in this model are the:

- meat and high protein group
- milk and dairy product group
- cereals and grain group
- fruit and vegetable group

Foods are classified into a particular group because of their vitamin and mineral content, as well as their carbohydrate, protein, and fat content. The Federal Government has established recommendations concerning how many servings from each group you should eat on a daily basis (refer to Table 16-1). Meeting these recommendations will adequately supply all of the essential vitamins and minerals required for an individual leading an active lifestyle (with the possible exception of the minerals iron and calcium). Although eating the recommended servings of the four food groups will ensure that all the essential vitamins and minerals an individual needs are supplied in adequate quantities, satisfying the recommendations will not necessarily ensure that every individual will be provided with an adequate level of caloric intake.

Your caloric requirements depend upon specific individual characteristics (e.g., age, gender, height, and weight), as well as specific program variables (e.g., the type, frequency, intensity, and duration of the regimen in which you participate). Most exercisers will require more calories than the minimum recommended number of servings will provide. A healthy way exercisers can obtain the extra calories they need is to increase the serving sizes of foods from both the cereal and grain group and the fruit and vegetable group, and the amount of non-animal high protein foods they eat.

Table 16-1. Recommended minimum number of servings from the Basic Four Food Groups with serving sizes.

Food Group	Recommended minimum number of servings			
	Teenagers	Adults	Pregnant women	Lactating women
Meat	2	2	3	2
Milk	4	2	4	4
Fruit-vegetable	4	4	4	4
Bread-cereal	4	4	4	4

Serving sizes

Meat: one serving is
2 ounces cooked, lean, boneless meat, fish, poultry or protein equivalent
2 eggs
2 slices (2 oz) cheddar cheese *
1/2 cup cottage cheese *
1 cup cooked dry beans, peas, lentils or soybeans
1 cup nuts
4 tablespoons peanut butter

Milk: one serving is
1 cup milk, yogurt, or calcium equivalent
1 slice (1-1/2 oz) cheddar cheese *
2 ounces processed cheese food *

Fruit-vegetable: one serving is
1/2 cup cooked or juice
1 small salad
1 orange
1/2 cantaloupe
1 medium potato

Bread-cereal: one serving is
1 slice bread
1 cup (1oz) ready-to-eat cereal
1/2 cup cooked cereal or pasta

* A serving of cheese can be used for either milk or meat group, but not both   *Modified from Williams, M.H. (1988).*

WHAT DOES EACH FOOD GROUP HAVE TO OFFER?

The cereal and grain group is an excellent source of carbohydrates, both complex and simple. It is also a good source of protein, vitamins, and minerals—particularly thiamin (B_1), iron (due to fortification), and niacin. Among the foods which are included in this group are breads, breakfast cereals, pastas, rice, tortillas, and taco shells. Foods that are made from oats, flour, or corn meal, such as pancakes or corn bread, are also included in the grain and cereal group.

The fruit and vegetable group provides many important vitamins and minerals. The composition of nutrients in different fruits and vegetables is extremely varied. For this reason it is important to select different fruits and vegetables throughout the week. In general, the fruit and vegetable group is an excellent source of the key vitamins A and C and also provides a good general supply of most other vitamins and minerals. Some fruits and vegetables that are particularly healthy choices are broccoli, spinach, carrots, bananas, and oranges.

Cheese, yogurt, cottage cheese, ice cream, and milk are all included in the milk and dairy product group. These foods not only are an excellent source of protein, but they also provide several important vitamins and minerals. Calcium is the most common mineral associated with this group, because milk and dairy products are the greatest contributor of calcium in the typical American diet. Calcium plays a vital role in the growth and maintenance of bones and teeth. It is important that you consume the recommended minimum amount of milk and dairy product servings each day, because your reliance upon calcium for the maintenance of healthy bones and teeth continues throughout your life.

The meat and high protein group supplies protein, niacin, iron, zinc, and thiamin. These nutrients are important for the maintenance of muscles, bones, red blood cells (the oxygen carrying component of blood), and healthy skin. Foods which are classified in this group include eggs, beef, pork, chicken, fish, luncheon meats, tuna, and hot dogs. Examples of high protein non-animal foods include legumes (beans), nuts, and peanut butter. These foods are included in the meat and high protein group because of their high protein and key nutrient content. Limiting your consumption of animal products to a moderate level—one to two servings a day—is recommended because such foodstuffs are commonly high in saturated fat and cholesterol. Choosing high protein, non-animal foods more often than animal products is recommended because such foods provide a greater variety of nutrients (including carbohydrates and fiber) and contain no cholesterol.

A fifth group, the "others" category, is often mentioned during discussion of the Four Food Group model. This group encompasses foods lacking in nutrients, such as alcohol, fats and oils, sweets, chips, crackers, soft drinks and condiments. Foods in the "others" category typically are high in calories, high in fat, high in sodium (salt), and low in beneficial nutrients. Foods from the "others" category should only be eaten after ensuring that the minimum number of recommended servings of each food group has been met in your diet. The "other" foods should only be eaten in moderation, as an adjunct to an already healthy balanced diet.

How To Evaluate A Day's Meals Using The Four Food Groups

The Four Food Group classification provides a straightforward and simple way to evaluate food intake and determine if your nutrient needs are being met. Evaluating the food intake of an individual based on the Four Food Groups involves keeping a record of the amount of all food and beverage consumed throughout the day. This record is then compared to what is recommended (refer to Table 16-2). If the recommended number of servings from a certain group is not ingested, the individual may not be acquiring an adequate amount of nutrients. Knowing the actual serving size will enable you to be better able to determine if your nutritional needs are being met. For example, one cup of milk constitutes a full serving of the milk and dairy product group, while two cups of cottage cheese is considered a serving.

A thorough evaluation of the sample one-day diet record illustrated in Table 16-2 indicates that this person did not consume enough calcium or riboflavin (the individual only had one dairy product serving) and had not ingested a substantial amount of vitamins and minerals. This particular shortcoming, for example, could have been supplied by two more servings of fruits and vegetables. To avoid intake deficiencies in the future, this individual could make dietary changes that might include choosing milk instead of a cola at lunch, eating a piece of fruit for a midday snack and eating a vegetable serving with dinner. Changes such as these are relatively small yet helpful ways which the individual can undertake to ensure that adequate amounts of all nutrients are ingested.

Table 16-2. Evaluation of a one-day diet record based on the Four Food Groups.

Food	Amount	Grain & Cereal	Fruit & Vegetable	Milk & Dairy	Meat & Protein	"Others" Group
Bran Flakes	1.5 cups	2				
Banana	1 medium		1			
Milk, 1%	1 cup			1		
Whole Wheat bread	2 slices	2				
Luncheon Meat	2 slices				1 (animal)	
Mayonnaise	1 tbsp.					1
Cola	1 can					1
Spaghetti	1 cup	2				
Tomato & Meat Sauce	1/2 cup 2 ounces		1		1 (non-animal)	
French Bread	1 slice	1				
Beer	1 can					1
TOTAL		7	2	1	2	3
Recommended amount		4	4	2	2	0
Serving difference		+3	-2	-1	0	+3

REDEFINING THE BASIC FOUR FOOD GROUPS

A new concept, the "Food Pyramid," has recently been developed and endorsed by the United States Department of Agriculture (1992) to replace the basic four food groups. Although this graphically illustrated pyramid has not been fully adopted or developed, its use is expected to begin in the near future—replacing the "Four Food Group" model. The message of the food pyramid is not much different than that of the four food group model. Both recommend approximately the same number of servings. The fundamental difference between the two models is distinguished by the emphasis of bread, cereals, rice, pasta, vegetables and fruits and the de-emphasis of animal and dairy products.

Since a pyramid cannot exist without a foundation, the bottom layer is built with breads, cereal, rice, and pasta to depict the relative importance of these foods. The pyramid recommends a varied combination (9-11 servings) for these foods each day. For its building materials, the second layer of the Pyramid relies upon vegetables (3-5 servings each day) and fruits (2-4 servings each day). The construction materials for the third layer are contained in two equal compartments. One of meat, poultry, fish, beans, eggs, and nuts (2-3 servings), and the other of milk, yogurt and cheese (2-3 servings). Although this layer is smaller and attempts to de-emphasize the use of animal products, the number of servings recommended is equal to or greater than that of the four food group model. The very small apex of the pyramid contains fats, sweets, alcohol, and oil—foods that you should consume in extremely limited amounts.

The food pyramid is based on a recommendation that you consume a minimum daily number of servings from each of the six food categories every day. It also is predicated on the suggestion that you focus more on building a strong, balanced foundation by emphasizing breads, cereals, rice, pasta, vegetables, and fruit as the major portion of your diet. As you continue to build your personal pyramid, you should eat a variety of foods that result in a strong, balanced, healthy diet.

Figure 16-1. The Food Guide Pyramid.

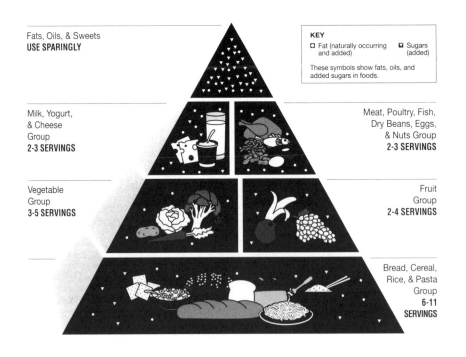

CARBOHYDRATE

Most physically active individuals realize that they should eat a diet rich in carbohydrates. Although they may know this, they often do not realize why this is important, or even of what a diet rich in carbohydrates would consist. Carbohydrates are an important means of replenishing your glycogen stores. Glycogen is your muscles' preferred source of fuel during aerobic exercise, because it is efficiently converted to energy. The availability of glycogen has been shown to influence the amount of exercise you can accomplish before fatigue occurs. This section of the chapter presents an explanation of the relationship between carbohydrate and glycogen, describes the importance of glycogen during exercise, and offers suggestions for increasing your dietary intake of carbohydrates.

GLYCOGEN AND CARBOHYDRATES AS FUEL

Carbohydrates are composed of complex and/or simple sugars that are readily converted into glucose once they are absorbed into the blood. The amount of glucose in the blood is strictly regulated to ensure that tissues dependent on blood glucose energy (e.g., the brain, heart and kidneys) have a constant supply of fuel. If your blood glucose concentration rises (as it does after eating carbohydrates), the excess glucose is stored as glycogen in your liver and muscles. Once your glycogen storage capacity has been met, the excess glucose is converted and stored as fat.

Blood glucose and liver glycogen are easily interconverted in your body because glycogen is made from linking glucose molecules together. If your blood glucose concentration decreases, glucose molecules are broken off from liver glycogen and reenter the blood stream. This control mechanism prevents large fluctuations in blood glucose levels from occurring and ensures that your dependent tissues are constantly supplied with energy.

Similar to liver glycogen, muscle glycogen is constantly utilized over the course of a day. Whereas liver glycogen supplies energy to organs and tissues, muscle glycogen provides energy exclusively to your working muscles. Muscle glycogen provides the best source of fuel during aerobic exercise because it is simply and readily converted to energy. Fat and protein are able to provide energy during exercise, but the process of their conversion to energy is much more complex than that of glycogen. The easy conversion of glycogen to energy helps optimize performance by decreasing the amount of work your body must do to produce energy.

The supply of muscle glycogen during vigorous exercise can last from 60 to 90 minutes depending on how much of this energy source was stored in your muscles prior to the onset of exercise. The amount of glycogen you store depends upon your level of daily carbohydrate and calorie replenishment and your level of fitness. As a general rule, the better trained an individual is, the more glycogen an individual can store. A non-exercising individual, who eats a proper diet and participates in normal daily activities, will not experience a depletion of muscle glycogen during a typical day even though muscle glycogen is constantly being used. Engaging in normal daily activities, as well as prolonged or intense exercise, however, will result in the greater utilization of glycogen for fuel, thereby depleting your glycogen stores. Exercisers have termed this depletion "hitting the wall" or "bonking" because it correlates with fatigue and exhaustion.

Low or depleted muscle glycogen stores at the onset of aerobic exercise, or glycogen stores that become low or depleted during exercise, can cut your workout short due to premature fatigue and exhaustion caused by a lack of sufficient fuel. Low or depleted muscle glycogen stores can limit the intensity at which you can exercise, or result in a tired and listless feeling the remainder of the day, or until your muscle glycogen stores are replenished. No exerciser wants to experience the symptoms of low or depleted muscle glycogen stores that can result in a compromised workout, or influence the outcome of a competition. Consequently, ensuring a sufficient intake of dietary carbohydrates should be a paramount concern of the physically active individual.

DIETARY CARBOHYDRATES

Your body must convert dietary carbohydrates into glycogen, because dietary glycogen does not exist. Since a single workout lowers your muscle glycogen stores, a daily intake of a sufficient amount of calories and carbohydrates is essential for the replenishment of muscle glycogen stores. Carbohydrates are found in a wide variety of foods in the form of starches and simple sugars. Starches are complex carbohydrates which exist in many foods. The grain and cereal food group, which includes foods such as bread, pasta, rice, cereals, and grains, is a good source of complex carbohydrates. Beans, peas, and certain vegetables (e.g., potatoes and corn) are also good sources of complex carbohydrates. Simple sugars are found in a variety of foods. In most instances, they provide the "sweet" flavor found in foods. Examples of nutritious foods containing simple sugars include fruit, fruit juices, and milk. In contrast, several foodstuffs from the "others" food group, such as sodas, sweet baked products, ice cream, chocolate, candies, and foods prepared with refined white sugar or honey, represent non-nutritious simple sugars..

Even though such products are high in simple sugars (which are carbohydrates), they are not the most appropriate choice for glycogen replacement. Consuming foods rich in simple sugars prior to working out can disturb your body's strict balance of blood glucose. Simple sugars are absorbed quickly into the bloodstream, causing a rapid increase in blood glucose. This increase, in turn, activates your body's mechanisms for regulating blood glucose levels so quickly that your blood glucose levels may actually swing too low. Interfering with this complex regulatory system may result in your having an inadequate level of fuel during exercise. For this reason, it is usually suggested that simple sugars should not be eaten for several hours prior to exercise. Complex carbohydrates, on the other hand, do not have the same impact on blood glucose as simple sugars. Complex carbohydrates are absorbed more slowly into your blood, thereby minimizing the risk of undesirable fluctuations in blood glucose levels. They also supply several important nutrients which are usually lacking in foods containing simple sugars.

INCREASING DIETARY CARBOHYDRATE

Each time you exercise, you are utilizing and relying upon stored muscle glycogen for fuel. This process results in lowered muscle glycogen storage at the end of a workout. Consuming a carbohydrate-rich diet will replenish your glycogen supplies to ensure adequate and/or optimal glycogen storage. Adopting a daily meal pattern rich in complex carbohydrates is the best way to replenish and maintain your glycogen stores. To increase the amount of complex carbohydrates in your diet, you should eat more servings from the cereal and grain food group, in addition to eating more beans and vegetables. These complex carbohydrate-rich foods efficiently replenish your glycogen stores and provide you with several other important nutrients.

Nutritious foods which are high in simple sugars, such as fruit, fruit juices and milk, are a much better choice than most "other" simple sugar rich foods. These foods not only provide nutrients, but their carbohydrate makeup is less likely to result in undesirable fluctuations in your blood glucose levels. For example, the simple sugars contained in milk and fruit are absorbed and converted to blood glucose quicker than complex carbohydrates. Foods high in simple sugars, however, are absorbed and converted to blood glucose more slowly than are the aforementioned examples of the sugar-laden "other" foods. Therefore, fruit, fruit juices, and milk provide a good source of carbohydrate to replenish your glycogen supplies. Animal foods from the meat and high protein food group contain little or no carbohydrates. As a result, it is very difficult to replenish your glycogen stores by eating steak, poultry, or fish. Several examples of carbohydrate-rich food choices are presented in Table 16-3.

Table 16-3. Carbohydrate-Rich Food Choices.

Complex	Not-So Nutritious Simple Carbohydrates
Bread, rolls, bagels, and English muffins (especially whole grain)	Products made with refined white sugar or honey
Whole grain breakfast cereals, pancakes, and corn bread	Sweet baked products, cookies, and cakes
Rice-brown, white, long or short grained	Sweetened fruit juices
Vegetables (especially potatoes and corn)	Ice cream and frozen yogurt
Cooked beans and peas	Chocolate and candy bars
Pasta and noodles	Carbonated beverages

Nutritious Simple Carbohydrates
Fruits and non-sweetened fruit juices
Dried fruits
Milk

By more frequently choosing complex carbohydrate and nutritious simple carbohydrate foods, or by substituting these choices for foods in the "others" category, you can easily increase the amount of daily dietary carbohydrates that you consume. You can increase the likelihood that you will have a diet which is high in complex carbohydrates by undertaking certain steps, including:

- Consuming a varied diet containing the recommended amount of servings from each food group.
- Consuming several additional servings from the cereal and grain group.
- Consuming extra fruits and vegetables in order to ensure that you ingest a sufficient level of calories.

PROTEIN

In recent years, many athletes have begun to better understand the fact that the role of dietary carbohydrate is more important as an energy source than dietary protein. This realization is not based on the assumption that protein is unimportant, but rather that as a fuel source during exercise, protein appears to have a very limited role.

Dietary protein is essential for many functions within your body. For example, it is a major component of muscle. It also serves as a structural basis for all of the enzymes and hormones which control the basic physiological functions in your body. It helps maintain the proper hydration level in your body. Finally, when needed, protein can act as a source of energy. Considering the important role protein plays in human functioning, consuming an adequate level of dietary protein is essential for all individuals—including athletes. The question arises, however, concerning whether an athlete or a physically active individual needs to consume more protein-rich foods than a sedentary person.

UNDERSTANDING PROTEIN RECOMMENDATIONS

The Recommended Daily Allowance (RDA) for protein provides a standard designed to ensure good nutrition for a healthy American adult and is based on the minimum daily amount of protein required for proper maintenance of body tissue. Since variability exists between individuals, the RDA recommendation includes a "safety factor" to ensure that almost all healthy people will be covered by this umbrella recommendation. The RDA for protein is 0.8 grams per kilogram (2.2 pounds) of body weight. This recommendation is basically useless for anyone besides an exercise scientist, physician, or registered dietitian. It is, however, what most researchers base their studies and conclusions on for determining if athletes require more protein. Most studies in this area have attempted to answer the question: "Do athletes require more protein than the RDA of 0.8 grams per kilogram body weight?" This is not a "user friendly" question for the general population. Even though the RDA for protein exists, individuals are unaware of the recommendation and would typically not know how to incorporate it into their lives, even if they were exposed to the RDA guideline for protein.

An analysis of the existing literature on the protein requirements of physically active individuals suggests that it would be more appropriate for such research to focus instead on the questions: "How much protein do athletes eat now?" and "Are they meeting their current needs for protein?" It appears that the data obtained by answering these two questions would be more applicable to the athletic population than the conclusions current research provides. National food consumption studies indicate that most Americans consume 1.5 to 2 times the RDA for protein. Specific studies calculating the actual dietary protein intakes of athletes have found intakes greater than 1.5 to 2 times the RDA. Comparison of what would be thought to be two extremes, football players and female ballet dancers, reveals similar results. The football players were shown to consume well over 2 times the RDA for protein, while the ballet dancers ingested greater than 1.5 times the RDA for protein.

Thus, even if the recommendation for the athlete may be greater, the average individual and the athlete are already consuming enough protein to ensure proper levels of consumption. One reason most exercisers are exceeding the RDA recommendation is because they have high caloric intakes. When more calories are consumed from a varied diet, increases in all nutrients occur—including protein. So even if active individuals require more protein, they are most likely already meeting the needs of their bodies.

PROTEIN FOODS

Foods in each of the four food groups provide protein (refer to Table 16-4). Obviously, the meat and high protein food group tends to provide the largest amounts of protein. Foods from the milk and dairy product group and cereal and grain group also supply an ample amount of protein. Fruits provide a relatively insignificant amount of protein to the diet. On the other hand, vegetables are a relatively good source of protein. According to the RDA, a 130-pound (59-kilogram) woman should consume 47 grams of protein daily, while a 154-pound (70-kilogram) man should consume 56 grams. This amount of protein (and more) can easily be provided by a varied, well-balanced diet, consisting of foods from each food group.

HOW MUCH PROTEIN DO ATHLETES REALLY REQUIRE?

Two issues should be addressed when discussing the protein needs of an athlete: protein as a source of fuel, and protein for building muscle mass. Research conducted in the early 1800s surmised that since muscles include considerable protein, then protein must be the preferred fuel for muscles, and that increases in muscle mass must come from extra dietary protein. It is now known that carbohydrate, in the form of muscle glycogen, contributes the primary fuel for muscle. It is also known that training is what builds and strengthens muscles, not simply extra dietary protein.

Even though scientists agree that protein is not the primary fuel or cause of increased muscle mass, they believe that protein plays an important secondary role during exercise that may increase an athlete's need for protein above the RDA. The American Dietetics Association's (ADA) most recent report on sports and nutrition recommended increased protein requirements only for individuals involved in intense aerobic training (greater than 70% $\dot{V}O_{2\,max}$). Even though ADA made the recommendation, it recognizes that the average American, including an athlete, consumes protein above this recommendation. The ADA does not support the notion that the protein needs of a competitive weight lifter are greater—all of the dietary protein a weight lifter may need is provided from a well-balanced diet. An individual who would like to add muscle bulk should focus on combining a sound resistance training program with a well-balanced diet.

Most scientists and dietitians agree that exercise does not increase the body's need for protein significantly. A few, however, believe that physically active

Table 16-4. Protein Content of Selected Foods.

FOOD	PROTEIN (grams)
Meat & High Protein Group	
Tuna, canned, drained 4 oz.	31.0
Chicken, 1/4 lb. cooked	31.0
Hamburger, 1/4 lb. cooked	31.0
Sirloin steak, 1/4 lb. cooked	27.0
Egg, 1 medium	6.0
Soybeans, 1/2 cup cooked	12.0
Peanut butter, 1 tbsp.	7.0
Most beans, 1 cup cooked	15.0
Milk & Dairy Product Group	
Milk, 1 cup	9.0
Cottage Cheese, 1/2 cup	14.0
Cheese, 1 slice	7.0
Ice cream, 1/2 cup	3.0
Yogurt, plain 1 cup	11.0
Cereal & Grain Group	
Spaghetti, 1 cup cooked	6.0
Rice, brown, 1 cup cooked	5.0
Rice, white, 1 cup cooked	4.0
Bread, 1 slice	3.0
Bagel, 1 whole	6.0
Fruit & Vegetable Group	
Broccoli, 1/2 cup cooked	2.0
Carrots, 1 large	1.0
Corn, 1 ear	4.0
Green peas, 1/2 cup cooked	4.0
Apple, 1 medium	0.3
Banana, 1 medium	1.0
Grapes, 1 cup	0.5

individuals have an increased need for protein. Peter Lemon, Ph.D., professor of applied physiology laboratory at Kent State University, is one of the most renowned advocates of the theory of an increased protein need for athletes. He recommends that athletes should consume between 1 to 1.5 times more protein than the established RDA. Since the average American, including an athlete, already consumes 1.5 to 2 times the RDA, it would appear as though athletes need not to increase their protein intake.

ARE THERE ANY RISKS ASSOCIATED WITH EXCESS PROTEIN CONSUMPTION?

Your body is unable to store extra protein. Protein consumed in excess of your body's needs is not used to build muscle but used for nonprotein bodily functions. If you consume protein in excess of your caloric and protein needs, the extra protein will not be stored as protein, but is converted to and stored as fat. As a result, if you consume large amounts of extra protein in addition to your regular diet, any weight gain would very likely be in the form of fat.

Potential for harm exists if protein is consumed in excess. The results are most likely to occur in the individual who consumes protein or amino acid supplements. Excess protein may lead to dehydration, because protein metabolism requires extra water for utilization and excretion (i.e., elimination) of its by-products. Since exercising individuals are already at an increased risk for dehydration (refer to the fluid balance section of this chapter), the additional strain of protein waste excretion may further encourage dehydration. Excess protein has also been shown to lead to an increase in the loss of urinary calcium. A chronic calcium loss, due to excess protein intake, is of particular concern because it increases the risk of osteoporosis, especially in women.

Young man's death raises question of safety

A healthy, athletic 23-year old male university student died of anaphylactic shock allegedly due to the body building amino acid supplement he ingested. Anaphylactic shock, caused by a severe allergic reaction to an allergen, is rare, but other mild allergic reactions to body building amino acid supplements may be common. One manufacturer of amino acid supplements previously claimed that their supplement "won't trigger common food allergies." The amino acid supplement this young man took did not trigger a common allergy, it triggered one that may have ended his life. It is advisable to avoid such protein and amino acid supplementation since the benefits of supplementation are yet undetermined, in addition to the fact that single amino acid supplements have not been thoroughly tested in human subjects, and, therefore, no margin of safety is available.

DIETARY FAT AND CHOLESTEROL

Research indicates that a diet high in fat and cholesterol can increase your risk for atherosclerosis (narrowing of the arteries), heart disease, and certain types of cancer. Atherosclerosis results when excess fat and cholesterol are deposited within your arteries, narrowing the passage for blood to flow through. If the passage becomes too narrow and blood flow is reduced significantly, anginal chest pain or a heart attack can occur. Decreasing the amount of dietary fat and cholesterol reduces your risk of coronary heart disease, aids in losing weight and increases the carbohydrate percentage in your diet.

BLOOD CHOLESTEROL

Two concepts should be understood when discussing cholesterol: blood cholesterol and dietary cholesterol. Blood cholesterol, measured by a clinician and expressed in milligrams per deciliter (mg/dl), is a factor which helps identify an individual's risk for heart disease. Dietary cholesterol is found only in foods of animal origin. As a preventive measure against the development of a high level of blood cholesterol, your dietary intake of cholesterol should be limited to less than 300 milligrams per day.

Although high blood cholesterol has harmful effects, cholesterol plays a vital and necessary role in proper human functioning. Cholesterol is involved in hormone production, cell wall structure development, and digestion. The amount of cholesterol in your blood is influenced by proper liver function, dietary cholesterol intake, exercise, body weight, and other yet to be identified influences. Problems arise when the concentration of cholesterol in your blood reaches unhealthy levels (refer to Table 16-5). When your blood cholesterol level reaches a certain point, the risk of harmful cholesterol and fat deposits forming in your arteries rises, increasing your chances of developing cardiovascular disease.

Table 16-5. Risk Classification Based on Total Cholesterol.

TOTAL CHOLESTEROL READING	CLASSIFICATION
<200 mg/dl	Desirable Blood Cholesterol
200-239 mg/dl	Borderline-High Blood Cholesterol
> or = 240 mg/dl	High Blood Cholesterol

Persons over the age of 20 should have their blood cholesterol levels checked at least once every five years. An annual recheck of blood cholesterol levels above 200 mg/dl is recommended. For individuals with cholesterol levels greater than 200 mg/dl, it is recommended that dietary changes, exercise, and lifestyle changes be the first measures adopted to help lower cholesterol levels. It is important that at-risk individuals consult with the proper health professionals before initiating any lifestyle or dietary changes for blood cholesterol reduction.

EXERCISE AND NUTRITION
• • •

Influencing Blood Cholesterol With Diet and Exercise

To avoid high blood cholesterol and its complications, adopting dietary preventive measures and exercising are top priorities. Adopting a low-fat diet with its prudent limitation of how much eggs, beef, pork, and other animal products you eat has been shown to be the best way for individuals to decrease the cholesterol content of their diets. One serving of an animal product per day from the meat and high protein food group, plus the avoidance of high fat processed foods and the consumption of nonfat or low-fat milk and dairy products, will help ensure that your dietary cholesterol intake is appropriately low. Engaging in an exercise program on a regular basis which adheres to the accepted exercise guidelines (refer to chapter 13) also has been found to produce desired changes in blood cholesterol profiles.

Limiting Dietary Fat

The American Heart Association recommends limiting your intake of dietary fat to less than 30% of your total calories. Most average Americans consume greater than 35% of their total calories from fat. One half of this dietary fat comes from animal products such as red meat (beef, pork, lamb, veal), poultry, fish and shellfish, separated animal fats (products fried in tallow or lard), dairy products (milk and cheese), and eggs. Some other contributors of fat in the diet include salad dressings and oils, most convenience foods, sweet baked products, and confections. Much of the fat and cholesterol we obtain is hidden in the foods we eat. Identifying foods high in fat and cholesterol is the key way to learn how to avoid them. Cholesterol is only found in animal foods and products. If an animal product is high in fat, it is usually high in cholesterol. As a general rule, meats and meat products and most processed and prepared foods—potato chips, crackers, frozen meals, cakes, and cookies—are high in fat. Tables 16-6 and 16-7 provide the calorie, cholesterol and percent fat of some common foods and note healthy low fat and low cholesterol alternatives (marked by *) to these choices.

Prepared foods, even though they are not animal products, can contain cholesterol depending on the type of fat or ingredient used. For example, potato chips fried in lard will contain cholesterol, while chips fried in vegetable shortening will not. It is important to note, however, that both these foods would be high in fat, since they were fried. Baked goods made with eggs (cakes and cookies) contain cholesterol from the egg yolk and are generally high in fat due to the butter, margarine, or oil included in the recipe. Whole milk and dairy products can also be high in fat and cholesterol. Alternative low-fat and nonfat products containing less fat and cholesterol, however, are available. Fresh and frozen fruits and vegetables (exceptions include avocados, coconuts, and olives) contain only small amounts of fat and should not be limited in an effort to reduce dietary fat intake.

The typical active American adult should limit the amount of dietary fat consumed both as a preventive health measure and a possible performance enhancer. A decrease in your consumption of fat will usually result in a healthy low-fat diet. A low-fat diet (less than 30% of calories coming from fat) is typically

Table 16-6. Calorie, Cholesterol, and Fat Content of Selected Foods.

Food	Amount	Calories	Cholesterol (mg)	% Fat
Fried Chicken	breast	260	95	75
Big Mac	1	570	85	55
Fried Fish	3 oz.	194	69	51
Steak	3 oz.	250	83	54
Baked Chicken*	breast	220	84	45
Baked Chicken w/out skin*	breast	175	85	20
Broiled Fish*	3 oz.	90	47	<1
Egg, whole	1 large	80	272	68
Egg, yolk only	1 large	63	272	80
Egg, white only*	1 large	16	0	0
Egg, substitute*	1/4 cup	96	1	66
Doughnut	1	105	0	34
Bran Muffin (small)*	1	100	0	27
Toast (dry)*	1 slice	80	0	7
Bagel (not egg)*	1	160	0	1
Granola	1/4 cup	125	0	29
Oatmeal*	3/4 cup	105	0	17
Bran Flakes*	3/4 cup	95	0	<1
Guacamole	1/4 cup	100	0	95
Salsa*	1/4 cup	10	0	0
Potato Chips	1 oz.	150	0	60
Peanuts	1 oz.	165	0	76
French Fries	1 pkg.	160	0	51
Chocolate Bar	1 bar	250	6	50
Tortilla Chips*	1 oz.	150	0	48
Popcorn (unbuttered)*	1 cup	25	0	<1
Apple (small)*	1 piece	60	0	0
Banana*	1 piece	90	0	0
Cream	1 tbsp.	37	13	97
Nonfat Evaporated Milk*	1 tbsp.	13	<1	<1
2% Milk	1 cup	125	18	36
Nonfat Milk*	1 cup	90	5	<1
Potato with Sour Cream	1 medium	270	10	17
Plain Potato*	1 medium	100	0	0
Butter	1 tbsp.	100	33	100
Margarine*	1 tbsp.	100	0	100
Clam Chowder	1 cup	165	22	38
Chicken Soup*	1 cup	75	3	60
Beer	12 oz.	145	0	0
Wine	3.5 oz.	72	0	0
Soda	12 oz.	150	0	0
Diet Soda	12 oz.	1	0	0

* *These are wiser choices of foods than the preceeding one(s).*

Table 16-7. Percent Fat Found in Common Foods.

	Fruits & Vegetables	Cereal & Grain	Milk & Dairy	Meat and High Protein Group			Combination & "Others" Foods
				Legumes & Nuts	Poultry & Fish	Red Meat	
Low in fat < 15% of calories coming from fat	Fruits: fresh frozen, canned, dried plain vegetables (no fat added), pure fruit juices	Grains & flours: barley, rice, corn, wheat, most breads & breakfast cereals, bagels, pita bread, corn tortillas, noodles & pasta	Nonfat (skim): milk, yogurt, cottage cheese	Dried beans & peas: garbanzo, lima, pinto, black, kidney, split peas, lentils, black-eyed	Egg whites, cod flounder, haddock, perch, tuna (in water), shrimp, scallops		Spaghetti with tomato sauce, mustard, soy sauce, catsup, sherbet, juice bars, soft drinks
Medium in fat 15-30% of calories coming from fat		Corn bread, flour tortillas, soft rolls, & buns, wheat germ, soda crackers	Low fat: yogurt, cottage cheese		Light meat of chicken and turkey (without skin), turkey breast, bass, catfish, crab, clams, fresh tuna, lobster	Completely trimmed: beef (round, tips, flank), pork, luncheon meats 0-2 grams fat/oz. (turkey 97% fat free, ham 94% fat free)	Frozen "diet" meals, beans in tomato sauce, animal cookies, ginger snaps, graham crackers, ice milk, frozen low fat yogurt
High in fat 30-50% of calories coming from fat		Biscuits & muffins, granola cereals, pancakes & waffles, snack crackers	Low fat milk (2%), most reduced calorie cheese, ice milk	Soybeans, tofu	Light meat of chicken & turkey (with skin), dark (without skin), turkey luncheon meat, salmon, tuna drained of oil, albacore	Completely trimmed: beef, veal, lamb, ham, Canadian bacon	Fish sticks, burritos, most frozen meals, hamburgers, pizza, spaghetti with meat, macaroni & cheese, french fries, cakes, candy bars, cookies, granola bars, doughnuts, ice cream
Very high in fat >50% of calories coming from fat	Avocado, olives, coconut	Snack chips, croissants, pastries	Whole milk, most cheeses, nondairy creamers, half & half, cream, ice cream	Most nuts & seeds, peanuts & peanut butter	Dark meat of chicken & turkey (with skin), whole eggs, ground turkey, anchovies, trout, tuna in oil	Partially trimmed meats: beef, veal, lamb, pork, spareribs, ground beef, sausages, most luncheon meats, hot dogs	Fried chicken, hot dogs, onion rings, potato chips, snack chips, nachos, cream soups, mayonnaise, salad dressing, chocolate, "gourmet" ice cream, butter, margarine.

Adapted from "Eating for a Healthy Heart," American Heart Association, Alameda County Chapter.

high in carbohydrates, fruits and vegetables, fiber, vitamins and minerals—all of which benefit an individual who exercises (since it helps maintain adequate levels of glycogen). A list of suggestions regarding how you can lower the amount of dietary fat you consume is discussed in Table 16-8.

LABEL READING FOR FAT AND CHOLESTEROL

Label reading to determine the fat content of food can be quite a tricky process. Labels can read 97% Fat Free, low fat, reduced fat, less fat, lean, lite, light, etc., and still be laden with fat. The wide array of label terminology confuses the consumer who often purchases products based on the label's claim regardless if it is truly lower in fat or not. An easy way to determine if a product is high in fat is to read the ingredients listed on the label. If a fat, oil, shortening, or meat is listed near the beginning or if several different fats are listed, then the product is generally high in fat.

The American Heart Association's recommendation that less than 30% of your calories should come from fat is far different from what labels frequently claim in their advertising text. To more accurately determine the amount of fat in a product, referring to the nutritional information on the label panel is most beneficial. Hopefully, this panel lists the number of calories and grams of fat per serving. By using these two numbers, the percent of fat contained in that food can be calculated. For example, a 2-ounce slice of luncheon meat which is labeled "80% Fat Free" derives more than half of its calories from fat:

Example of Label "80% Fat Free Luncheon Meat"	
Serving size	2 oz.
Calories	145
Fat (g)	10
Carbohydrate (g)	0
Protein (g)	14

The number of fat grams should be multiplied by nine (because fat supplies nine calories per gram) to convert the fat grams to calories. The resultant number is then divided by the total number of calories to calculate the percent of calories from fat:

$$\frac{\text{Fat (g) x 9 calories per gram of fat}}{\text{Number of calories}} = \text{the percent of calories derived from fat}$$

For the aforementioned example of "80% Fat Free Luncheon Meat"

$$\frac{\text{10 g of fat x 9 calories per gram of fat}}{\text{145 calories}} = \text{62 percent calories from fat}$$

This "80% Fat Free" product derives 62% of its calories from fat. The average consumer would expect the product to contain 20% fat because of the "80% Fat Free" claim (80% + 20% = 100%). However, "80% Fat Free" represents the percent fat free per unit weight which is different from the percent of calories. The American Heart Association's recommendation of less than 30% dietary fat is based on calories, not weight. Thus, this "80% Fat Free" product is far greater than the 30% or less recommendation and would be considered high in fat. Label reading is essential to avoid the confusion caused by the deceptive claims of food manufacturers.

Definitions for the claims manufacturers make are not consistent from product to product because two different federal agencies regulate the terminology. The United States Department of Agriculture (USDA) supervises labels on meat products, most poultry products and eggs, while the Food and Drug Administration (FDA) supervises most other foods. Some overlap of which agency is responsible occurs. In addition, some foods are regulated by the state in which they are sold. With different agencies regulating different products, it seems impossible to know what the claim on the label really means. Among the definitions of some common food label terms and the respective agency responsible for regulating the use of a specific term are the following:

• *Leaner/Lower Fat/Less Fat (USDA)*
  May be used if there is at least a 25 percent reduction in fat content as compared to the original product.

• *Lite/Light/Lightly (FDA & USDA)*
  USDA policy indicates these terms may be used if there is a 25% reduction in fat as compared to the original meat or poultry product. These words are commonly used to refer to calories and sodium, and the same 25% reduction guidelines can be applied. FDA policy, which regulates the use of these terms, is somewhat meaningless, because few standards exist. These policies are deceiving to the consumer, especially with a product such as "extra light" olive oil. This claim refers to the color and extraction method used; it has nothing to do with a reduction in calories or fat.

• *Low Calorie (FDA & USDA)*
  Products containing no more than 40 calories per serving; be sure to determine if the serving size is reasonable.

• *Low Fat (FDA)*
  Refers to most milk and dairy products. The product must have a fat content by weight of less than 2% (for low fat milk, this is still 35% of its calories from fat).

• *Low Fat/Lean/Extra Lean (USDA)*
  These terms can be used on meat and poultry products (except ground beef and hamburger) that are not more than 10% fat by weight. The term "extra lean" may be used when a product is no more than 5% fat by weight (except

ground beef and hamburger). For ground beef and hamburger, the terms "lean" and "extra lean" require the product to be less than 22.5% fat by weight, compared to regular ground beef at 30% fat by weight.

• *No Cholesterol or Cholesterol Free (FDA)*
  Food contains less than two milligrams cholesterol and no more than 5 grams total fat per serving.

• *Low Cholesterol (FDA)*
  Food contains fewer than 20 milligrams of cholesterol per serving and no more than 5 grams total fat per serving.

• *Reduced Cholesterol (FDA)*
  Foods must have at least a 75% reduction in cholesterol from the original product. The amount of cholesterol in the original and improved product must be listed.

Table 16-8. How to Make a "Fat" Difference in Your Diet.

---

1. **Read the labels.** Check the serving size on the nutritional label, and then identify the number of grams of fat per serving. Compare brands, and select the product with the least amount of fat.

2. **Limit your intake of added fats.** Butter, Margarine, salad dressings, and cooking oils have about 10 grams of fat per tablespoon. Use a low-fat or a nonfat substitute instead. Many reduced-fat commercial products are currently on the market.

3. **Eat lean meats.** Substitute lower-fat cuts of meat for those high in fats. Ask your butcher for advice if needed.

4. **Eat poultry instead of red meat.** Chicken and turkey usually have less fat than beef or pork. Poultry-based luncheon meats and ground meat are also lower in fat than their beef and pork counterparts.

5. **Trim and skin your meat.** Remove all visible fat from meat and poultry prior to cooking. Also, remove the skin from poultry.

6. **Limit your portions of meat.** Limit your intake of meat and poultry to less than three ounces per serving—six ounces per day.

7. **Eat more fish.** Most fish are lower in fat, especially saturated fat, than are red meats and poultry.

8. **Eat water-packed tuna.** Tuna packed in water has substantially less fat and calories than oil-packed.

9. **Eat low-fat frozen dinners.** If you eat frozen dinners, buy frozen dinners that have a maximum of 10 grams of fat per serving; some frozen dinners have as few as six to seven grams of fat.

10. **Eat low-fat dairy products.** Be heart-healthy selective when eating all dairy products. For example, use nonfat (skim) milk or 1% milk instead of whole or 2%. Use nonfat or low-fat yogurt instead of whole-milk yogurt or sour cream. Eat nonfat frozen desserts instead of ice cream. If you eat cheese, eat cheese that has less than five grams of fat per ounce.

11. **Eat vegetable protein foods.** Dry beans and peas are low in fat and high in both protein and soluble fiber (which reduces your blood cholesterol level).

12. **Limit your intake of nuts and seeds.** Although nuts and seeds have protein and fiber, both are high in fat.

13. **Eat complex carbohydrates.** Replace foods high in fat with non- or low-fat starchy foods such as pastas, whole-grain breads, rice, vegetables, and cereals.

14. **Eat fruits and vegetables.** Eat at least five to six servings a day of fruit and vegetables—both are high in essential vitamins, minerals, and fiber.

15. **Eat low-fat breads and cereals.** Some breads (e.g., croissants) and cereals (e.g., granola) are high in fat (often saturated fat). Read the label and select low-fat alternatives (e.g., bagels) accordingly.

16. **Limit your intake of fried foods.** Eat foods that have been baked, broiled, grilled, poached, steamed, microwaved, or roasted instead of fried. Battered and breaded foods that have been deep-fried are very high in fat.

17. **Use vegetable coating sprays.** Coat your non-stick skillet with a vegetable spray instead of oil, butter, or margarine.

18. **Use unsaturated fats for cooking.** Unsaturated fats (monounsaturated and polyunsaturated) are found primarily in vegetable oils (such as peanut, olive, canola, sunflower, and corn). Replacing unsaturated fats for saturated fats has been found to reduce cholesterol levels in some individuals.

19. **Limit your intake of sauces and gravies.** Most sauces and gravies should be avoided because they are made with fat. Instead, eat natural juices, fat-skimmed broth, and vegetable salsas.

20. **Limit your intake of chocolate.** Substitute cocoa, which has less fat, for chocolate.

Unfortunately, the existing terminology for labeling is not particularly helpful when trying to select foods which are low in fat and cholesterol. Reading the list of ingredients is the first step to determining if a product is low in fat. The next step is to calculate the actual percentage of fat using the equation which was discussed earlier in this section. In general, if less than 30% of a food's calories are from fat, it is considered to be a good choice. This does not mean a food with greater than 30% of its calories coming from fat should never be eaten. Rather, this food should be eaten in moderation or with a low-fat food to balance out the total fat percentage of your diet.

Weight Management

Approximately 25% of the adult American population is considered to be obese. Yet, more than 50% of American adults feel they have a weight problem. Billions are spent annually on diet books, diet pills, diet drinks, etc. We live in a weight-conscious society that has produced people who are willing to try almost anything to lose weight. Unfortunately, the commonly employed methods of weight loss tend not to be either physiologically sound or safe.

Weight loss occurs when an individual is in a negative caloric balance. A negative caloric balance can be achieved by either reducing calorie intake through dietary measures or increasing caloric expenditure through physical activity. Weight loss that occurs only by severe calorie restriction can result in the breakdown of muscle tissue for energy and limited amounts of fat loss. The less muscle tissue you have, the lower your metabolic rate will be. Thus, the more weight individuals lose through dieting alone, the more their metabolic rates will decline and the greater their tendency to regain the weight they have lost.

Weight charts are commonly used to provide individuals with an idea of what an appropriate weight might be for them. Yet body composition, as measured by percent fat, is a much better indicator of whether you need to lose weight. As a result, a weight chart should only be used as a guide to what you should weigh—not as an absolute ideal. For example, a six-foot male weight lifter who has only 8% body fat, yet weighs 230 pounds due to his large amount of muscle mass, would be considered to be (at a minimum) 40 pounds overweight according to standard height-weight charts. In fact, however, the man would, in all likelihood, be extremely fit and should not consider losing weight to merely fall within a reference weight range.

It is important to keep in mind that weight gain does not occur in a day or a week. Accordingly, it is not realistic to expect weight loss to occur that quickly. The combination diet-exercise approach to weight reduction tends to produce a rate of weight loss of about one to two pounds per week (the rate of weight loss recommended by most experts), meaning it will take you longer to reach your desired goal. Statistics indicate, however, that weight which is lost in this manner is much less likely to be regained.

Dietary Changes for Weight Management

Extremely restricted diets, whether they involve dietary regimens that strictly control caloric intake, liquid diets or diets in which the consumption of only a few types of food is allowed, should be avoided due to the potentially harmful effects they can have on your body. The fundamental basis for a sound diet should begin with meeting the minimum number of servings recommended by the Four

Food Group model. This guideline ensures that you will consume a minimum level of calories and nutrients each day. Once the base dietary pattern following the Four Food Groups has been established, individuals with higher caloric needs can add additional servings and still lose weight. High calorie foods do not have to be eliminated from your diet completely. Eating smaller portion sizes or consuming high calorie foods less often will make any dietary modifications easier to incorporate into your lifestyle. Reducing the total amount of fat in your diet is another worthwhile dietary strategy for weight reduction.

Dietary fat intake is of primary concern for anyone desiring to lose weight since fat contains nine calories per gram, while carbohydrates and proteins only contain four calories per gram. For example, switching from 2% milk to nonfat milk results in a calorie savings of 35 calories per cup due to the elimination of fat. It becomes quite clear that reducing dietary fat will have a significant effect upon your ability to reduce the total number of calories that you consume.

WHY IS EXERCISE IMPORTANT?

Exercise is the only reasonably safe and effective method for increasing caloric expenditure. An individual can expect to burn 200-300 calories during a 30-minute bout of moderately intense aerobic exercise (refer to chapters 13 and 17 for more detailed exercise prescription information). In addition, exercise has been shown to help individuals maintain their amounts of lean tissue and possibly their resting metabolic rates. A recent survey published in the American Journal of Clinical Nutrition revealed that 90% of maintainers (individuals who lose weight and keep it off) exercise on a regular basis, while only approximately one-third of relapsers (individuals who lose weight only to regain it) were physically active. Rather than simply promoting immediate weight loss, exercise helps to ensure that weight loss is permanent. Finally, it is important to remember that exercise can greatly improve your health regardless of its effect on body composition. ❑

BIBLIOGRAPHY •

1. Berning, J.R., Steen, S.N. (Eds). *Sports Nutrition for the 90s: The Health Professional's Handbook.* Gaithersburg, MD: Aspen Publishers, Inc., 1991.
2. Clark, N. "Fueling up with carbs: How much is enough?" *Phys Sportsmed* 19(8):68-69, 1991.
3. Franklin, B.A., Rubenfire, M. "Losing weight through exercise." *JAMA* 4:244, 1980.
4. Lemon, P.W.R. "Protein and exercise: Update 1987." *Med Sci Sports Exerc* 19(5):S179-S190, 1987.
5. Marcus, J. *Sports Nutrition, Sports and Cardiovascular Nutritionists.* Chicago, IL: The American Dietetics Association, 1986.
6. McCathy, P. "How much protein do athletes really need?" *Phys Sportsmed* 17(5):170-175, 1989.
7. Pennington, J.A.T. *Food Values of Portions Pommonly Used.* New York, NY: Harper & Row, 1989.

8.   Slavin, J.L., Lanners, G., Engstrom, M.A. "Amino acid supplements: Beneficial or risky?" *Phys Sportsmed* 16(3):221-224, 1988.

9.   Smith, N.J., Worthington-Roberts, B. *Food for Sport.* Palo Alto, CA: Bull Publishing Company, 1989.

10.   Whitney, E.N., Hamilton, E.M.N. *Understanding Nutrition*, 4th Ed. New York, NY: West Publishing Company, 1987.

11.   Williams, M.H. *Nutrition for Fitness and Sport*, 2nd Ed. Dubuque, IA: Wm. C. Brown Publishers, 1988.

CHAPTER 17

· ·

EXERCISE &
WEIGHT CONTROL

by

Thomas P. Sattler, Ed.D.
and
Julie E. Mullen, M.S.

• • •

At a recent health and fitness seminar, a panel of experts from a local hospital fielded nutrition questions from the audience. An elderly gentleman asked, "Should I eat more tomato soup or chicken soup to help me lose weight and stay energetic?" A panel member quickly responded, "Your consumption of the appropriate nutrients is predicated on your current physiological status, caloric requirements, fat composition, and the efficiency of your metabolic system." The elderly gentleman shook his head and said, "Thank you, but do I eat more tomato soup or chicken soup?"

Americans are continually barraged with nutrition and weight management information as new research, diets, and exercise programs emerge daily. Although prevalent, this information is often confusing, complicated, or even contradictory. This chaos is leading many people to make serious, even life-threatening, mistakes in pursuit of the ultimate goal—weight loss.

Americans currently eat five to ten percent fewer calories than 20 years ago, yet weigh approximately five pounds more. In the United States, 50 million men and 60 million women aged 18-79 are overfat, including more than 12 million who are considered severely obese. A startling one out of five children aged five to 17 is obese. Obesity is now considered an epidemic in this country. Furthermore, at any given time, approximately 20 million adults in the U.S. are dieting to lose weight and another 20 million think that they should be. In their zealous quest for thinness, more people are suffering from eating disorders such as anorexia nervosa and bulimia. In addition, it is estimated that Americans annually spend more than 30 billion dollars on diet books, products, and services.

How did Americans reach this point? The answer is equivocal. Obesity can be caused by several factors, including genetics, hyperphagia (eating too many calories), a high-fat or high-sugar diet, a sluggish metabolic rate, and a sedentary lifestyle. Hyperplastic obesity is caused by an abnormal increase in the number of fat cells during the first year of life and puberty. An individual of normal weight has about 25 to 30 billion fat cells, while an obese person can have as many as 42 to 106 billion fat cells. With so many reservoirs for fat, it is easy for fat to accumulate.

Hyperplastic obesity is rare. Most Americans suffer from hypertrophic obesity in which the number of fat cells is normal, but the size of the cells increases up to 40 percent due to greater fat deposits. Contrary to popular belief, obesity in this country seems to primarily be the result of a sedentary lifestyle, not due to overeating. Research shows that obese people don't necessarily eat more than their healthy weight counterparts. They simply move less and, therefore, burn fewer calories and store more fat. As they store more fat, the size of their fat cells expands.

Many people who are overfat (but not obese) constantly struggle to lose weight as well. American culture's high premium on thinness has made dieting a way of life for a large segment of the adult population. Because our society imposes such an unrealistic model for the "desirable" physique, many people will try virtually anything to attain a physiologically impossible standard. The demand for quick fixes has encouraged promises of immediate weight loss through nutritionally worthless plans such as fasting, the semi-starvation diet, the all-grapefruit diet, the high protein-low carbohydrate diet, the high fat-low carbohydrate diet, or even the wood pulp regimen—several of which have been found to cause serious health problems. Admittedly, it is challenging to know what to believe.

In reality, all of their tireless efforts to fit into smaller pants haven't helped the vast horde of dieters shed the pounds and keep them off. As a point of fact, <u>DIETING JUST DOESN'T WORK</u> for most people. Ninety percent of all dieters regain the lost weight within one year and 99 percent within five years. Many are trapped by the "yo-yo" syndrome in which they repeatedly lose and regain the same weight plus some more. The weight loss industry is flourishing simply because no diet gimmick or special food ultimately is successful at long-term weight maintenance.

The only permanent way to effectively lose weight and keep it off is to swear off diets forever. Instead, all individuals should commit to a lifetime of sound nutritional practices and regular exercise. They should forget promises of instant weight loss and accept that successful weight control requires time, discipline, and perseverance. Although it sounds difficult, the results far outweigh the endless frustration of repeatedly losing and regaining the same pounds.

EXERCISE AND WEIGHT CONTROL

• • •

UNDERSTANDING THE BASICS

CALORIES, METABOLISM, AND ENERGY BALANCE

Proper weight control requires an understanding of calories, metabolism, and energy balance. Calories are a measure of the fuel or energy value of food. When food is broken down in digestion and used to create energy, your body produces heat. The more calories a particular food contains, the more potential energy available for your body and the more heat that is produced when that food is digested and used for fuel. If you eat lots of high calorie foods and don't use the energy, your body stores this energy for future use in the form of fat.

Metabolism is the process of breaking down food and converting nutrients into fuel to supply energy. Metabolic rate is a quantitative measure of how fast you digest food and burn calories through activity and muscular work. Because your muscles use 90 percent of the calories that you consume, the more muscular tissue that you have and the more you use your muscles (i.e., the more active you are), the higher your metabolism. The greater your metabolism, the greater your caloric needs. As a consequence, highly active individuals can eat more food than their sedentary counterparts because they require more calories to fuel their muscles. Because athletes, for example, have a higher level of metabolism, they tend to burn calories faster than inactive people.

How do calories and metabolism apply to weight loss? Weight control is predicated on the energy balance equation in which calories consumed (through food) must be equal to calories expended (through activity). When you eat and burn up the same number of calories daily, your energy level is balanced. As a result, your existing level of weight is maintained. By contrast, you gain weight when you eat more calories than you expend—a situation many individuals find themselves in due to overindulgence and inactivity. Over a period of time, if you cumulatively eat 3500 more calories than you use, you will gain one pound of fat. By the same token, to lose weight, you must eat less than your body requires. One approach to achieve such a negative balance is to eat less; the other is to increase your caloric expenditure level through exercise. When you consume fewer calories than you use, your body will rely on stored fat and/or muscle to produce energy. Once you start using body fat or muscle for energy, you will begin to lose weight. Similar to weight gain, for every 3500 calories that you are in deficit, you'll lose one pound.

THE IMPORTANCE OF MAINTAINING BLOOD SUGAR

If weight loss is this simple, why do so many individuals fail in their efforts to "win the losing game?" Unfortunately, many individuals rely on weight loss approaches that are fundamentally flawed. For example, many dieters tend to limit their intake of fluids so they don't retain water weight. These individuals fail to realize that water weight loss doesn't cause a change in their physique and will be regained immediately when they ingest fluids again.

Many dieters also reduce their caloric intake level by skipping meals or cutting back on their intake of carbohydrates. Skipping meals or limiting carbohydrates causes your blood sugar level to plummet. Over time, when your blood sugar level drops severely, your body thinks it is starving and doesn't know when it will be fed again. To protect itself from starvation, your body actually conserves fat. The longer your blood sugar level is low, the more efficient your body becomes at storing food as fat and holding onto existing fat.

If you severely restrict your intake of calories, eventually your body will burn muscle tissue to help supply energy. Because lean body mass (LBM) affects your metabolic rate, using muscle for energy (and thereby losing it) causes your metabolism to fall, thereby actually slowing your rate of caloric expenditure. With a decreased rate of metabolism, your caloric needs decline. As a consequence, the process of losing weight and keeping it off becomes much more difficult— even though you reduce your level of caloric intake. In response to fewer calories, your body adapts to protect itself by automatically lowering your metabolic rate. In addition, cutting calories without incorporating exercise into your weight management program further depresses your level of metabolism. Without the "boost" that exercise provides to your metabolic rate, you continue to burn calories more and more slowly, eventually resulting in plateaus—a condition that frequently plagues many dieters.

After you've dieted for a while, what happens when you step on a scale? Often, you are lighter due, in large part, to the fact that you have lost water and muscle weight. You have, however, lost <u>very little</u> fat weight. It is important to remember that weight loss is not necessarily fat loss. In many instances, while you may appear to be lighter, you actually may be proportionally fatter.

This area of misplaced optimism is a point where many dieters go wrong. In their excitement about achieving a lower number on the scale, they immediately and incorrectly assume that they have lost fat. In reality, they may have set themselves up for failure (i.e., not being able to keep the weight off) by metabolizing LBM instead of fat, thereby lowering their resting metabolic rate. Keep in mind that in order to lose weight and keep it off effectively, you must focus on losing fat, not muscle.

IDEAL BODY WEIGHT: THE CONCEPT

Perhaps, the most commonly used method for assessing whether individuals are within their ideal body weight ranges are height-weight tables. Unfortunately, a number of problems exist with using height-weight tables to determine ideal body weight. For example, the body weights in the tables are considered to be desirable only on the basis that they had a positive correlation with longevity for the population studied—they do not take in account the health problems that are frequently associated with obesity. The members in the main group ever investigated for this purpose were subscribers to Metropolitan Life Insurance. Obviously, however, this particular group of individuals is not representative of the general population (in fact, few minorities or individuals of lower socioeconomic status were included). Furthermore, the body weights of these individuals were only measured once (if at all—since many individuals verbally reported their body weights and were never actually weighed). The information regarding the applicants' body weights was only obtained at the time that the individuals initially applied for the life insurance. No information was obtained regarding changes in body weight or the development of health problems after the insurance policies were initially purchased. These problems aside, the fundamental weakness of height-weight tables is that they do not assess body composition (i.e., the relative amount of body fat that comprises total body weight).

Because the relative percentage of body fat of your body has more important implications concerning your health and functional capabilities than does your body weight, many health/fitness professionals surmise that a specific ideal body weight can be established once an individual's percent body fat is known. Such a conclusion is a somewhat shortsighted view for a number of reasons. Since all of the available techniques for measuring body composition only provide an estimate of percent body fat, the resulting calculations are subject to error. For example, hydrostatic (underwater) weighing, the accepted "gold standard" for analyzing body composition, has a standard error of approximately plus or minus two to three percent. The more commonly employed techniques such as skinfold measurements and bioelectrical impedance have standard errors of approximately plus or minus five to eight percent.

Unfortunately, even if your percent body fat could be accurately and precisely assessed, additional information would be needed to determine your ideal body weight. How much body fat you have may not matter as much as where it is located on your body.

Findings from recently conducted studies indicate that the location of fat deposits on your body influences the ease of your ability to lose weight, and increases your risk of developing a number of health-related problems. Scientists have classified where the fat is deposited on your body into two basic categories: male-pattern (graphically depicted as apple-shaped) and female-pattern (graphically depicted as pear-shaped). Despite their illustrative names, each type of fat pattern can occur in both sexes, although men usually tend to be "apples" and women typically are classified as "pears." "Apples" characteristically deposit high amounts of fat in the abdominal and trunk regions, while "pears" deposit high amounts of fat in the hip, buttocks, and thigh regions.

The waist-to-hip ratio (WHR) is a simple, yet accurate, method for determining your personal distribution pattern for body fat. Waist-to-hip ratio is determined by dividing your waist circumference by your hip circumference. Waist circumference is defined as the smallest circumference between the rib cage and belly button. Hip circumference is defined as the largest circumference of the hip-buttocks region. Men with WHR values exceeding 1.00 are considered "apples," while women with WHR values above 0.80 are considered "apples."

Available evidence indicates that individuals with fat distributed on the upper body (apples) are highly prone to "the deadly quartet" of risk factors for coronary heart disease—high blood pressure, type II (non-insulin dependent) diabetes, elevated levels of triglycerides (hypertriglyceridemia), and low levels of high density lipoproteins ("good cholesterol") in the blood. The greater your exposure to these four factors, the higher your risk of heart disease. All news is not bad for "apples," however. Research has shown that weight loss (particularly fat loss) tends to be easier for "apples," because they benefit from the high turn-over rate of abdominal adipocytes (fat cells). Unfortunately, for individuals classified as "pears," weight loss is more difficult because those adipocytes which are located in the hip, buttock, and thigh regions do not easily relinquish their fat—a fact to which many "pears" who have attempted to lose weight can readily attest.

IDEAL FOR WHAT?

To determine your ideal body weight, you shouldn't rely solely on a bathroom scale, height-weight tables, or percent body fat measurements. What represents a safe, realistic, and perhaps more importantly attainable body weight for you will depend (to a large extent) on the following factors:

- *Medical History.* Your current medical history, to include a thoughtful review of your personal health risk factors should be taken into account when attempting to define your ideal body weight. For example, if your blood pressure is elevated, a modest weight reduction could be quite beneficial. Extra body mass means that your heart must work harder to pump blood through miles of extra capillaries that feed the extra tissue. Type II diabetes and blood lipid-lipoprotein profiles are further examples of medical conditions that can be positively affected by weight loss.

- *Family History.* Body weight, like most other physical characteristics, is strongly influenced by genetic factors. If your parents and siblings are extremely overweight, it is highly unlikely that you will ever be "model-thin". As unfair as such a judgment might at first appear, such a limitation should be kept in mind when establishing your ideal body weight goals.

- *Body Fat Distribution.* As previously stated, body fat located in your upper body region is very risky in terms of your health. If you possess a high amount of upper body fat (as determined by your WHR), you should consider losing weight (specifically body fat) through a combined program of sensible eating and exercise.

- *Functional Ability.* If your existing body weight inhibits your ability to (1) effectively and efficiently perform your activities of daily living and (2) comfortably engage in the recreational pursuits of your choice it is probably not at an ideal level.

Set Point Theory

Many nutritional and weight control experts hypothesize that your overall level of body weight and level of relative body composition can be affected by a number of conditions, particularly by a factor referred to as the set point. Proponents of the set point theory claim that the body has an internal control mechanism which is located deep within the hypothalamus of the brain that drives the body to maintain a particular level of body fat. When the amount of fat you have stored in your body falls outside the set point range (either increases or decreases), your brain makes the necessary adjustments in both your appetite and your metabolic rate until the amount of fat you have stored falls once again within the set point range. Accordingly, this physiological feedback mechanism determines the amount of fat your body sustains. A higher set point results in more fat stored, while a lower set point causes less fat to be stored.

All factors considered, dieting tends to increase your set point, because it usually results in the loss of LBM which causes a concomitant decrease in your metabolic rate. Over time, this process often leads to the "yo-yo" syndrome in which perpetual dieters continue to eat too few calories and, in the absence of resistance exercise, to significantly reduce their levels of LBM. As a result of the effect that their diminished level of LBM has on their metabolic rate, they also continue to store more body fat. Faced with a succession of higher set points, these individuals tend to encounter more difficulty losing weight with each successive diet. Over time, they tend to repeatedly lose and regain the same pounds.

According to proponents of the set point theory, the most effective way to lower your set point—and therefore your levels of stored fat—is through exercise. Research has shown that the best program of exercise for sound weight management is one that combines both aerobic exercise and strength training.

Losing the right "Weigh"

Preparing Your Mind

A careful examination of the evidence clearly indicates that because diets don't produce long-lasting results, they should be shunned forever. No matter how appealing their promises, almost all diets appear to be doomed to fail eventually. Diets are something individuals go on and off, and far too often when individuals go off a diet they end up heavier than they were initially.

The key issue that needs to be addressed is, without following a strict diet, how do you lose weight? In reality, the answer is straightforward: successful weight control begins with a lifetime commitment to nutritionally sound, balanced eating habits and a physically active lifestyle. Before trying to lose weight, you should abandon the notion that your weight management efforts will involve temporary measures on your part. To lose weight and keep it off (the really difficult part of weight control), you must be willing to incorporate permanent changes in your eating habits and physical activity level. Although this approach may sound somewhat intimidating, you should remember that the benefits of such a lifestyle change far outweigh the costs. Most importantly, your health will improve. You'll have more energy. You'll also feel better about yourself. You'll lower your risk of developing a wide variety of medical conditions. Finally, if you're like most people who are successful in their weight control efforts, you'll enjoy life more.

Making a long-term commitment to weight control often involves behavioral changes. While many theories exist about how to properly change your behavior, keep in mind that the process essentially involves substituting alternative behaviors for some of the strongest habit patterns in your daily life. The process takes time. The best way to approach the task is to identify elements of your eating and exercise habits that need to be changed and then institute a program to affect that change—one small step at a time.

Certainly, the first step in changing your behavior is to identify and evaluate your current eating habits and physical activity patterns. In order to develop habit awareness, most experts recommend keeping a diary. Such a diary is essential to providing a basis on which to determine which specific behavior(s) contributed to your present weight problem. You should keep a journal for a week in which you faithfully record every morsel of food and beverage you consumed and every physical activity you performed (walked up four flights of stairs, washed and folded three loads of laundry, stood on your feet seven hours at work, exercised for 20 minutes on the StairMaster® 4000 PT® exercise system, etc.). Your diary should also include the times of day you ate and were physically active. Such information may be helpful in identifying how to expand the total amount of time that you exercise or how to eliminate extracurricular eating (i.e., snacking).

After the week has ended, you should carefully review the information in your diary or bring it to a professional for help. A registered dietitian, for example, could help you analyze your nutrient and caloric intake, identify triggers that may stimulate eating (coffee breaks, television, restaurants) and evaluate your overall level of energy expenditure. For example, if your diary entries show that you are eating a lot of high-fat foods such as doughnuts, french fries, and chocolate, you can make the necessary adjustments in your eating habits. By the same token, if your diary points out that you tend to nibble endlessly while watching television, you can either change the environment around your television (i.e., make food less accessible, find something else to do while watching tv, etc.) or change your leisure habits so that you reduce the time spent watching television. Finally, your diary may show that you're far too inactive to achieve your weight control goals. For example, if you sit at a desk all day and then spend your evenings on the couch, you'll never be able to lose your desired amount of fat weight and keep it off.

DEVELOPING A PLAN AND PUTTING IT INTO ACTION

If your weight control goal is to take unwanted fat weight off and keep it off, you must eat sensibly and exercise regularly. Only by adhering to a sound diet and exercising on a regular basis can you ensure that your efforts will be successful. Knowing what constitutes a sensible diet and a sound exercise program is critical to achieving maximum results.

1. *Eat Sensibly.* A sound diet for weight reduction will be relatively low in calories (according to the American Dietetic Association guidelines, your diet should never fall below a level of approximately 10-12 calories per pound of your current body weight) and yet provide all nutrients essential to normal bodily functioning, contain foods that appeal to individual taste, and can be easily incorporated into an individual's lifestyle. A sensible diet will, and must, foster new, healthier (e.g., limiting fat consumption, avoiding fried foods, reducing salt intake, etc.) eating habits that can be maintained over the long-haul.

   One of the first steps in deciding what to eat is to determine how much (calorie-wise) you should eat to affect your desired fat loss. The simplest way for calculating what your daily caloric intake should be is to multiply your present weight (in pounds) by 15 calories (12 calories to meet your minimum basal needs, plus three calories to account for your physically active lifestyle). For example, a 150-pound individual needs 2250 calories daily to sustain that person's body weight. The next step would be to reduce the daily maintenance total by 250 calories— the amount necessary to achieve a one-pound weight loss per week when it's combined with a program to burn an additional 250 calories a day through exercise (giving you a net negative caloric balance of 500 calories daily). Because a pound of body fat has 3500 calories (7 x 500 = 3500), you'll lose one pound a week—a moderate rate of loss that is more likely to be sustained than a "quick-fix" approach.

   Accordingly, if the person in the example maintains a caloric intake of 2000 calories daily, that individual will lose one pound weekly. Although decreasing your caloric intake by only 250 calories (the equivalent of eliminating one slice of pizza from your diet daily) may not seem like much, research suggests that more drastic reductions may have negative consequences. For example, if you reduce your intake too much, you won't be providing yourself with enough energy to support an active lifestyle. Furthermore, you greatly diminish your chances of sticking with your new eating regimen. More ominously, over time extremely large cuts in your caloric intake may cause your body to metabolize muscle tissue instead of fat. As a guideline, keep in mind that the American Dietetic Association strongly recommends that your daily caloric intake never fall below 1000-1200 calories.

Once you determine how much you should eat to achieve your weight control goals, the next step is to identify what you should eat. As a basic rule of thumb, your diet should be high in complex carbohydrates and low in fat. A comprehensive overview of what constitutes a nutritionally sound diet is presented in the next chapter of this text.

In order to enhance your efforts to keep from eating too much, you should consider restructuring your eating habits to include the following possible steps:

- Limit yourself to one portion. Have your food served on your plate in the kitchen, not family-style at the table. After taking one portion, wrap up and store leftovers immediately to discourage nibbling.
- Have your food served on small platters so it doesn't look as if you are depriving yourself.
- Eat more slowly. Take smaller bites, chew your food longer and put down your utensils between bites. It takes at least 20 minutes for the satiety center in your brain to trigger a feeling of fullness. By that time, most people have finished their portions and are beginning seconds.
- Forget about being a committed member of the "clean plate club" and stop eating when you're full. Use any leftovers wisely (i.e., for a potluck dinner, as donations to feed those in need, or as a meal for your pet).
- Try to focus only on eating during a meal. Break any habit you may have of reading, watching television, opening mail, or talking on the phone while eating. If you sit down and concentrate on your meal, you increase the likelihood that you will enjoy your food and that you won't eat past the point of being full.
- Keep high-fat foods out of your place of residence entirely. If those with whom you live insist that you have high-fat items at home, try to keep them out of sight so that you aren't tempted every time you open the cupboard or refrigerator. Likewise, don't keep dishes of candy, nuts, or other treats in a convenient place where you can nibble on them.

One final factor relating to the precept of sensible eating involves your frequency of meals. How often you eat can impact on whether you compromise your commitment to eating sensibly. By keeping your blood sugar level at an adequate level, eating frequently can help you prevent (or at least minimize) the onset of those hunger pangs which often drive even the most well-intentioned individual to snack or binge. Research suggests that if you want to maintain a balanced level of blood sugar, you should eat at least three regular meals or five to six mini-meals daily. The point to remember is that skipping meals or eating almost all of your daily calories in one meal can hinder your efforts to lose body fat.

2. *Exercise Regularly.* Eating sensibly is only one component of a sound weight management program. For successful, lifelong weight control, sensible eating and regular exercise go hand-in-hand. Proper exercise will impact on your weight control efforts in a number of ways. The more you exercise on a regular basis, the faster your body will burn calories. In addition, strength training exercise can either help you build muscle tissue or, at a minimum, counter the tendency for a severely calorie-restricted diet to cause a significant loss of muscle along with the fat. Also, keep in mind, that exercise can improve your physical appearance, even if you don't lose a significant amount of weight. Because muscle is more dense than fat, you can look more fit and trim without changing your total body weight. While, in general, any physical activity you enjoy will help promote some degree of weight loss, an exercise program that combines aerobic conditioning and strength training represents the best form of exercise for weight control.*

One major factor that often hinders the efforts of individuals to integrate exercise into their weight control efforts is the alarmingly high amount of misinformation that exists concerning the relationship between exercise and weight management. Most of the misconceptions relating to the impact of exercise on weight control often result in either unhealthy practices or unrealistic expectations. Ultimately, these unhealthy practices have a negative impact on the type and magnitude of the results that you achieve from your efforts to successfully manage your fat weight.

Accordingly, it is in your best interest to know as much as possible about the role that exercise plays in helping you achieve your weight control goals. Sound information can help you approach weight management with an open mind regarding the need for, and the beneficial consequences of, participating in physical activity on a regular basis. Among the more popularly held myths and misconceptions are the following:

• **Myth: Performing aerobic exercise at a low rather than a high intensity promotes a greater loss of body fat.**
   Fact: It is true that the lower the intensity level at which you exercise, the more the body prefers to use fats, rather than carbohydrates as fuel. Unfortunately, this physiological actuality has led many individuals to mistakenly believe that because the body utilizes a greater percentage of fat as fuel during aerobic exercise at a relatively low level of intensity, such exercise is more effective for fat loss than high-intensity exercise. These individuals ignore a very important fact. The "absolute" amount of fat calories burned during high-intensity exercise tends to be equal to, or greater than, the num-

---

* *For information on how to develop exercise programs for aerobic conditioning and strength training, refer to chapters 7, 8, and 13 in this text.*

ber burned during low intensity exercise, even though the "percentage" of calories burned from fat is higher during low-intensity exercise. Keep in mind that you lose weight and body fat when you expend more calories than you consume, not because you burn fat (or anything else) when you exercise. By the same token, all other factors considered, the most positive feature of low-intensity aerobic exercise is that it is well-tolerated by most individuals.

- **Myth: Aerobic exercise suppresses your appetite.**
  Fact: The vast majority of studies which have attempted to investigate the relationship between exercise and appetite have demonstrated that your level of caloric intake is usually unchanged or slightly increased in response to long-term aerobic exercise training. Your energy intake, however, is usually increased below your increase in energy expenditure. This results in a negative energy balance (i.e., energy expenditure greater than energy intake) and, additionally, a loss of body weight and body fat. Some evidence exists that if you vigorously exercise before you eat, you will actually eat less because of an increase in body temperature and an alteration in hormone levels (i.e., catecholamines). The centers for the thermoregulatory system, appetite, and sleep lie right next to each other in the brain stem. When you affect one, you tend to affect the others.

- **Myth: The more you sweat, the more fat you lose.**
  Fact: If you exercise in extreme heat or humidity, or in "rubberized" clothing, you certainly will sweat profusely and lose weight. Any resultant weight loss, however, represents primarily lost water, not lost fat. When you replenish your body fluid stores by eating and drinking, those lost pounds return almost as fast as they left originally. Another problem with attempting to create a "new" you through perspiration loss involves the fact that you expose yourself to the risk of heat injury if you exercise vigorously in extreme heat or in rubberized clothing—both of which preclude safely controlling internal (core) temperature by preventing sweat from evaporating. Keep in mind that how much you sweat is not a good barometer of how much energy you're expending. Perspiring is more dependent on such factors as temperature, humidity, body composition, and individual variability.

- **Myth: You can burn fat from specific regions of the body by exercising those areas.**
  Fact: Contrary to what you may want to believe, the phenomenon of "spot reduction" has absolutely no factual basis. When you exercise, you utilize energy produced by metabolizing fat from all of the regions of your body—not just the specific muscles involved in the exercise. Performing sit-ups, for example, will build abdominal muscle strength and endurance, but will not trim fat off your abdominal region any more rapidly than off your buttocks or thighs.

- **Myth: Aerobic exercise causes your resting metabolic rate to stay elevated for a long time after a workout.**

Fact: In general, the available scientific data indicate that the amount of energy expended after an aerobic workout tends to be very small. The number of calories burned during the recovery is dependent upon the intensity and the duration of the workout. Following exercise of unusual intensity and duration, your metabolic rate may remain elevated for as long as 24 hours—but at a point that is just barely above your resting baseline level. In general, approximately 15 extra calories are burned during recovery for every 100 calories expended during the exercise bout.

- **Myth: Muscles will turn to fat when you stop exercising regularly.**
  Fact: Muscles cannot turn to fat. Muscle and fat (adipose) are two separate and distinct tissues. They simply do not have the physical capability of changing from one type of tissue to another. In reality, muscles have the unique property of "use it or lose it." If you don't use a muscle, it will literally waste away (atrophy). This process is perhaps best illustrated when someone has to wear a cast on a broken leg. When the cast is eventually removed, the relatively unused leg muscles are considerably smaller than they were prior to the injury. If muscle could turn into fat, you should see a veritable "fat ball" when you take the cast off an injured limb, not a significantly atrophied set of leg muscles.

- **Myth: Aerobic exercise effectively offsets the decrease in lean body mass often associated with dieting.**
  Fact: An analysis of the available data indicates that, in general, the combination of a conventional aerobic exercise program with a calorically restricted diet does little (if anything) to help you preserve lean body mass during weight reduction. It is important to keep in mind that the less lean body mass you have, the lower your resting metabolic rate. As a result, it is more likely that you will regain some, or all, of the weight you lose if you only exercise aerobically. On the other hand, if you engage in exercise designed to improve your muscular fitness level at the same time you are losing weight, you enhance the likelihood that you will be able to maintain your level of lean body mass. The optimal exercise prescription for sound weight management is one that combines aerobic conditioning and strength training. Such a prescription allows you to expend a relatively large number of calories, while simultaneously preserving or increasing your level of lean body mass.

- **Myth: Strength training will cause your muscles to substantially increase in size (and weight), thereby effectively offsetting any fat loss you may achieve.**
  Fact: Despite opinions to the contrary, little likelihood exists that strength training will cause your musculature to hypertrophy. Considerable evidence suggests that less than 20 percent of the male population and very few women can develop large muscles even if they wanted to, regardless of what protocol they follow. Of the six primary factors that affect how "big" your muscles can get, you ef-

fectively can control only one of those factors (how much of a demand you place upon them). The other factors are genetically determined. As a result, in the absence of taking growth hormones or using anabolic steroids, your chances of obtaining large muscles from strength training are not high. Keep in mind that whatever your weight control goals, strength training can help by preserving your level of LBM and, thereby, maintaining your resting metabolism.

A Case Study

Mary Smith, a 40-year-old secretary, is 5'3" and weighs 140 pounds. She has 30 percent body fat and a sedentary lifestyle (no regular exercise), although she is a member of a local health/fitness club. Her diet log shows that she usually skips breakfast or grabs a sweet roll and coffee with cream. She drinks coffee all morning to keep her going. Lunch and dinner are often high-fat selections from fast food restaurants. Her assessed need for daily caloric intake is about 2100 calories (140 times 15 calories).

- Mary wants to reduce her body fat to 22 percent. She calculates her estimated ideal weight by first finding her fat-free body weight. Her fat weight equals 42 pounds (140 times .3). Therefore, her fat-free body weight equals 98 pounds (140 minus 42). To determine her ideal weight, she divides this fat-free body weight by her ideal percentage of fat-free weight (i.e., 1.0 minus her goal body fat percentage). So, Mary divides 98 pounds by .78 (1.0 minus .22) and gets 126 pounds. Therefore, her objective is to lose 14 pounds to achieve her ideal body fat of 22 percent.
- Mary reduces her current intake of calories by 250 for a daily total of 1850. She starts eating a breakfast of water or juice, a bagel, fruit, and/or cereal. She now limits herself to only two cups of coffee each morning. To avoid going to fast food restaurants, Mary brings her lunch to work and carries lean meat sandwiches on whole grain bread, fruit, soups, pretzels, salads and water, iced tea, or juice. For dinner, she tries to prepare meals each weekend to freeze for weeknights. This way, Mary can quickly heat up pasta, chicken breasts or fish. To stay away from the vending machine, she stashes snacks at her desk, including dry cereal, fruit, cut-up vegetables, and graham crackers. At home, she now has skim milk (instead of whole), fat-free salad dressings, low fat cheeses and reduced fat crackers. Occasionally, she will eat frozen yogurt for her sweet tooth.
- Mary begins a daily exercise program at her health/fitness club. Three days a week, she exercises on either a StairMaster 4000 PT exercise system or a Spinnaker™ 3600 RC™ recumbent exercise cycle for 20 minutes, followed by a five-minute workout on the Gravitron® 2000 AT™ in order to develop her upper body muscles. Two days a week, she works out on the StairMaster CardioSquat™ and Kayak™ machines for 30 minutes combined.
- After nine weeks into her program, Mary has lost 15 pounds (part from

a decreased level of caloric intake and part from a dramatically increased level of caloric expenditure by exercising) and her body fat is now 22 percent. She feels energized, looks better, and is motivated to maintain her new healthy eating and exercise habits even beyond achieving her estimated ideal body weight.

Weighing The Consequences

In summation, the most appropriate approach for achieving permanent weight loss is a sensible diet combined with a program of sound exercise that includes both aerobic conditioning and strength training. While such a weight management "game plan" may not produce as rapid a weight loss as the more popularly promoted, very low-calorie diets (VLCD), it will provide you with a medically sound and effective strategy for "winning the losing game." Almost without exception, VLCD, largely as a result of their detrimental effects on resting metabolic rate, set individuals up for weight regain and, in their eyes, failure—just ask anyone you know who has ever gone through the roller coaster experience of yo-yo dieting. A sensible diet-exercise approach to weight reduction tends to produce a rate of weight loss of about one to two pounds per week (the rate of weight loss recommended by most experts). Although it might take you somewhat longer to reach your desired weight-management goal, any weight lost in this manner tends to be truly lost, not momentarily misplaced. ❏

BIBLIOGRAPHY •

1. American College of Sports Medicine. Position Statement on Proper and Improper Weight Loss Programs. *Med Sci Sports Exerc*, 15(1):9, 1983.
2. American College of Sports Medicine. *Resource Manual for Guidelines for Exercise Testing and Prescription*, 2nd ed. Philadelphia, PA: Lea & Febiger, 1993.
3. Anderson, R., Brownell, K.D., Haskell, W.L. *The Health & Fitness Club Leader's Guide*. Dallas, TX: American Health Publishing Co., 1992.
4. Anspaugh, D., Hamrich, M.H., Rosato, F.D. *Concepts and Applications: Wellness*. St Louis, MO: Mosby Yearbook, 1991.
5. Bennet, W., Gurin, J. *Dieter's Dilemma*. New York, NY: Basic Books, 1988.
6. Bowers, R.W., Fox, E.L. *Sports Physiology*, 3rd ed. Dubuque, IA: Wm. C. Brown Publishers, 1992.
7. Brody, J. *Jane Brody's Nutrition Book*. New York, NY: Bantam Books, 1988.
8. Brooks, G.A., Fahey, T.D. *Exercise Physiology: Human Bioenergetics and Its Applications*. New York, NY: Macmillan Publishing Co., 1985.
9. Bryant, C.X., Peterson, J.A. "How much should you weigh?" *Fit Manag* 8(12):24-26, 1992.
10. Clark, N. *Nancy Clark's Sports Nutrition Guidebook*. Champaign, IL: Leisure Press, 1990.
11. Heyward, V. *Advanced Fitness Assessment and Exercise Prescription*. Champaign, IL: Human Kinetics Books, 1991.
12. Howley, E.T., Franks, B.D. *Health/Fitness Instructor's Handbook*, 2nd ed. Champaign, IL: Human Kinetics Publishers, 1992.

13. McArdle, W.D., Katch, F.I., Katch, V.L. *Exercise Physiology: Energy, Nutrition, and Human Performance*, 3rd ed. Philadelphia, PA: Lea & Febiger, 1991.

14. Miller, D.K., Allen, T.E. *Fitness: A Lifetime Commitment*. New York, NY: Macmillan Publishing Company, 1990.

15. Nieman, D.C. *Fitness and Sports Medicine: An Introduction*, 2nd ed. Palo Alto, CA: Bull Publishing Co., 1990.

16. Polivey, J., Herman, C.P. "Diagnosis and Treatment of Normal Eating." *J Consul Clin Psych*, 55(5), 20, 1987.

17. Van Itallie, T.B. "Topography of body fat: Relationship to risk of cardiovascular and other diseases." In *Anthropometric Standardization Reference Manual*. Lohman, T.G., Roche, A.F., Martorell, R. (Eds.). Champaign, IL: Human Kinetics Books, 1988.

18. Whitney, E.N., Hamilton, E.M.N. *Understanding Nutrition*, 4th ed. New York, NY: West Publishing Co., 1987.

CHAPTER 18

$\bullet \bullet$

EXERCISE AND WOMEN'S ISSUES

by

Robyn M. Stuhr, M.A.
and
Rosemary Agostini, M.D.

• • •

*T*he number of women taking advantage of the opportunities to engage in physically demanding activities, both recreational and in the job force, has increased dramatically since 1972—the year that Congressional legislation mandating equal opportunity for females in all areas of education (including athletics) was enacted. A partial review of the achievements of women in the last 20-plus years illustrates how pervasive and far-reaching this growth has been. During the 1980s, two American women reached the summit of Mt. Everest. A woman recently took first place in a national ultra-marathon race, beating both her female and male competitors. Increasing numbers of women are becoming fire fighters, police officers, construction workers, etc. The effects of Title IX have been demonstrated in the strength, power, agility, and inherent beauty of women participating in the athletic arena.

As more women train and push their bodies to higher limits, however, several important medical issues need to be addressed. Specific areas of concern include the female triad—disordered eating, amenorrhea, and osteoporosis; exercise and pregnancy; exercise and menopause; and musculoskeletal injuries. This chapter provides information that will help women, and the individuals who train them, to design medically sound physical conditioning programs.

THE FEMALE TRIAD

Unfortunately, for some athletic women a risk exists that they may develop one or more of three medical disorders, collectively known as the female triad. The female triad refers to the inter-relatedness of three medical disorders: disordered eating, amenorrhea, and osteoporosis. Young women, driven to excel in their chosen sports and pressured to fit a specific body image (e.g., leanness, low percent body fat, or lower weight) in order to attain their performance goals, place themselves at risk for the development of disordered patterns of eating. Such eating behavior may lead to menstrual dysfunction and, subsequently, premature osteoporosis. Alone, each disorder is a significant medical concern, but, collectively, the potential for more serious health consequences and a higher risk of mortality exists.

EATING DISORDERS AND EXERCISE

Disordered eating refers to the spectrum of abnormal patterns of eating, including behaviors such as the following:

- Bingeing, purging or both
- Food restriction
- Prolonged fasting
- Use of diet pills, diuretics, laxatives
- Inappropriate thought patterns such as preoccupation with food, dissatisfaction with one's body, fear of becoming fat, and a distorted body image

Anorexia nervosa and bulimia nervosa are at the extreme end of the spectrum of disordered eating. Anorexia nervosa is the syndrome of self-imposed starvation and distorted body image. One percent of the general female population suffers from this disorder, and up to nearly seven percent of the population of ballet dancers and gymnasts. Some anorectic women are indistinguishable from high performance athletes. It is essential that you seek professional help if you feel any possibility exists that you might have anorexia nervosa, since it can be fatal. Bulimia nervosa is the syndrome of secretive binge eating episodes followed by self-induced vomiting, fasting, and purging with laxatives and/or diuretics. It affects up to 10% of college-aged students. It can lead to problems with blood electrolytes (hypokalemia, which is low potassium levels), erosion of the teeth, tears in the esophagus, and digestive problems. Again, seek professional help if you think that you may be suffering from bulimia. Although many athletes do not meet strict diagnostic criteria for anorexia nervosa or bulimia nervosa, they may exhibit similar behaviors and thought patterns, placing them at a significantly increased risk for the development of the serious endocrine, metabolic, skeletal, and psychiatric disorders which are often observed in these conditions.

EXERCISE AND MENSTRUAL FUNCTION

Menstruation is the cyclic discharge through the vagina of blood or tissue from the nonpregnant uterus. A normal menstrual cycle ranges from 21 to 36 days. Most women start their menstrual periods by age 16. If your period has not started by that age, or your cycles are shorter than 21 days or longer than 36 days, you should consult your doctor.

Women who engage in intense training may stop having their periods altogether. While the absence of your period may appear to present less of a hassle than fussing with pads, tampons, cramps, etc., it is very important to find out why you are not having a cyclic menstrual period. Two to five percent of the general female population and up to 43% of athletic women do not have menstrual periods—a condition known as amenorrhea. Amenorrhea, however, is not exclusive to athletes; other factors have also been found to cause amenorrhea, including pregnancy, very early menopause, anorexia nervosa, and certain types of tumors.

The cause of exercise-induced amenorrhea is still not fully understood, but contributing factors include excessive weight loss/thinness, age, a previous history of menstrual abnormalities, and diet—not to mention the intensity, duration, and frequency of exercise. The incidence of amenorrhea is particularly high in participants in gymnastics, distance running, ballet, and figure skating. Amenorrhea can, however, occur in any sport.

Why all the concern about amenorrhea? Research beginning in the 1980s has linked amenorrhea to low estrogen levels. Because estrogen is essential for developing and maintaining normal bone health, low levels can reflect serious deficits. Your basic skeleton—calcium deposition in the bone—is laid down by age 35. Theoretically, therefore, if you don't deposit adequate levels of calcium in your bones as a young woman, you may develop osteoporosis (i.e., decreased bone mass and increased susceptibility to fractures) at a relatively earlier age. Worse yet, your case of osteoporosis may be even more severe than normal. Regrettably, osteoporosis affects over 30 million Americans annually.

A more common form of menstrual dysfunction is oligomenorrhea, which is infrequent menstruation of two or more months between cycles. The precise cause of menstrual irregularities is unknown. Amenorrhea and oligomenorrhea are not permanent conditions. In fact, in most highly active women normal menstrual functioning returns one-to-two months after decreasing their levels of physical activity. If amenorrhea persists, you should undergo a thorough hormonal and gynecological evaluation and, if necessary, receive medical treatment.

Perhaps the most common type of menstrual problem is premenstrual syndrome (PMS). Premenstrual syndrome is believed to be caused by a hormonal imbalance—either an excess in estrogen or a deficiency in progesterone. An alternative theory concerning the etiology of PMS has identified the gradual withdrawal of endorphins (opiate-like proteins found in the nervous system) as contributing to PMS. Premenstrual syndrome encompasses a variety of emotional, behavioral, and physical symptoms. Due to the large variability in onset during the menstrual cycle, duration of symptoms, and severity of symptoms, the identification of an appropriate treatment for PMS is often difficult. Non-pharmacologic treatments that have been shown to be effective include exercise, smoking cessation, weight loss, stress reduction/relaxation therapy, minimizing alcohol intake, and a diet high in protein but low in sodium and sugar. If these non-drug therapies are ineffective for you, you should consult your gynecologist for treatment.

Osteoporosis

Osteoporosis refers to premature bone loss and inadequate bone formation, resulting in low bone mass, microarchitectural deterioration, increased skeletal fragility, and an increased risk of fracture. The areas of the body which are most commonly affected by osteoporosis are the hip, wrist, and vertebrae (e.g., compression fractures). Osteoporosis affects over 20 million people in the United States. Research has found that, relatively speaking, women suffer more severely from osteoporosis than men. Women, in general, are at high risk, with older women, Caucasian women, and menopausal women particularly susceptible. Other risk factors include smoking, excessive alcohol consumption, a diet low in calcium, anorexia, amenorrhea, and steroid use.

Any condition or action which reduces the level of calcium in your bones increases your risk of osteoporosis. Factors which have been shown to decrease calcium absorption include smoking, consuming caffeine or alcohol, lactose (milk) intolerance, and high fiber intake. Treatment includes calcium supplements— 1000 mg per day in menstruating women, 1500 mg in menopausal or nonmenstruating women. The best source of calcium, however, is food. Eight ounces of milk or four ounces of cheese provides 200 mg of calcium. Tums or oyster-based calcium is also helpful. A practical guideline is that active women who ingest under 2000 calories daily should supplement their diet with calcium and iron. Amenorrheic and post-menopausal women may wish to consult their physicians regarding the possible benefits (and risks) of hormone replacement therapy. Sunlight and low-impact weight-bearing (e.g., walking, independent step-action stair climbing) or weight-loading (e.g., strength training, Crossrobic™ training) exercise also help keep your bones healthy. It is important to keep in mind that recent evidence suggests that exercise alone is not a sufficient stimulus to prevent the loss of bone mass after menopause. Exercise in combination with estrogen replacement therapy and adequate calcium intake (1500 mg/day), however, has been shown to effectively protect against post-menopausal related bone loss. As a preventive measure, women should be encouraged to exercise and eat a nutritious diet during the critical years between adolescence and early middle-age (35) when bone mass is being laid down.

Exercise During Pregnancy*

Many women want to continue exercising during pregnancy. They are often perplexed, however, by warnings that exercise during pregnancy may be harmful, or by open-ended suggestions to simply "use common sense" when deciding whether to exercise during this important time in their lives. Should pregnant women exercise? To answer this question, three critical issues need to be addressed: Is it safe for a woman who is pregnant to exercise? If so, what types

---

*Editors Note: The material contained in this section is adapted from "Active Pregnancy", an article which appeared in Fitness Management 9 (11): 36-42, 1993.

of exercise modalities and exercise prescriptions are appropriate for a pregnant woman? Finally, what benefits does exercising offer a pregnant woman and the developing fetus?

Without question, the most important factor which must be considered when designing and implementing an exercise program for a pregnant woman is safety. An exercise program must not subject either the expectant mother or her fetus to undue harm or risk of injury. In order to ensure that a pregnant woman can safely engage in a medically sound exercise program, two steps are essential. First, she must be evaluated to determine whether any possible contraindications exist to her exercising. Next, if she is cleared to exercise, she should engage in an exercise program that places particular emphasis on precautionary measures that have been incorporated into the exercise regimen to ensure that the program addresses her special needs as an expectant mother.

CONTRAINDICATIONS FOR EXERCISE DURING PREGNANCY

Prior to initiating or maintaining an exercise program, a pregnant woman must be evaluated for contraindications or signs that she should not exercise. The American College of Obstetricians and Gynecologists (ACOG) provides a list of absolute and relative contraindications for aerobic exercise during pregnancy. Absolute contraindications include coronary heart disease, ruptured membranes, premature labor, multiple gestation, vaginal bleeding, placenta previa, incompetent cervix, history of three or more spontaneous abortions or miscarriages. Relative contraindications include hypertension (high blood pressure), anemia or other blood disorders, thyroid disorders, diabetes, palpitations or irregular heart rhythms, breech presentation in the last trimester, excessive obesity, extreme underweight, history of precipitous labor, history of intrauterine growth retardation, history of bleeding during present pregnancy and an extremely sedentary lifestyle. Women possessing absolute contraindications should not exercise, while those with relative contraindications may exercise with their physician's approval (these women, however, should be enrolled in closely supervised exercise programs). Physicians are the only individuals qualified to evaluate the aforementioned contraindications. A pregnant woman who does not have an obstetrician or physician should not be allowed to participate in an exercise program.

PRECAUTIONARY MEASURES

The numerous physiological changes which occur during pregnancy require special adjustments in an exercise program for the expectant mother. Exercise programs developed for pregnant women should always place particular design emphasis on precautionary measures to avoid placing the mother or her fetus at risk.

One potential threat (especially during the first trimester of pregnancy) to the safety of the developing baby is exercise-induced fetal hyperthermia (i.e., increased temperature in the uterus). Heat stress is known to cause fetal growth retardation in animals. Exercise is associated with a rise in both maternal and fetal body core temperature. The fetus usually maintains a body core temperature of 0.5 - 1.0^{0}C above that of the mother, and has no means of dissipating heat; therefore, the fetus must depend entirely on the mother's thermoregulatory abilities. By adhering to four relatively basic guidelines, a pregnant woman who exercises can ensure she does not place herself and her fetus at risk for heat injury. First, make sure that she is adequately hydrated. This objective can be accomplished by consuming copious amounts of fluid (just short of feeling bloated) thirty minutes before exercise, and drinking beyond the point of thirst cessation during the recovery period. Second, keep the intensity of her exercise regimen at the low end of the intensity range (50-60% of maximal exercise capacity) since this precautionary measure will decrease the heat load generated by the exercise and reduce the strain placed on a pregnant woman's thermoregulatory mechanisms. Third, never wear clothing that is impermeable to water (e.g., the synthetic stretch fibers often worn during aerobic dance), because they prevent the evaporation of sweat from the skin (the body's chief heat loss mechanism), thereby increasing the risk of heat injury. Fourth, and perhaps most importantly, be particularly sensitive to the existing environmental conditions at the time of the exercise bout, since temperature and relative humidity can greatly influence both the degree of heat stress and the body's ability to effectively respond to the heat stress. As a general rule, a pregnant woman should refrain from exercising when the ambient temperature is greater than 80^{0}F and, concurrently, the relative humidity exceeds 50%.

Prolonged (greater than five minutes) exercise performed in a supine (lying face-up) position, may be problematic for some pregnant women. When an expectant mother is in a supine position, the excess weight of her fetus may obstruct venous return (the flow of blood back to the woman's heart). Therefore, after the fourth month of pregnancy, the ACOG recommends that exercise not be performed in a supine position. Signs and symptoms of obstructed blood flow include lightheadedness, dizziness, or syncope (fainting).

Relaxin, a hormone which loosens some of the joints, ligaments and tendons within the body (particularly within the pelvic region), is present in high amounts during the last trimester of pregnancy. Thus, most women are generally more flexible during pregnancy than at any other time in their lives. This increase in joint and connective tissue laxity may increase the potential for joint injury. Pregnant women should, therefore, not overstretch or perform exercises in a ballistic (i.e., jerky, bouncy) manner. The aim of flexibility programs during pregnancy should not be to improve joint range of motion, but rather to relieve muscle cramping or soreness and relax the lower back region in order to alleviate the pain which is generated from the lordostic pressure on the spine.

Finally, it is important that pregnant women carefully monitor their diets to make sure that they consume adequate amounts of carbohydrates to meet the demands of both exercise and their fetus. Fortunately, most pregnant women have little difficulty eating enough to meet the energy demands of exercise.

Once a pregnant woman has been medically cleared to exercise, it is essential that every effort possible be taken to ensure that her exercise program is well-rounded and safe. The two major components of physical fitness that should be considered for inclusion in a comprehensive pre-natal exercise program are aerobic fitness and muscular fitness.

AEROBIC CONDITIONING

The ACOG has established guidelines (refer to Table 18-1) for aerobic exercise during pregnancy and the postpartum period that are based on many of the aforementioned theoretical concerns. These advisory instructions are intended to be suitable for all pregnant women regardless of their basic level of physical fitness. Many leading authorities, however, believe that the ACOG guidelines are too conservative and that a more appropriate exercise prescription for a pregnant woman would be one that is more individualized. These experts feel that decisions related to the type, intensity, duration, and frequency of exercise should be made according to a woman's current fitness level, the stage of her pregnancy, and her personal interests.

It appears that some exercise activities are more suitable than others for a pregnant woman who is just beginning an exercise program. The most suitable aerobic exercises for the newly exercising pregnant woman are low-impact activities such as walking, swimming, cycling and independent-action stair climbing. Women accustomed to running prior to pregnancy can safely continue to do so provided that they "listen to their bodies". All factors considered, the most appropriate form of aerobic exercise for a pregnant woman is the one that she most enjoys and can safely perform.

The fundamental purpose of exercise during pregnancy is to maintain or improve fitness. Thus, the intensity, frequency, and duration at which exercise is prescribed for a pregnant woman should be adjusted slightly downward. An appropriate level of exercise intensity for a pregnant woman is 50% of maximal oxygen uptake, or resting heart rate plus 50%-60% of the difference between resting and maximal heart rate. If, however, a pregnant woman is unable to comfortably carry on a conversation while exercising (a.k.a. the "talk test"), she should reduce her exercise work rate. The "talk test" tends to err on the side of conservatism and can be very helpful in ensuring that the intensity of an exercise bout is not excessive for a particular individual at a particular moment in time. As far as exercise frequency and duration are concerned, it is suggested that a healthy pregnant woman exercise at least three times per week (non-consecutive days) for 20-30 minutes per session. Some examples (e.g., Joan Benoit Samuelson) exist of women who are able to engage in more intense, more frequent and longer bouts of exercise. It is the opinion of many experts that an individualized exercise prescription is safer and more effective for the vast majority of pregnant women. Over the course of their pregnancies, most women appear to spontaneously adjust the intensity, duration, and/or frequency of their workouts to appropriate levels (e.g., most women tend to naturally exercise at lower intensities and for shorter durations during the latter stages of pregnancy).

Table 18-1. American College of Obstetricians and Gynecologists (ACOG) Recommendations for Exercise in Pregnancy and Postpartum*

1. During pregnancy, women can continue to exercise and derive health benefits even from mild-to-moderate exercise routines. Regular exercise (at least three times per week) is preferable to intermittent activity.

2. Women should avoid exercise in the supine position after the first trimester. Such a position is associated with decreased cardiac output in most pregnant women; because the remaining cardiac output will be preferentially distributed away from splanchnic beds (including the uterus) during vigorous exercise, such regimens are best avoided during pregnancy. Prolonged periods of motionless standing should also be avoided.

3. Women should be aware of the decreased oxygen available for aerobic exercise during pregnancy. They should be encouraged to modify the intensity of their exercise according to maternal symptoms. Pregnant women should stop exercising when fatigued and not exercise to exhaustion. Weight-bearing exercises may, under some circumstances, be continued at intensities similar to those prior to pregnancy, throughout pregnancy. Non-weight-bearing exercises, such as cycling or swimming, will minimize the risk of injury and facilitate the continuation of exercise during pregnancy.

4. Morphologic changes in pregnancy should serve as a relative contraindication to types of exercise in which loss of balance could be detrimental to maternal or fetal well-being, especially in the third trimester. Further, any type of exercise involving the potential for even mild abdominal trauma should be avoided.

5. Pregnancy requires an additional 300 kcal/d in order to maintain metabolic homeostasis. Thus, women who exercise during pregnancy should be particularly careful to ensure an adequate diet.

6. Pregnant women who exercise in the first trimester should augment heat dissipation by ensuring adequate hydration, appropriate clothing and optimal environmental surroundings during exercise.

7. Many of the physiologic and morphologic changes of pregnancy persist four to six weeks postpartum. Thus, pre-pregnancy exercise routines should be resumed gradually based upon a woman's physical capability.

* American College of Obstetricians and Gynecologists: *Exercise During Pregnancy and the Postpartum Period (Technical Bulletin #189)*. Washington, DC: ACOG, 1994.

STRENGTH TRAINING

Many women would like to continue strength training during pregnancy, but are somewhat hesitant due to the seemingly inconsistent and diverse opinions available on the subject. In recent years, however, a growing number of professionals from the medical and exercise science communities have tendered specific advice for pregnant women interested in strength training. Most experts agree that based upon the limited data available, proper strength training poses little risk to either the mother or the developing fetus. As a matter of fact, strength training may be very beneficial for a pregnant woman. For example, proper strength training can provide a pregnant woman with an enhanced level of muscular fitness necessary to compensate for the postural adjustments that typically occur during pregnancy. Accordingly, the maintenance of improved posture should help lessen a pregnant woman's likelihood of experiencing low back pain. The performance of activities of daily living should also be relatively easier for a pregnant woman with an improved level of muscular fitness.

Authorities on the subject, however, are relatively quick to point out that strength training is not advisable for all women or all pregnancies. Available research suggests that the following recommendations regarding strength training and pregnancy are appropriate:

- Women having any of the ACOG contraindications for aerobic exercise during pregnancy should not participate in strength training.
- Women who have never strength trained should not participate in an unsupervised strength training program during pregnancy.
- No ballistic exercise movements should be employed during the last trimester of pregnancy.
- Women should be encouraged to breathe normally during strength training, because oxygen delivery to the placenta may be reduced during any act of breath holding (i.e., the performance of a Valsalva maneuver).
- Maximal lifts and heavy resistances should be avoided since they may expose the joints, connective tissue, and skeletal structures of an expectant woman to excessive forces. An exercise set consisting of at least 12-15 repetitions without undue fatigue should ensure that the resistance level is not too great during any particular strength exercise.
- A strength training workout consisting of a single set of a series of exercises, collectively involving all of the major muscle groups of a woman's body, should be performed two times per week.
- As a training effect occurs, it is recommended that overload be achieved initially by increasing the number of repetitions and, subsequently, by increasing the amount of resistance lifted.
- Strength training on machines is generally preferred over using free weights because machines tend to require less skill and can be more easily controlled (i.e., all factors considered, they're safer).
- If a particular strength exercise produces pain or discomfort, it should be discontinued and an alternative exercise should be performed.
- A pregnant woman should immediately consult her physician if any of the following warning signs or complications appear: vaginal bleeding, abdominal pain or cramping, ruptured membranes, elevated blood pressure or heart rate, or lack of fetal movement.

Limited research has shown that strength training can be an integral part of a balanced exercise prescription for a pregnant woman. It would appear that strength training can help a pregnant woman to more effectively manage many of the various rigors of pregnancy. Research also suggests that strength training may not be appropriate for every pregnant woman. Consequently, training prescriptions for those pregnant women who choose to engage in a strength training program should be individualized where appropriate. As a general rule, those individuals involved in designing strength training programs for pregnant women should always be conservative in their approach to manipulating the various strength training variables.

NEVER SETTLE FOR LESS

Scientific evidence exists that exercise can, and will, enhance the well-being of pregnant women. Among the more commonly cited benefits of exercising during pregnancy are the following: it reduces the severity and frequency of back pain associated with pregnancy by helping pregnant women maintain better body posture; it provides a psychological "lift" which helps counteract the feelings of stress, anxiety, and/or depression which can accompany pregnancy; it helps control weight gain; it improves digestion and reduces constipation; and it produces a greater energy reserve for meeting the requirements of daily life.

In summary, an exercise program can and should be undertaken during pregnancy. Controversy still exists, however, regarding the safety and efficacy of vigorous exercise during pregnancy. A good indicator of an appropriate exercise prescription is that the woman be fully recovered within 15-20 minutes after the completion of the exercise bout. Table 18-2 provides a listing of signs and symptoms which should prompt a pregnant woman to stop exercising and consult the physician who is monitoring her pregnancy. A knowledgeable exercise specialist, working closely with the woman's physician, can make exercise a safe (for both the mother and the fetus), productive, and enjoyable endeavor.

Table 18-2. Reasons to Discontinue Exercise and Seek Medical Advice

1. Any signs of vaginal discharge
2. Sudden swelling of the ankles, hands, and face
3. Persistent, severe headaches and/or visual disturbance; unexplained spells of faintness or dizziness
4. Swelling, pain, and redness in the calf of one leg (phlebitis)
5. Elevation of pulse rate or blood pressure that persists after exercise
6. Excessive fatigue, palpitations, chest pain
7. Persistent contractions (>6 to 8/hour) that may suggest onset of premature labor
8. Unexplained abdominal pain
9. Insufficient weight gain (<1.0 kg [2.2 lbs]/month during last two trimesters)

Adapted from Wolfe, et al. "Prescription of aerobic exercise during pregnancy." *Sports Med* 8:273-301, 1989.

Exercise and Menopause

Menopause, commonly referred to as the "change of life," represents the point in time that the cessation of menstrual function occurs. Women typically stop menstruating between the ages of 45 and 55. A gradual decline in reproductive function tends to characterize the 10-15 years preceding the final menstrual period. Hot flashes are perhaps the earliest sign that a woman is going through menopause. Additional signs and symptoms of menopause may include any or all of the following: vaginal dryness, a reduced sex drive, urinary incontinence (a problem with urine leakage), weight gain, anxiety, depression, and irritability. These alterations can be very unpleasant and disconcerting for many women.

Women in the post-menopausal stage undergo several important hormonal changes—most notably, a reduction in serum estrogen levels. The inability of the ovaries to produce estrogen during menopause results in significant physiological changes. The loss of estrogen, for example, causes a decrease in the absorption of minerals (e.g., calcium) by the bones. Lower levels of calcium, an important nutrient, cause the bones to become less dense and weakened, a condition which is collectively known as osteoporosis. Estrogen deficiency may also place post-menopausal women at a higher risk for heart disease because of its effect on blood lipid-lipoprotein profiles. Specifically, low serum estrogen levels have been associated with elevated lipid levels (cholesterol and triglycerides) and reduced levels of high-density lipoprotein (HDL-C—the "good" type of cholesterol carrier that plays a cardioprotective role).

Exercise has been found to have positive effects on several of the menopausal symptoms. For example, exercise promotes bone mineralization, which helps retard the progression of osteoporosis. Anecdotal evidence and limited research suggest that exercise can also decrease the number and severity of hot flashes. Exercise has also been shown to improve self-image and feelings of confidence, decrease anxiety and depression, and positively contribute to energy levels, quality of sleep, and the management of stress in menopausal women.

Post-menopausal women are often instructed to perform pelvic floor (Kegel) exercises. Kegel exercises are designed to improve the tone of the muscles, ligaments, and fascia known as the pelvic floor. The pelvic floor controls urination and defecation, enhances the sexual response to orgasm and provides support to the pelvic organs. Many women are unaware that they have muscles in this area which can be strengthened just like their biceps or quadriceps.

Why should a woman pay attention to this small group of muscles? Millions of women are affected by stress urinary incontinence. Stress urinary incontinence is the involuntary loss of urine during physical exertion or activities such as laughing, sneezing, or coughing. Unfortunately, many women consider incontinence an inevitable consequence of childbirth and aging, which it is not. Active women of all ages report experiencing incontinence. This can be particularly bothersome when it occurs during physical exertion. In fact, some women stop exercising, change their choice of activity or begin wearing a protective pad instead of seeking medical advice or beginning a program of Kegel exercises. Strengthening the pelvic floor muscles can provide these women with needed support and control (refer to reference #17 for detailed information on how to perform Kegel exercises).

MUSCULOSKELETAL PROBLEMS

Injuries appear to be *sport specific* rather than *sex specific*. This statement refers to the fact that injury types and rates are similar for men and women in the same sport, but different for individuals in different sports. One injury-related problem that seems more common in women than men is patellofemoral stress syndrome (pain around and behind the knee cap). Research suggests that this musculoskeletal condition may occur more frequently in women because they have disproportionately wider hips than men. The recommended program for treating this problem includes strengthening the quadriceps (particularly the vastus medialis, the medial portion of the quadriceps muscle), stretching the quadriceps and the hamstrings, and checking for (and correcting) excessive pronation (check to see if there is excessive wear on the lateral portions of the heels on your shoes) or fallen arches in the foot.

Certain women are particularly at-risk for developing stress fractures. Stress fractures are pathological fractures, partial or complete, that occur as a result of recurrent microtrauma. Factors that may predispose women athletes to stress fractures include amenorrhea, anorexia nervosa, low estrogen levels, and low calcium intake. To reduce your risk of stress fractures, you should (hopefully) have normal menstrual periods, limit your volume of exercise (i.e., frequency, intensity, and duration), and eat a well-balanced, calcium-rich diet.

The third trimester of pregnancy represents a time when a woman is at an increased risk for ligamentous and musculoskeletal injuries. Relaxin, a hormone that loosens all the joints, ligaments, and tendons in the body (particularly within the pelvic region), is present in high amounts during the latter stages of pregnancy. Thus, most women will be more flexible during pregnancy than at any other time in their lives. This increase in joint and connective tissue laxity concomitantly increases the potential for joint injury. As a result, pregnant women should avoid overstretching or performing exercises in a ballistic (i.e., jerky, bouncy) manner.

A final concern for active women with regard to injury is breast-related problems that can occur during exercise. Excessive breast movement may cause pain by straining the supporting fascial attachments called Cooper's ligaments. Motion between the breast and a woman's brassiere or shirt can cause sore and/ or bleeding nipples (i.e., jogger's nipple). Abrasions resulting from bra strap fasteners, straps, and underwires are also relatively common occurrences. These problems can be alleviated by the use of a good sports brassiere. A good sports bra should have the following basic design features:

- Judicious placement of seams
- Wide nonelastic shoulder straps
- Breathable fabrics (mesh, cotton/poly blend)
- Seamless cups
- Ample armholes
- Covered hooks or fasteners (if present)
- Little vertical stretch compared with horizontal stretch (for dressing/comfort)

The point to remember is that the selection of a brassiere to wear while exercising is a very personal matter. Each woman should select a sports bra that feels most comfortable for her and permits the least movement of her breasts.

We've Come a Long Way

Exercise can and should be an integral part of a woman's lifestyle. As discussed in this chapter, several special medical considerations exist for physically active women. These special concerns should be taken into consideration for women participating in exercise programs. Fortunately, more and more information is becoming available, and health and fitness professionals are now better equipped to design and supervise exercise programs specifically for women. The key is to seek help from a qualified professional when you have questions regarding exercise and fitness. We have come a long way, but we still have a long way to go. ❑

BIBLIOGRAPHY •

1. American College of Obstetricians and Gynecologists. *Exercise During Pregnancy and the Postpartum Period (Technical Bulletin #189)*. Washington, D.C.: ACOG, 1994.
2. Bachmann, G. "Prevention of menopausal sequelae." *N Engl J Med* 10(2):359-369, 1991.
3. Blair, S., et al. "Physical fitness and all-cause mortality: A prospective study of healthy men and women." *JAMA* 262:2395-2401, 1989.
4. Bo, K., Maehlum, S., et al. "Prevalence of stress urinary incontinence among physically active and sedentary female students." *Scand J Sports Sci* 11(3):113-116, 1989.
5. Bolen, J. "Depression." *Medical & Orthopedic Issues of Active and Athletic Women*. Philadelphia, PA: Hanley & Belfus, pp. 213-216, 1994.
6. Bryant, C.X., Peterson, J.A. "Active Pregnancy." *Fitness Management* 9(11): 36-42, 1993.
7. Chalmers, J., Ho, K.E. "Geographical variations in senile osteoporosis: The association with physical activity." *J Bone Joint Surg* 52:667-675, 1970.
8. Clapp, J.F. "A clinical approach to exercise during pregnancy." *Clin Sports Med* 13(2):443-458, 1994.
9. Clark, N. *Sports Nutrition Guidebook*. Champaign, IL: Leisure Press, 1990.
10. Fletcher, G., et al. "Statement on exercise: Benefits and recommendations for physical activity programs for all Americans." *Circ* 86(1):340-344, 1992.

11. Help for Incontinent People. P. O. Box 544, Union, South Carolina 29379, 800-Bladder.

12. Johnson, M. "Disordered eating." *Medical & Orthopedic Issues of Active and Athletic Women.* Philadelphia, PA: Hanley & Belfus, pp. 141-151, 1994.

13. Kulpa, P. "Exercise during pregnancy and post-partum." *Medical & Orthopedic Issues of Active and Athletic Women.* Philadelphia, PA: Hanley & Belfus, pp. 191-199, 1994.

14. Lemcke, D. "Osteoporosis and menopause." *Medical & Orthopedic Issues of Active and Athletic Women.* Philadelphia, PA: Hanley & Belfus, pp. 175-182, 1994.

15. McMurray, R., Mottola, M., Wolfe, L., Artal, R., et al. "Recent advances in understanding maternal and fetal responses to exercise." *Med Sci Sports Exer* 25(12):1305-1321, 1993.

16. Marshall, L. "Clinical evaluation of amenorrhea in active and athletic women." *Clin Sports Med* 13(2):405-418, 1994.

17. Nattiv, A., Agostini, R., Drinkwater, B., Yeager, K. "The female athlete triad." *Clin Sports Med* 13(2):405-418, 1994.

18. Noble, E. *Essential Exercises for the Childbearing Year,* 3rd ed. Boston, MA: Houghton Mifflin, 1988.

19. Wolfe, L.A., et al. "Prescription of aerobic exercise during pregnancy." *Sports Med* 8:273-301, 1989.

CHAPTER 19

• •

EXERCISE
AND THE
ENVIRONMENT*

by

W. Larry Kenney, Ph.D.
and
George Havenith, Drs.

• • •

Understanding how your body responds and adapts to a variety of environmental conditions that can be present during exercise is critical to ensuring that you remain safe when you engage in physical activity. This chapter focuses on those specific responses and adaptations of your body to several commonly encountered environmental stressors (high heat and humidity, cold, altitude, and air pollution) that affect your exercise performance capability.

HIGH HEAT AND HUMIDITY

Of the many environmental factors which can impact your opportunity to engage in safe and effective exercise, none is as potentially life—and health—threatening as heat stress. Preventing heat-related problems by properly adjusting your exercise program to account for the effects of hot ambient temperatures involves a commonsense approach based on an understanding of how your body physiologically responds to heat. While few documented heat-related standards exist for recreational or clinical exercise environments, industry's experience in dealing with heat stress issues can provide important insight into such matters.

In industrial settings, heat stress has received considerable attention worldwide because of its potential impact on worker productivity, health, and safety.

---

* Note: Some of the material contained in this chapter is adapted from "Considerations for preventive and rehabilitative exercise programs during periods of high heat and humidity," an article which appeared in *The Exercise Standards and Malpractice Reporter* 3(1):1-7, 1989.

While no promulgated standard exists for heat stress evaluation and decision making, several proposed standards regarding this matter exist in the United States and across the world, which provide quantitative information that can be directly applied to an exercise setting. In the U.S. alone, standards for heat stress have been proposed by the National Institute for Occupational Safety and Health (NIOSH), the American Conference of Governmental Industrial Hygienists (ACGIH), the American Industrial Hygiene Association (AIHA), and the U.S. Armed Forces. These organizations all have proposed standards aimed at preventing body temperature from rising excessively during physical exertion, mitigating the deleterious effects of dehydration, etc. Based upon accurately assessing the environmental conditions and the intensity of physical activity, these standards can be easily adapted to an exercise setting (both indoor and outdoor). While various standards differ slightly in their approach, they typically provide two cut-off points: "action limits" above which specific actions should be taken, and "ceiling limits" above which exercise should not be attempted without somehow changing the environment.

EVALUATION OF THE ENVIRONMENT

When trying to make decisions about the thermal environment, it is important that you evaluate all aspects of the environment which impact your ability to exercise safely. Not only are temperature and humidity important, but air movement and (when exercising outdoors) solar radiation also play a major role. One single temperature which takes all the effects into account is the "wet-bulb globe temperature" or "WBGT." WBGT is a single temperature index which is dependent upon air temperature, humidity, solar radiation, and wind velocity, and, as a result, represents a composite measure of the impact of the environment on exercising subjects.

WBGT can be measured using relatively simple low-cost instrumentation or can be calculated from data available from local weather services. Three measurements are combined into the WBGT calculation: air temperature, natural wet-bulb temperature (measured by placing a wetted wick over the thermometer bulb), and globe temperature (the temperature inside a copper globe painted flat black). Indoors, WBGT is calculated as WBGT = (0.7 times natural wet-bulb temperature) + (0.3 times globe temperature) and can be expressed as either ^{0}C or ^{0}F. Outdoor WBGT is calculated as (0.7 times natural wet-bulb) + (0.2 times globe temperature) + (0.1 times air temperature).

BASING EXERCISE DECISIONS ON WBGT

It is important to remember that, even in industry, no enforced standards exist concerning heat stress. Accordingly, the recommended cut-off points presented in this section are meant to serve only as helpful guidelines in deciding such issues as "when it is too hot to exercise," "how long exercise should last under certain conditions," etc. For exercise programs and individual exercise prescription, the criteria document proposed by NIOSH [under the Occupational Safety and Health Act of 1970 (Public Law 91-596)] in 1972 and revised in 1986 can be easily adopted.

Figures 19-1 and 19-2 graphically illustrate the NIOSH's theory regarding what constitutes an appropriate approach to evaluating heat stress. Both figures define several distinct limits concerning when it is safe to exercise which are based on exercise intensity (expressed here as energy expenditure per hour) and ambient WBGT (in both °C and °F). Two sets of limits are proposed, including one set for heat-unacclimatized persons (the Recommended Alert Limit or RAL) and one for heat-acclimatized persons (the Recommended Exposure Limit or REL). Each figure also reflects a proposed "ceiling limit" (C)—a level above which probably no one should exercise unless the environment can be changed. Secondly, several action limit lines are included on each graph for intermittent exercise of varying durations.

Figure 19-1. Recommended Heat-Stress Alert Limits
Heat-Unacclimatized Individuals.

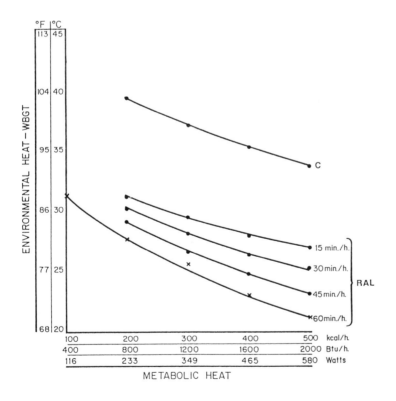

C = Ceiling Limit
RAL = Recommended Alert Limit
* For "standard individual" of 70 kg (154 lbs.) body weight and 1.8 m² (19.4 ft²) body surface.
(Based on information from DHHS NIOSH Publ. No. 86-113)

Figure 19-2. Recommended Heat-Stress Exposure Limits for Heat-Acclimatized Individuals.

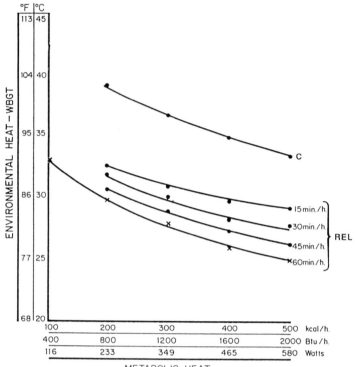

C = Ceiling Limit
REL = Recommended Exposure Limit
* For "standard individual" of 70 kg (154 lbs) body weight and 1.8 m² (19.4 ft²) body surface.
(Based on information from DHHS NIOSH Publ. No. 86-113)

While it takes some practice in using such guidelines to decide when it is safe to exercise, they, in fact, provide a numerical index for making appropriate decisions about your exercise environment. Probably the most important question you may be confronted with is how to deal with an environment which is below the ceiling limit, but above the RAL or REL (whichever applies). This area represents environmental conditions in which exercise can still be performed, but with an increased risk to the participant. In such cases, the following actions are recommended:

- *Change the environment.* If the exercise area cannot be cooled to an appropriate WBGT by means of fans or air conditioning, change the exercise site to one with an environment that meets the WBGT requirements; move to a shaded area or an area with greater air movement.
- *For the session, decrease the exercise intensity.* Similar to cooling the environment, lowering the intensity represents another way of staying within

an acceptable temperature/intensity zone. Ways to accomplish this, while still getting a training effect, include sufficiently slowing the pace of the exercise bout, adding rest cycles to a routine, etc. Perhaps the most useful technique for identifying and maintaining a safe level of exercise intensity involves the proper use of target heart rate (unchanged from cool conditions). Exercise heart rate is increased about one bpm for every degree Centigrade above 25^0C and two bpm for every mm Hg above 20 mm Hg water vapor pressure. Strict adherence to a scientifically determined target heart rate will cause an appropriate decrease in intensity.

Heat acclimation

One of the best methods for decreasing your risk of developing a heat illness or injury is to gradually acclimate yourself to exercising in hot environments. Through this process, your heart rate and body temperature at a given exercise intensity decrease, your sweating rate increases, and your sweat becomes more dilute. It has been estimated that as much as 25% of the apparently healthy population may be heat intolerant in an unacclimated state, with that number decreasing to about two percent after thorough acclimation. The best method of acclimation is to exercise aerobically in a hot environment. The first such session may last as little as 10-15 minutes for safety reasons and gradually increase in duration to 20-60 minutes. It takes most healthy people 10-14 days to fully acclimate to hot environments, although illness and alcohol consumption have been shown to slow this process.

It should also be noted that the benefits of heat acclimation are lost quite rapidly when an individual stops exercising in the heat. In general, with each two days of abstaining from heat exposure, one day of acclimation is lost. Thus, after three to four weeks without heat exposure, an individual should be considered unacclimated. After even short periods without heat exposure (weekends, short periods of illness) risks during heat exposure due to de-acclimation can be substantial.

Fluid Intake

Along with heat acclimation, adequate hydration is a critical factor in preventing adverse side effects of exercise when the temperature and/or humidity is high. Progressive dehydration occurs during exercise when sweating is profuse. As little as a two percent reduction in your body weight during exercise can result in impaired temperature regulation. Furthermore, a four percent decrease in body weight translates into a six percent decrease in maximal aerobic capacity and a 12% reduction in exercise time to exhaustion.

You should take steps to ensure that fluids are readily available so that you can drink before, during, and after exercise. All individuals should be encouraged to drink as much water as is physically comfortable 15-30 minutes prior to exercise, a cupful (6-8 ounces) of water at 15-minute intervals during exercise, and more water than their sense of thirst dictates after exercise. This latter point is especially applicable if you are over the age of 60, since research has shown a decreased thirst sensitivity to body hydration status in elderly persons.

The fluid should be cold (45-55°F) and, palatable; and with a few exceptions, water is the replacement drink of choice. Little need exists to replace electrolytes lost during most exercise sessions, since these small decrements are typically replenished when the next meal is eaten. For participants on a restricted salt diet, their physician should be consulted with regard to salt balance. Unless the exercise bout lasts in excess of 90 minutes, little or no advantage can be attained by consuming commercially marketed sports drinks.

INDIVIDUALS AT RISK

The guidelines presented in this chapter are based on the assumption that the exercise participant does not have any overt disease or condition which may increase the likelihood of a heat illness or injury. Among the factors that can raise your risk of incurring heat-related problems are the following: hypertension (alters the control of skin blood flow), diabetes (neuropathies may affect sweating and/or skin blood flow), aging (alters peripheral cardiovascular and sweating responses), various drug regimens (including diuretics, beta-blockers, alpha-agonists, and vasodilators), alcohol use (causes vasodilation and enhances dehydration), obesity, and a prior history of heat illness or difficulty acclimating to heat. It is in your best interest to be as knowledgeable as possible about the effects of each of these factors on temperature regulation (for more information refer to item 8 in the bibliography).

MANAGEMENT PLAN FOR FACILITIES

In order to be prepared to deal with real or expected periods of hot weather, fitness facilities should develop and implement a standardized management plan for handling stress. Among the topics which should be included in such a plan are:

1. An increase in the level of medical screening and surveillance of exercise participants.
2. An evaluation of all aspects of the facility's thermal environment, preferably using WBGT as a criterion measure.
3. An approved decision-making flowchart concerning heat stress issues, which is based on proposed standards such as NIOSH, ACGIH, AIHA, etc., and tailored to your clientele and exercise setting.
4. A policy of strongly encouraging exercise participants to gradually acclimate to heat stress.
5. Making cold, palatable fluids readily available, and instituting a plan for increasing the fluid intake level of exercise participants before, dur-

ing, and after exercise (schedule drink breaks for the entire exercise group).

6. Take steps to make exercise participants more knowledgeable about heat stress, including early signs and symptoms of heat illness (chills, light-headedness, dizziness, piloerection, nausea, etc.).

7. Emergency procedures, for handling heat illness, which have been incorporated into the overall emergency plan for the facility.

COLD

The winter months signal the advent of cold weather for most areas. Cold temperatures, however, are not an adequate reason for individuals to dramatically alter their aerobic training efforts—even if they prefer to exercise outdoors. Similar to exercising in extreme heat, you can safely exercise in the cold, provided that you adhere to a few commonsense guidelines. Such guidelines are applicable to all of your alternatives for exercising aerobically outdoors in the cold, including jogging, cross-country skiing, and ice skating.

HOW DOES THE BODY RESPOND TO THE COLD?

Before you identify what you personally can do to adapt to cold weather conditions, you should first consider how your body responds to the cold. Essentially, your body responds physiologically to cold weather in two primary ways: increased metabolic rate and increased tissue insulation.

Changes in metabolic rate can be elicited either voluntarily (by exercising) or involuntarily (shivering thermogenesis). Thermogenesis involves the production of heat in your body by means of shivering (and to a smaller degree, sympathetic chemical excitation). Shivering results from "cold" signals to the hypothalamus which in turn sends nonrhythmic impulses to the anterior motorneurons of the skeletal muscles throughout your body. Contrary to most individuals' perception of the process of shivering, these impulses do not cause the muscles to actually shake. Rather, they prompt the muscle spindle stretch reflex mechanism to oscillate. At a certain point, shivering begins and heat production rises. During maximal shivering, your body can increase the amount of heat it produces to as high as four to five times normal.

Before your body alters its metabolic rate, however, its initial response to the cold is to constrict blood vessels. Except for your head, this constriction occurs in the surface blood vessels in most of the peripheral areas of your body (hence the term peripheral vasoconstriction). When blood is literally sidetracked from the surface areas of your body into the deeper blood vessels, the net effect of the process of vasoconstriction is to increase the relative insulative level of surface tissues. When blood is shunted away from a person's skin, the "insulative thickness" of the surface tissues is increased. In turn, the rate of heat loss decreases.

Exercise Responses To The Cold

Under most circumstances, cold weather should not present a significant problem for anyone who wants to exercise outdoors. Cold ambient air, for example, does not pose a particular danger to your respiratory passages. By the time that inspired air reaches the bronchi in your lungs, the air is warmed to a temperature sufficiently high to be safe. Humans can breathe air at temperatures as low as -35^0C (-31^0F) without a detrimental effect; however, in individuals who have angina, breathing cold air may interfere with their ability to recognize anginal pain. Using a scarf to cover your nose and mouth will pre-warm and pre-humidify the air.

As long as your body core temperature is kept relatively normal, and sufficient clothing is worn to keep the surface areas of your body relatively warm, your capacity to exercise will not be impaired. Your maximal ability to take in, transport, and utilize oxygen (maximal oxygen uptake) and the oxygen cost of submaximal exercise are generally unaffected by the cold. Your heart rate may be slightly lower while exercising in the cold, but this is not a universal finding. Stroke volume (the amount of blood pumped by the heart per beat) tends to be higher at low exercise intensities, but is unaffected by cold at higher workloads. Cardiac output (the amount of blood pumped by the heart on a per minute basis) is not changed.

If your core temperature and muscle temperature fall below normal, your maximal aerobic capacity and cardiovascular endurance may be reduced. A cool muscle has a decreased ability to generate force for a given cross-sectional area of muscle fibers. Therefore, in order to maintain force, more fast twitch fibers must be recruited, resulting in a greater reliance on anaerobic glycolysis and, perhaps, more lactic acid production. Thus, your ability to perform activities that require dynamic muscle strength and power may be negatively affected by cold weather.

Fortunately, the process of maintaining your body core temperature at normal levels and of insulating the exterior surface area of your body against the cold elements is not particularly difficult. As was discussed previously, under almost all conditions, your body produces sufficient heat to maintain its core temperature. Aerobic exercise makes it easier for your body to regulate its core temperature on a more voluntary basis. During exercise, more than 75% of the energy produced by your working muscles is converted to heat, which elevates core temperature. During moderate and intense exercise, sufficient heat is generated to maintain core temperature. At low intensities of exercise, however, core temperature could begin to fall after one hour of exercise in cold weather were it not for the onset of involuntary thermogenesis.

Insulating your body against the cold by wearing sufficient clothes involves common sense. Clothing traps warm air next to your skin and decreases heat loss by conduction and convection. It is important that you wear water repellent outer clothing (to prevent soaking from rain or snow) and inner clothing which allows sweat to evaporate. Wet or damp clothing transfers heat away from your body up to 20 times faster than dry clothing. Accordingly, the best clothing for exercising in the cold is that which protects your body from the cold, while still allowing sweat to evaporate. In recent years, significant progress has been made in the development and manufacture of cold weather exercise clothing. Clothing made of GORE-TEX™ fabric, for example, is lightweight and provides adequate protection from the environmental stressors, yet still permits water (perspiration) to evaporate.

Most experts suggest wearing several layers of clothing so that the articles can be removed—a layer at a time—as you become warmer while exercising (due to increases in metabolic heat production). In general, the following guidelines are recommended with regard to clothing:

- Avoid heavy, bulky garments.
- Use up to four layers of clothing in severe weather.
- Wear an absorbent, non-irritating material for the first layer of clothing.
- Wear socks made of an absorbent, breathable material.
- Protect your hands—wear cotton or wool gloves.
- Wear a hat—large amounts of heat can be lost from an uncovered head.
- If necessary, keep your facial area warm—preferably with a wool scarf.

How Cold Is Too Cold?

Under most conditions, it will not be too cold for you to exercise outdoors provided you dress properly. In a few circumstances, however, the relative temperature will be such that exercising outdoors would be ill-advised. The most common way to express relative temperature is the wind chill index. Ambient temperature alone is not always a valid indication of "coldness." Because wind exacerbates heat loss by increasing the degree to which the warmer insulating air layer which surrounds your body is continually replaced by the cooler ambient air (collectively, it increases the convective heat loss), wind can have a substantial cooling effect on your body. For example, the combination of a -9.4^{0}C (15^{0}F) temperature with 30 MPH winds produces the equivalent temperature of -32.2^{0}C (-26^{0}F). The measure used to quantify these equivalent temperatures is the wind chill index. Individuals who plan to exercise in cold weather should consult a wind chill index table (see Table 19-1) to ensure that the cooling effect of the wind—in concert with the ambient air temperature—does not place them in a potentially unsafe environment for working out. As a rule of thumb, any wind chill temperature of less than minus twenty degrees Fahrenheit should be viewed with caution and greater than minus seventy degrees Fahrenheit is potentially quite unsafe.

The key to safely exercising out-of-doors is to be prepared. Bundle up—in layers. Use common sense. Unless the wind chill index dictates otherwise, don't let the elements interfere with the benefits and joy of exercising.

Wind Speed (mph)	Thermometer Reading (°F)										
	50	40	30	20	10	0	-10	-20	-30	-40	-50
	(Equivalent temperature [°F])										
5	48	37	27	16	6	-5	-15	-26	-36	-47	-57
10	40	28	16	4	-9	-24	-33	-46	-58	-70	-83
15	36	22	9	-5	-18	-32	-45	-58	-72	-85	-99
20	32	18	4	-10	-25	-39	-53	-67	-82	-96	-110
25	30	16	0	-15	-29	-44	-59	-74	-88	-104	-118
30	28	13	-2	-18	-33	-48	-63	-79	-94	-109	-125
35	27	11	-4	-20	-35	-51	-67	-82	-98	-113	-129
40*	26	10	-6	-21	-37	-53	-69	-85	-100	-115	-132
	Minimal Risk				Increasing Risk				Great Risk		

Table 19-1. Wind Chill Index.

* Wind speeds greater than 40 MPH have little additional effect.

HYPOTHERMIA DURING WATER SPORTS

A risk of hypothermia is also present at higher ambient temperatures, when people are active in water-related sports (e.g., swimming or [wind] surfing). Water exposure results in an increase in heat loss of up to 25 times that in air environments. During the swimming sessions of triathlons, when water temperatures are 18-19°C (64-66°F), 10%-30% of contestants have body core temperatures below 35°C (95°F). At such temperatures, both physiological and psychological effects of the cooling can be expected. Similar problems may also occur during the cycling period after the swimming session, due to an "after drop" in body core temperature during the first 10 minutes of cycling. The risk of hypothermia for novice windsurfers is relatively high. Regular dips in cool water, with subsequent evaporation of the moisture when standing on the board, in combination with physical exhaustion, may create a substantial risk of hypothermia.

ALTITUDE

The relative altitude where you exercise can also have an effect on your body. As altitude increases, barometric pressure decreases and the air becomes less dense. The percentage of oxygen in the air stays fairly constant (20.93%) with changing altitude, but due to the declining barometric pressure, the partial pressure of oxygen (pO2) declines. At sea level, pO2 is 159 mm Hg, at 5,300 feet (Denver, Colorado), it is reduced to 132 mm Hg; and at 14,100 feet (Pikes Peak), it is as low as 94 mm Hg. A consequence of the reduction in pO2 is that hemoglobin saturation is decreased (i.e., less oxygen is carried by the arterial blood), and the amount of oxygen available at the cellular level is diminished. This reduces maximal oxygen uptake ($\dot{V}O_{2\,max}$) and concomitantly limits your physical working capacity (PWC). The reduction in $\dot{V}O_{2\,max}$ and PWC is directly proportional to the increase in altitude. At very low pO2's (< 100 mm Hg), mental and motor performance may also be impaired. Problems with judgment result in a higher risk of being in an accident.

Changes in performance capabilities begin to manifest themselves at approximately 5,000 feet (1,524 meters). For example, activities such as sprinting or long jumping tend to be enhanced at altitude—a performance improvement that likely results from the fact that your body has to overcome less resistance (since the air is less dense) while it is in flight. It appears, however, that the more aerobic an activity is, the more it will be negatively affected by altitude. As a rule, the higher the altitude, the larger the decrement in aerobic performance. Since less oxygen is present in your blood at high altitude, your heart beats more frequently to deliver a sufficient amount of oxygen to your working muscles. As a result, when you are exercising at a high altitude, you must reduce the intensity of your exercise bout in order to stay within your training heart rate range.

When you remain at high altitude for extended periods, acclimatization occurs. This is achieved by an increase in red blood cell production, thereby increasing oxygen transport capacity. An improved muscle vascularization and increased cellular oxidative capacity also occurs. $\dot{V}O_{2\,max}$ and PWC typically do not reach levels seen at sea level, however.

Many people experience some form of acute mountain sickness (AMS) after about six hours at high altitude. Symptoms such as a severe headache, lassitude, nausea, indigestion, and sleep disturbances are observed in some individuals at levels of 7,000 feet, and are quite common above 10,000 feet. At these higher altitudes, more severe symptoms such as brain or lung edema can occur. As a result of modern transportation (airplanes, cable cars, or mountain ascents by automobile), ascent times have decreased and incidences of mountain sickness have increased. A rule of thumb for the prevention of AMS is: rest one day at 7,500 feet and another day for each additional 2,000 feet increase in altitude. In addition, it is advisable to sleep at a lower altitude than where you reside during the daytime—"climb high, sleep low." If you experience AMS, the rule is as follows: mild symptoms, stop ascent until the symptoms disappear; more severe symptoms, descend to a lower altitude.

An additional factor which coincides with an increase in altitude is a change of climate. In general, with every 1,000 feet, ambient temperature decreases 2^0C. Thus, additional risks of cooling (wind chill and hypothermia) are present. In addition, the risk of dehydration is higher at altitude. Water loss is increased and water intake is often reduced due to limited availability. The former is due to both the decrease in the amount of water vapor in the air with altitude (increased evaporation) and increased diuresis (urine production). Thus, you should drink more than normal (> 2.5 liters/day) when at altitude. Finally, at altitude the amount of UV-radiation is much stronger than at sea level. As a result, you should take precautions with respect to sunburn and snow blindness.

AIR POLLUTION

A vast number of people involved in exercise and sports inhabit densely populated urban areas where they are increasingly confronted with problems related to air pollution caused by traffic and industry. During times of temperature inversion or when air movement is low, air pollutants can reach concentrations that can severely impede physical performance. The most common air pollutants are: carbon monoxide, sulfur oxides, nitrogen oxides, ozone, peroxy-acetyl-nitrate, aerosols, soot, dust, and smoke. The effect of these pollutants is, in part, related to their penetration into the body.

As they are inhaled, the main effects of air pollutants are on the respiratory tract. The nose removes large particles and highly soluble gases very effectively (e.g., 99.9% of inhaled sulfur dioxide is removed in the nose), but smaller particles and agents with low solubility pass easily. During exercise, where mouth breathing plays an important role, this air filtration process is much less efficient, and more pollutants reach the lungs. With respect to the short-term effects of pollutants on exercise performance, the main problems are irritation of the upper respiratory tract, respiratory discomfort, and reductions in the oxygen transport capacity of the blood.

Carbon monoxide (CO) emissions in urban areas are greater than emissions of all other pollutants combined. CO primarily affects exercise performance through its strong (200 times stronger than that of oxygen) capacity to bind to hemoglobin (COHb) in the blood, thereby reducing the blood's capacity to transport oxygen to the tissues. Very high levels of COHb are needed to produce reductions in submaximal exercise performance. Therefore, under realistic outdoor conditions, CO effects only become evident when maximal exercise performance is at issue. For example, maximal oxygen uptake is reduced at COHb concentrations above 4.3%. During prolonged exposure to heavy traffic, COHb concentrations of 5% have been observed. In persons with cardiovascular impairment, problems may occur during submaximal exercise at lower concentrations of COHb (2.5%-3%).

Sulfur oxides (SOx), mainly in the form of sulfur dioxide, exert their influence through irritation of the upper respiratory tract, which can cause reflexive bronchoconstriction and increased airway resistance. Nose breathing strongly reduces this effect compared to mouth breathing. For submaximal exercise, the threshold level before pulmonary function is compromised is between one and three parts per million (ppm). For maximal exercise, no cut-offs are as yet available. For asthmatics, the threshold values for eliciting a bronchoconstrictor response are lower (0.2-0.5 ppm of SO_2).

Of the nitrogen oxides (NOx), only the effect of nitrogen dioxide (NO_2) has been studied in humans. Acute exposure to high concentrations of NO_2 (200-4000 ppm) is extremely dangerous and has resulted in several deaths. During submaximal exercise, no effect of NO_2 levels up to 1-2 ppm has been observed, but effects of higher concentrations and/or its effects during maximal exercise have not been studied.

Another pollutant which may create a health risk is ozone (O_3). During light to moderate submaximal exercise lasting several hours, exposures to 0.3-0.45 ppm O_3 have resulted in decrements in pulmonary function and increased subjective discomfort. For more intense levels of exercise, the respiratory discomfort can become severe and thereby limit performance. Ozone has also been associated with eye irritation, general respiratory discomfort, and nausea.

Effects of aerosols on physiological function are usually caused by their effect as an airway irritant. The most common aerosols are sulfates (minimal adverse effects), sulfuric acids (minimal effect unless prolonged exposure, larger particles, and/or high ambient humidity), nitrate aerosols (minimal effect), and saturated and unsaturated aldehydes (e.g., formaldehyde, acrolein, and crotonaldehyde) are also irritants with minimal effect.

The effects of minute particles of soot, dust, and smoke on exercising humans have not been evaluated. Generally, particulate inhalation results in bronchoconstriction. The penetration of these particulates in the respiratory system is related to the size of the particle. Below three microns, they can reach the alveoli; between three and five microns, they usually settle in the upper respiratory tract; and above five microns, they are not able to enter the respiratory tract. Thus, particles smaller than five microns can cause pulmonary inflammation, congestion, or ulceration. Exercise, by increasing respiratory rate, may aggravate the contamination of the lungs.

The presence of more than one pollutant—which is generally the case in most smog conditions—usually has a more powerful effect on the body. Also, an interaction of air pollution with other environmental stressors (e.g., heat, cold, and altitude) may occur. For example, additive effects have been observed for heat stress and carbon monoxide, peroxy-acetyl-nitrate, and ozone. Low relative humidity enhances adverse health effects of ozone, whereas high relative humidity may enhance the untoward effects of sulfur dioxide and nitrogen dioxide. Low ambient temperature can, through breathing cold air, result in reflexive bronchoconstriction, especially in asthmatic individuals. For such individuals, the presence of a pollutant in the air they breathe has an even stronger effect than the sum of the two separate effects (i.e., cold and pollution. Finally, high altitude interacts with carbon monoxide. Both stressors limit the oxygen transport capacity of the blood and, thus, create cumulative adverse effects on exercise performance. Pollutants originating from cigarette smoking should also be avoided prior to and during exercise. The pollutants present in cigarette smoke have been shown to have a deleterious effect on exercise performance. When combined with smog, the effects of cigarette smoke are obviously compounded.

When exercise is to be performed in a high pollution area, valuable information may be acquired from local meteorologists. In order to minimize potential problems, you should carefully plan your activities, taking into consideration daily and seasonal fluctuations in pollution:

- Avoid exercise during rush hours (the CO level peaks during rush hours).
- Avoid high cigarette smoking areas prior to and during exercise.
- Avoid combinations of high temperature, humidity, and air pollution (high heat and humidity potentiate the deleterious effect of air pollution).
- Limit the amount of time spent in high pollution areas to a minimum (physiological effects of air pollution are both time and dose dependent).
- Be aware of seasonal variations in ozone levels. The ozone level is usually low in winter, increases during summer with a daily peak around 3 p.m., and reaches maximal peak values in early autumn. ❏

BIBLIOGRAPHY •

1. Adams, W.C. "Effects of ozone exposure at ambient air pollution episode levels on exercise performance." *Sports Med* 4:395-424, 1987.
2. American Conference of Governmental Industrial Hygienists. "Threshold limit values for chemical substances and physical agents in the workroom environment with intended changes." ACGIH, Cincinnati, 1979.
3. American Industrial Hygiene Association. "Heating and cooling for man in industry," 2nd Ed. AIHA, Akron, 1975.
4. Balke, B. "Variations in altitude and its effects on exercise performance." In *Exercise Physiology*. Falls, H. (Ed). New York, NY: Academic Press, pp. 240-265, 1968.
5. Brooks, G.A., Fahey, T.D. *Exercise Physiology: Human Bioenergetics and Its Applications*. New York, NY: John Wiley & Sons, 1984.
6. Hage, P. "Air pollution: adverse effects on athletic performance." *Phys Sportsmed* 10:126-132, 1982.
7. Horvath, S.M. "Exercise in a cold environment." *Exerc Sport Sci Rev* 9:221-263, 1981.
8. Kenney, W.L. "Physiological correlates of heat intolerance." *Sports Med* 2:279-286, 1985.
9. National Institute for Occupational Safety and Health. "Criteria for a recommended standard . . . occupational exposure to hot environments." (DHHS NIOSH Publ. No. 86-113), U.S. Department of Health and Human Services, Washington, DC, 1986.
10. Pierson, W.E., Covert, D.S., Koenig, J.Q., et al. "Implications of air pollution effects on athletic performance." *Med Sci Sports Exerc* 18:322-327, 1986.
11. Powers, S.K., Howley, E.T. *Exercise Physiology: Theory and Application to Fitness and Performance*. Dubuque, IA: Wm. C. Brown Publishers, 1990.
12. Sawka, M.N., et al. "Hydration and vascular fluid shifts during exercise in the heat." *J Appl Physiol* 56:91-96, 1984.
13. Sutton, J.R., Jones, N.L. "Exercise at altitude." *Ann Rev Physiol* 45:427-437, 1983.
14. Triservices Document. "Prevention, treatment, and control of heat injury." *US Army TB Med* 507, 1980.

CHAPTER 20

EXERCISE ADHERENCE:
IMPLICATIONS FOR ADULT
FITNESS AND CARDIAC
REHABILITATION PROGRAMS

by

Barry A. Franklin, Ph.D., Susan Haapaniemi, M.S.
Kirk Hendrickson, B.S., and Linda Terrien, R.N., B.S.N.

• • •

Since the 1970s, the American public has displayed a heightened awareness of the important role that regular physical activity plays in the promotion of a healthy lifestyle and the avoidance of chronic disease. Among the factors which reflect this change in attitude toward exercise has been the extraordinarily high levels of exercise equipment sales, which reached $2.075 billion in 1991. Recent studies have shown that exercise offers significant health benefits for all Americans, including those who, for whatever reason, choose to engage in vigorous exercise. Expectations are that these new, more positive attitudes towards regular physical activity will continue to grow, as additional scientific information is obtained.

Regular aerobic exercise is widely promoted in the prevention and treatment of several "chronic" health problems. Exercise training, for example, decreases the rate-pressure product and perceived exertion during standard submaximal work loads and increases the maximal oxygen uptake ($VO_{2\ max}$) by approximately 20% ± 10%. Aerobic exercise training also helps control diabetes, obesity, blood lipid abnormalities, as well as lowers blood pressure. Conversely, sedentary living is now recognized as a major risk factor for the development of coronary artery disease.

Despite the preventive and therapeutic value of physical activity, few Americans exercise on a regular basis. Only 22% of American adults engage in leisure time activity at the level recommended for health benefits; in addition,

24% are completely sedentary, and 54% would benefit from more activity. Dropout rates among those who voluntarily enter physical conditioning programs are generally highest in the first three months, increasing to approximately 50% by 12 months (refer to Figure 20-1). Thus, it appears that exercise is not unlike other health-related behaviors (e.g., medication compliance, smoking cessation, weight reduction) in that typically half of the individuals who initiate a behavior change will maintain that change, regardless of the specific type of program or the initial health status of the individuals.

Figure 20-1. Relationship between the dropout rate (%) and the duration of exercise training (months) in 7 studies with a total of 734 healthy adults and 14 studies with a total of 3,887 cardiac patients. Widely differing definitions of "exercise dropout" in these studies may have contributed to the variability in results.

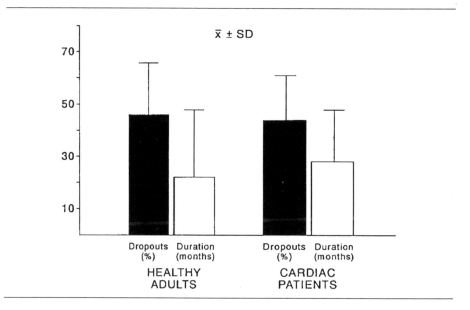

The primary factors associated with poor exercise adherence include cigarette smoking, blue collar occupation, lack of recreational exercise, and an inactive occupation. The noncompliance rate appears to increase progressively, from 59% in the presence of smoking alone, to 95% when all four factors are present. Additional characteristics of the early exercise dropout are shown in Table 20-1 and include obesity, low socioeconomic status and increased physical strength. Psychological traits that predict exercise dropout proneness include Type A personality, depression, anxiety, low self-motivation, hypochondriasis, low ego strength, and extreme introversion or extroversion.

According to Prochaska and DiClemente, interventions designed to empower clients/patients to initiate and maintain lifestyle modifications should be based on their particular stage of readiness for change (refer to Figure 20-2). For example, while the "precontemplator" may need consciousness raising, the "con-

Table 20-1. Variables Predicting the Exercise Dropout.

Personal Factors	Program Factors	Other Factors
Smoker	Inconvenient	Lack of spouse support
Inactive leisure time	time/location	Inclement weather
Inactive occupation	Excessive cost	Excessive job travel
Blue-collar worker	High-intensity exercise	Injury
Type A personality	Lack of exercise variety	Medical problems
Increased physical strength	(e.g., running only)	Job change/move
Extroverted	Exercises alone	
Poor credit rating	Lack of positive feedback	
Overweight and/or overfat	or reinforcement	
Poor self-image	Inflexible exercise goals	
Depressed	Low enjoyability ratings	
Hypochondriacal	Poor exercise leadership	
Anxious		
Introverted		
Low ego strength		

templator" may require a critical analysis of the advantages and limitations of changing behavior versus remaining status quo. Similarly, exploring alternative action plans, providing specific instructions (how to's), offering positive personal feedback, and halting recidivism, may be employed for the determination, action, maintenance, and relapse stages, respectively. It is important, however, to recognize that deviations from serial progression, that is, either temporary or permanent exits, are most likely to occur during the determination and maintenance phases.

Physicians and allied health professionals can use several interventions that are applicable to this model to enhance exercise adherence. The purposes of this chapter are: (a) to present educational and motivational strategies to the exercise leader or adult fitness program director who is vitally interested in stimulating interest and enthusiasm among program participants; (b) to summarize the advantages and limitations of different program settings or models, specifically group versus home-based exercise training; and (c) to review the value of continuing education through workshops and certifications to reinforce the knowledge and proficiency standards, responsibilities, and behavioral strategies of the good exercise leader.

EDUCATION

Education plays a critical role in enhancing client/patient adherence to preventive and rehabilitative exercise programs. The goal of education is to foster competence—which has been defined as "knowing what we're doing, why it works, and doing it on purpose." Education stressing the "hows" and "whys" of exercise should serve as an integral part of a physical conditioning program and include substantive information on body mechanics, energy expenditure, exercise prescription, the importance of warming up and cooling down, exercise myths and misconceptions, guidelines on appropriate exercise clothing and shoes, nutrition, and the effects of environmental stressors (e.g., heat, humidity, cold, etc.) on exercise performance. Participants should also be cautioned against practices that counteract the benefits of exercise and/or may be potentially hazardous (proscriptions), such as exercise during illness, taking cold or very hot showers immediately after a workout, cigarette smoking, alcohol consumption, ingestion of heavy meals immediately before or soon after exercise, and infrequent high-intensity exercise bouts.

Effective participant education is predicated on several fundamental principles of learning. It is important to realize that learning styles may vary from one participant to another. Some people respond to visual material, while others more easily grasp phonetic (auditory), tactile, or kinesthetic stimuli. Optimal learning and retention occurs when information is presented in a variety of formats, and reinforced on a regular basis.

Education should also include individualized instruction. This helps to ensure that participants receive customized learning opportunities that are tailored to their specific needs. The educational curriculum should provide interactive learning that allows participants to ask questions and to "learn by doing." Accordingly, the instructional program should place sufficient demand on the participant to cause him or her to feel a direct emotional interaction with the materials.

These principles are reflected in surveys of individual's learning preferences. One-on-one interaction is generally the learning method of choice, followed by slides and movies, books and pamphlets, and group discussions, respectively. The least-preferred method of learning is one of the most common—the lecture. These responses agree with the principle that people learn best when they are actively involved in the learning process, as opposed to being passive recipients of information.

The same general learning principles can be applied to the adult fitness or cardiac rehabilitation program. The educational component should ideally begin with an individualized or small-group introductory meeting. This provides a foundation for the entire educational process, when overall goals are reviewed, and participants receive an orientation to the program. Next, the staff should work to mutually establish specific goals and approaches for the participant. While many persons may have similar goals, varied benefits of the program may be emphasized for different individuals. For example, one client may focus on diet and exercise for the reduction of body weight and fat stores, while another may seek to improve physical work capacity. Mutual goal setting is especially important, because it reduces the potential for resistance and dropout, fosters participants' self-worth and empowerment, and ensures that the clients' needs are being met.

An individual interview also provides an opportunity to identify the client's developmental state, coping techniques/defense mechanisms, belief systems and values, social support systems, expectations (realistic or unrealistic), and stage of readiness for change (refer to Figure 20-2). In a one-on-one session, personalized material, such as the exercise prescription, can be explained at a pace that is compatible with the participant's learning ability. Moreover, individual counseling allows for considerable interaction and immediate feedback in an environment that is less threatening than a large group setting. Among cardiac patients, "being embarrassed" is often cited as a key barrier to getting information. Individualized sessions can be invaluable in minimizing these concerns.

Figure 20-2. Progressive stages of readiness for behavior change, with specific reference to temporary and permanent exits and relapse. (From Prochaska and DiClemente).

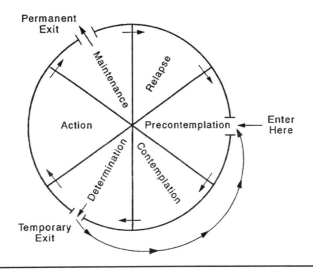

In some programs, participants are assigned to a staff member who oversees their involvement on an ongoing basis, from orientation to exercise sessions, educational activities, assessment, and general problem-solving. This approach—known as primary care—has proven to be quite successful in enhancing patients' retention of information, as well as ensuring satisfaction. It is, however, not always compatible with the complexities of staff scheduling. Alternative approaches to education and counseling are provided in the following sections.

SLIDE PRESENTATIONS

Slide presentations accommodate both visual and auditory learning styles in a group setting. In addition, question-and-answer periods permit interaction with, and clarification from, professional staff. Combining slides with a lecture results in increased comprehension, compared to a lecture alone (which is the least-preferred method of learning). Care should be taken, however, to avoid an overemphasis on statistics and complex graphs, figures, tables, and charts. To this end, it is recommended that at least every third or fourth slide be a picture or cartoon which serves to reinforce a salient point.

MINI-LECTURES AND/OR QUESTIONS OF THE DAY

Usually conducted during or immediately after an exercise session, these require less time (generally 2-10 minutes) than formal group lectures, and allow for immediate feedback from professional staff. Mini-lectures are best suited to subject matter that is focused or limited in scope, and are primarily used to reinforce information that has previously been presented.

BOOKS AND PAMPHLETS

Every program should have a variety of written materials that are readily available to participants. Such materials are especially well-suited to the independent visual learner. However, when providing client and family instructive materials, it is important to use those written by physicians or allied health professionals for national guidelines and associations (refer to Table 20-2).

Table 20-2. National Educational Programs and Guidelines.

National Institutes of Health
National Cholesterol Education Program
American Diabetes Association
American Lung Association
American College of Sports Medicine
American Heart Association
American Cancer Society
National Weight Control Resource Directory
Sports and Cardiovascular Nutritionists of the
   American Dietetic Association
National Heart Attack Alert Program

NEWSLETTERS

Newsletters can be informative, customized vehicles for providing health and fitness information in the context of a specific program. The level of difficulty and subject matter can be easily tailored to the needs and interests of the participants. Authors may include professional staff, student interns, or the clients themselves. Newsletters can also incorporate other motivational techniques, such as announcements and awards.

BULLETIN BOARDS

Like mini-lectures, bulletin boards can be used to highlight focused information. Also, the visual nature of a bulletin board contributes to the multi-media aspect of an educational curriculum. Bulletin boards can be readily altered, making them an excellent way to reinforce information and communicate regular updates on fitness and health. They can also increase group cohesiveness and camaraderie when participants are encouraged to provide educational, personal, and humorous contributions.

MODELS

Anatomical diagrams and models are especially valuable educational tools for the kinesthetic learner. The availability of these for independent study, as well as during individual and group instruction, provides customized, private learning opportunities, and enhances overall comprehension.

VIDEOS

The escalating use of videos by the general public makes this an attractive educational option. To capitalize on the recent proliferation of VCRs, a video library should be part of a comprehensive program. Videos give participants the opportunity to learn independently in the privacy of their homes, at a convenient time. Also, family members can be simultaneously educated.

GUIDED PRACTICE

Practice, or hands-on learning, is perhaps the most fundamental and effective means of grasping and retaining information. Learning is the process whereby knowledge is created through the transformation of experience. True understanding does not occur until the participant has a chance to experience the concept. Accordingly, a participant may appreciate the significance of the target heart rate concept and the importance of accurately palpating pulse when they face the challenge of modulating the appropriate exercise intensity.

Regardless of the format in which information is delivered, it is critical to ensure that it is understandable. Ninety percent of all patient educational materials are above the average U.S. reading level (8th grade). If participants can't comprehend the information, they won't comply. Thus, all written materials should be assessed for reading difficulty. This can be done with simple formulas that consider the number of syllables in the text, and the average sentence length. If appropriate materials cannot be obtained, existing materials should be rewritten in a simpler style. For example, complicated text can be modified by substituting commonly used words for medical terminology. Conversely, the teaching of medical terminology can be incorporated into the curriculum, so that participants can comprehend the material.

In conclusion, educational programs that are geared toward developing competence should serve to enhance exercise adherence. Programs should be structured and include a variety of materials to accommodate diverse learning styles, reading abilities, areas of personal interest, and learning preferences. There should also be opportunities for individual instruction and feedback, regular reinforcement of materials, and methods for evaluating outcomes.

MOTIVATION

In addition to educating people about exercise, it is necessary to motivate them to act. Motivation is a crucial factor in program effectiveness, safety, and long-term adherence. Programmatic and related factors affecting exercise adherence are shown in Figure 20-3. Unfortunately, the negative variables often outweigh the positive variables that contribute to sustained participant interest and enthusiasm. Such an imbalance can decrease the effectiveness of the program and lead to a decline in adherence. Since the magnitude of the conditioning response varies directly with the frequency of participation, poorly motivated subjects (infrequent exercisers) are generally training failures. Conversely, overly motivated or competitive subjects often overestimate their capacities and are thus frequently subject to orthopaedic injury, musculoskeletal soreness, or both. Thus, the dropout rate of poorly or overly motivated participants may be high.

Figure 20-3. Variables affecting adherence to exercise training programs.

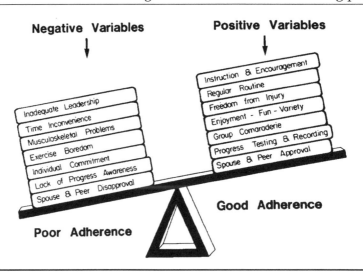

Research and empirical evidence suggest that certain program modifications and motivational strategies may enhance participant interest, enthusiasm, and long-term adherence. These include:

- **Recruit physician support of the health-fitness program.** Recent studies indicate that the single most important factor determining patients' participation in exercise appears to be a strong recommendation from their primary care physician. Simple physician counseling has also been shown to be highly effective in motivating patients to make other significant lifestyle changes (e.g., smoking cessation).
- **Provide exercise facilities and locker rooms that are appropriately maintained.** One of the first things program participants notice is the cleanliness of the equipment and facilities. Comfortably bright lights,

light-colored walls, and bright carpets all suggest a clean environment. In addition, the facility should have a good ventilation system and control over temperature and humidity. Regular maintenance and calibration of all exercise equipment should be standard procedure.

- **Clarify individual needs to establish the intrinsic motive to exercise.** An initial semi-structured interview allows staff to determine exactly what the client hopes to gain from the exercise program. During this interview the fitness leader should clarify individual needs and expectations, and establish a schedule to monitor progress and reassess goals.

- **Emphasize short-term goals.** According to Rejewski and Kenney, goal setting should be viewed much like climbing a ladder, with an emphasis placed on reasonable distances between rungs. Clients should be oriented toward short-term objectives that are specific, clearly defined, and realistically attainable. The key is to draw the participants' focus to the process, rather than the final objective, for example, a body weight of 160 pounds or a cholesterol level under 200 mg/dl.

- **Minimize injury/complications with a mild-to-moderate intensity exercise prescription.** Oftentimes, novice exercisers become discouraged due to muscular soreness or injury from increasing the activity dosage too abruptly. Excessive intensity (>90% $\dot{V}O_{2\,max}$), frequency ($\geq$ 5 days/week) or duration ($\geq$ 45 minutes/session) of training offer the participant little additional gain in aerobic capacity ($\dot{V}O_{2\,max}$), yet the incidence of orthopedic injury increases substantially (refer to Figure 20-4). Attention to warm-up, proper walking or running shoes, and training on appropriate terrain (i.e., avoiding hard and uneven surfaces) should aid in decreasing attrition due to injury. A recommended prescription for beginners is to exercise approximately 30 minutes every other day, at a perceived exertion of 11 to 13 (refer to Figure 20-5). Recent studies, however, have shown similar training effects in subjects who completed three 10-minute bouts of moderate intensity exercise per day versus those who performed one "continuous" exercise bout of 30 minutes. Finally, participants should be counseled to discontinue exercise and seek medical advice if they experience premonitory signs or symptoms, including abnormal heart rhythms (palpitations), chest pain or pressure, or dizziness (refer to Figure 20-6).

- **Encourage group participation.** Group commitments tend to be stronger than those made independently. The encouragement of the group often provides the incentive to continue during periods of decreasing interest. Poorer long-term adherence has been reported in programs where an individual exercises alone, compared to those that incorporate group dynamics. Most people (9 out of 10) prefer group, as opposed to individual exercise. Apparently, social reinforcement through camaraderie and companionship are potent motivators related to increased exercise adherence.

- **Emphasize fun and variety in the exercise program.** The type of physical activity program has also been shown to influence long-term exercise adherence. Regimented calisthenics readily become monotonous and boring, leading to poor exercise adherence. Similarly, persons who

Figure 20-4. Relationship between frequency and duration of exercise training, percentage of improvement in aerobic capacity ($\dot{V}O_{2\,max}$), and the incidence of orthopaedic injury. Above an exercise duration of 30 minutes/session, or a frequency of three sessions/week, additional improvement in $\dot{V}O_{2\,max}$ is small, yet the injury rate increases disproportionately. (Adapted from Pollock, M.L.).

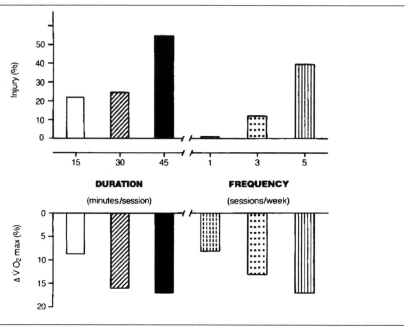

initiate home-based stationary cycle ergometer training, often fail to persist with their exercise program. Physical conditioning regimens that are most successful are those that are pleasurable and offer the greatest diversification.

The "Games-As-Aerobics" approach provides an ideal complement to a walk-jog format. The approach differs from many standard intervention or rehabilitation programs in that it maximizes the pleasure principle. It is predicated on the belief that people seek activities that provide fun and repeated success as opposed to the pain and discomfort associated with some traditional programs. Stretching and flexibility movements are frequently camouflaged in the form of individual or partner activities, games, and relays. Exercises are modified to incorporate ball passing and other movement skills for variety. Fitness leaders may also use hula hoops, medicine balls, jump ropes, elastic bands, parachutes, aquatic facilities, progressive resistance devices, and other contemporary exercise equipment (refer to Figure 20-7) to diversify their programs.

Figure 20-5. Perceived exertion scale with descriptive "effort ratings." (From Borg, G.)

Figure 20-6. Warning signs and symptoms that require medical review and temporary cessation of exercise training.

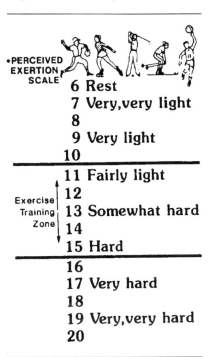

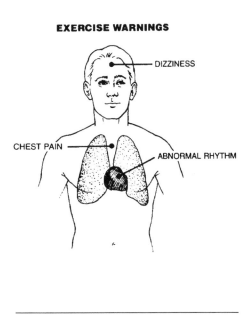

- **Incorporate effective behavioral and programmatic techniques into the physical conditioning regimen.** Exercise adherence is enhanced through "personalized" positive feedback to participants, as well as through longer time-based distance goals, established by the exerciser. Research has also demonstrated the effectiveness of self-management strategies, including behavioral contracting and goal setting, in improving exercise adherence. One clear advantage of these techniques is that the participant plays a major role in the planning.
- **Employ periodic fitness testing to assess the participant's response to the training program.** Favorable physiologic adaptations to chronic endurance exercise include a decreased heart rate, blood pressure and perceived exertion during submaximal exercise, increased physical work capacity and $\dot{V}O_{2\,max}$, reduced body weight and fat stores, and an improved serum lipid/lipoprotein profile. Such changes are powerful motivators that produce renewed enthusiasm and dedication.

    We have employed both submaximal and maximal exercise testing to assess serial changes in cardiorespiratory fitness. Submaximal testing is particularly easy to administer and requires no physician supervision. The initial or baseline exercise test protocol is followed, facilitating a comparison of the heart rate, blood pressure, and rating of

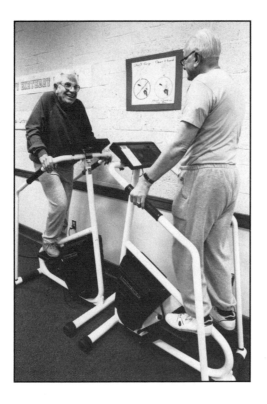

Figure 20-7. Exercise training facility at William Beaumont Hospital, Beaumont Rehabilitation and Health Center, Birmingham, Michigan. Participants have access to sophisticated exercise equipment in a mini-gymnasium, including a variety of arm and leg ergometers, treadmills, rowing machines, cross-country skiing devices, progressive resistance equipment, and vertical climbing systems (pictured). A swimming pool serves as an added option.

perceived exertion (RPE; 6-20 scale) at standard submaximal work rates (refer to Figure 20-8). The endpoint of the test is that work rate at which the upper limit of the prescribed heart rate range has been achieved.

- **Include the spouse, family members, and/or friends in periodic functions.** The attitude and support of those with whom an individual interacts frequently helps determine whether or not that person will participate in and adhere to an exercise program. A participant's spouse, as well as family and friends, can play significant roles in this regard. The importance of this influence became evident in one study that showed that the husband's adherence to the exercise program was directly related to the wife's attitude toward the program (refer to Figure 20-9). Of those men whose spouses had a positive attitude toward the exercise program, 80% demonstrated good-to-excellent adherence and only 20% exhibited fair-to poor-adherence. In contrast, when the spouse was neutral or negative, 40% showed good-to-excellent adherence and 60% demonstrated fair-to-poor adherence. These findings suggest that program counseling and educational gatherings, including both participants and spouses, will help to reduce misunderstandings and create and maintain positive attitudes that support exercise adherence.

- **Use progress charts to record exercise achievements.** The importance of immediate, positive feedback on reinforcement of health-related behaviors is well documented. A progress chart that allows participants to document daily and cumulative exercise achievements (e.g., mile-

Figure 20-8. Comparison of heart rate, blood pressure, and ratings of perceived exertion (RPE) at standard submaximal work loads during mini-testing versus baseline or initial exercise testing. Extrapolation of the mini-test heart rate/work load (METs) relationship facilitates estimation of the maximal oxygen consumption, expressed as METs.

| Workloads | Mini-Test | | | Initial Test (Pre-conditioning) | | |
	Heart Rate	Blood Pressure	RPE	Heart Rate	Blood Pressure	RPE
Rest	64	106/74		59	120/78	
2.0 mph 0% grade	68	122/70	6	94	130/78	11
3.0 mph 0% grade	76	132/74	7	113	158/78	14
3.0 mph 2.5% grade	80	136/80	9	120	170/78	15-16
3.0 mph 5.0% grade	86	142/78	9-10	125	182/78	17
3.0 mph 7.5% grade	98	146/82	12			
3.0 mph 10% grade	106	148/80	13-14			

Estimated Peak Mets After Phase II
Exercise Program - From mini test results

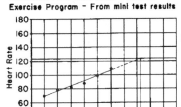

Maximum METS before exercise program

5

Maximum METS after exercise program

9 - 10

age) can facilitate this objective. One example is the computerized exercise session progress report system at the Aerobics Center in Dallas, Texas. The system provides exercisers with an updated record of the number of "aerobic points" they have earned, the miles they have run, and related training accomplishments. A practical alternative, however, is a progress chart which allows the participant to record his or her daily workout mileage. If the chart is strategically placed near the running track or locker room, it becomes a matter of pride to motivate individuals to "increase" their exercise totals.

• **Include an optional recreational game to the exercise program format.** The standard warm-up, endurance, and cool-down sequence used in most adult fitness programs offers little in terms of fun or variety. A recreational game should be used to complement this format. Game modifications which serve to minimize skill and competition and maximize participant success are particularly important. For example, volleyball played allowing one bounce of the ball per side, facilitates longer rallies and provides additional fun, while minimizing the skill level required to appreciate the game. Many team games and individual sports can be modified in a similar fashion. Through such modifications, the

Figure 20-9. Relationship of wives' attitudes to husbands' adherence to an exercise training program. (Adapted from Heinzelman, F. and R.W. Bagley).

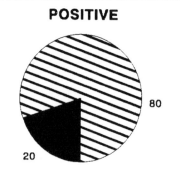

POSITIVE

80

20

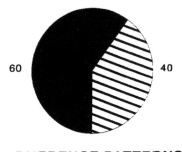

NEUTRAL OR NEGATIVE

60

40

ADHERENCE PATTERNS

Excellent or good
Fair or poor

leader is better able to emphasize the primary goal of the activity: enjoyment of the game for its own sake.

- **Play music during exercise sessions.** Appropriate background music may mask general fatigue and stimulate participants to exercise more energetically. This belief was substantiated in our survey of 114 recreational joggers, 99 of whom (87%) indicated a preference for background music during their training. Many felt that inspiring music aided their workout, whereas others noted reductions in their perceived exertion at any given pace. The recent proliferation of headsets further attests to the efficacy of this exercise accessory.

- **Establish regularity of workouts.** If individuals start their workouts at the same time each day, they will accept them as part of their routine schedule, and exercise will become habitual. Availability of morning and evening sessions should serve to further increase the compatibility of an exercise commitment with the varied schedules of participants.

- **Recognize participant accomplishments through a system of rewards.** Peer recognition is another powerful motivator. Recognition of lifestyle, health, or exercise achievements can be made in the form of inexpensive trophies, plaques, ribbons, certificates, or "iron-on" insignias. To this end, an annual awards ceremony or banquet is recommended.

- **Provide qualified, enthusiastic exercise leaders.** Although numerous variables affect exercise adherence, perhaps the single most important is the exercise leader. Exercise leaders should be well-trained, compassionate, sensitive, empathetic, tactful, innovative, and enthusiastic. Table 20-3 lists recommended behavioral strategies of the good exercise leader. Workshop and certification offerings by the American College of Sports Medicine and other professional associations serve to promote "quality control," knowledge and proficiency standards for program personnel.

Table 20-3. Behavioral Strategies of the Good Exercise Leader.

1. Show a sincere interest in the participant. Learn why clients have gotten involved in the program, and what they hope to achieve.
2. Remove as many initial barriers to participation as possible. If cost, distance, child care, or other factors make it difficult for the client to attend, help them find ways to get around them.
3. Be optimistic and enthusiastic in your instruction and guidance, and project a positive helping attitude.
4. Develop a personal association with each participant.
5. Learn participants' names and greet them by shaking hands.
6. Consider the reasons why adults exercise (i.e., health, rehabilitation, recreation, weight loss, social, personal appearance) and allow for individual differences by providing the client with choices.
7. Don't overlook the importance of caring follow-up. Call or send a note if someone fails to show up for an appointment, or with successive unexplained absences. A phone call after your initial meeting can sway a contemplator toward joining your program.
8. Practice what you preach. Participate in the exercise sessions yourself.
9. Honor special days (e.g., birthdays) or exercise accomplishments with t-shirts, ribbons, or certificates.
10. Attend to orthopaedic and musculoskeletal problems.
11. Counsel participants on proper foot apparel and exercise clothing.
12. Introduce "first-time" exercisers on the gymnasium floor.
13. Reinforce participants by providing them with frequent feedback on their appearance and lifestyle alterations. Personal feedback which helps to track progress toward goals is ideal. Use this time to also assess potential recidivism and intervene accordingly.
14. Use goal setting as a motivational tool. Build on areas of client perceived interest, "How would he/she like to be different?"
15. Show your optimism. This creates a positive self-fulfilling prophesy where the participant succeeds largely because of your belief that he/she can persevere.
16. Give clear and concise information. Listen, summarize, and clarify to make sure that your communications have been correctly understood.

PROGRAM MODELS: GROUP VERSUS HOME

Participation in a supervised, gymnasium-based adult fitness or cardiac rehabilitation program is not always feasible. Such programs may be associated with inconvenient hours, increased costs, and extended travel time. One study, in fact, showed that patients undergoing gymnasium-based exercise training spent more time in their cars going to and from the program than patients in a home-training comparison group spent on their cycle ergometers.

For many participants, unsupervised home exercise may be a reasonable alternative to promote weight management, enhance psychological status, and improve functional capacity, especially if a training partner can be recruited.

Advantages of home-training programs include lesser cost, increased convenience, and the promotion of independence and personal responsibility for health and fitness needs. Such programs can also be as effective as supervised programs in improving functional capacity for low, moderate, and high risk patients. Drawbacks, however, include the limited means of teaching clients (patients) necessary principles and proscriptions for exercise, the lack of opportunity to counsel and encourage lifestyle changes for coronary risk reduction, and the lack of medical surveillance, emergency care, and peer support. Several program modifications have been proposed to overcome these limitations, including regular telephone contact with staff and transtelephonic exercise electrocardiographic monitoring for those at intermediate and high risk for future cardiac events.

In a recent, provocative editorial, DeBusk suggested that the current gymnasium-based cardiac rehabilitation model suffers from the following shortcomings: a) difficulty in distinguishing its effects from those of standard physicians' care; b) lack of support by physicians; c) inconvenience of the group format; and, d) relatively low participation rates (<15% of all eligible patients). Nevertheless, considerable data demonstrate the safety, efficacy, and cost effectiveness of this model. Moreover, supervised programs can provide emergency support for patients and ongoing surveillance information for referring physicians (refer to Figure 20-10). Group programs are appropriate for the wide range of medically complex patients eligible for cardiac rehabilitation services, including those with concomitant neurologic, vascular, orthopaedic or pulmonary conditions. Supervised preventive and rehabilitative programs also facilitate education about exercise and coronary risk reduction, provide variety and recreational opportunities, offer staff guidance and peer support, and enhance the potential for adherence and safety.

In summary, contemporary models must be developed to ensure that apparently healthy adults and patients with heart disease can more easily participate in comprehensive, exercise-based programs of primary and secondary prevention. The challenge for those developing these models is to incorporate techniques to facilitate optimal adherence and overcome many of the current limitations of home and group programs, while maximizing their benefits.

Continuing Education and Training
For Exercise Program Personnel

The emergence of exercise as an accepted intervention in preventive and rehabilitative programs has created the need for educating and training allied health professionals, including nurses, physical and health educators, exercise physiologists, and physical therapists. Although numerous professional organizations have responded through the sponsorship of conferences, establishment of committees, and development of educational materials, perhaps the most significant efforts in this area have been through the American College of Sports Medicine (ACSM).

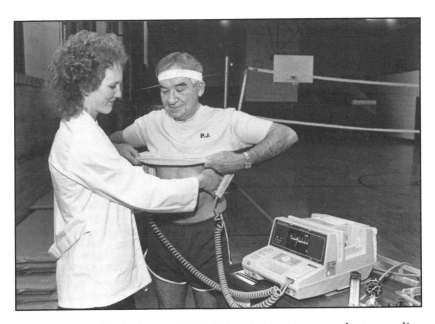

Figure 20-10. Technique of obtaining instantaneous electrocardiographic rhythm strips with defibrillator paddles during outpatient cardiac exercise programs. Changing patterns of signs or symptoms may often herald a deterioration in clinical status, impending cardiovascular complications, or medical emergencies.

The ACSM has published "position stands" concerning the recommended quantity and quality of exercise for developing and maintaining fitness in healthy adults and patients with coronary artery disease. In addition, it has developed guidelines for exercise testing and prescription for these populations. Paralleling the evolution of the guidelines has been the development of workshops and a certification process incorporating both written and practical examinations for individuals involved in the administration of graded exercise testing and training programs.

Currently, the ACSM offers two primary categories of certification: the Health and Fitness Track and the Clinical Track. Progressive degrees of knowledge, skills, and competencies exist within each of the certification levels. Moreover, individuals certified at a given level are responsible for the knowledge and proficiency requirements of the level(s) below their attained level of certification.

The Health and Fitness Track is designed primarily for persons working in programs of a preventive nature (i.e., for healthy individuals or those with controlled medical conditions). Three levels of certification, in hierarchical order, are offered in this track: Exercise Leader, Health Fitness Instructor, and Health Fitness Director, respectively. These individuals typically work in corporate or community-based recreational settings (e.g., fitness centers, YMCAs, Jewish Community Centers).

The Clinical Track is designed for professionals who are primarily responsible for working with at-risk or diseased individuals, particularly those with cardiovascular or pulmonary problems. In addition to working in corporate or community settings, these individuals may work in hospital or clinic-based rehabilitation programs. Three progressive levels of certification are also offered in this track: Exercise Test Technologist, Exercise Specialist, and Program Director.

The ACSM's *Guidelines for Exercise Testing and Prescription* details the recommended/required experience and educational backgrounds for these certifications. Specific learning objectives are outlined to aid in preparation for both the written and the practical examinations. Continuing education credits and current cardiopulmonary resuscitation training are required to maintain certification on an ongoing basis.

The American Heart Association offers certification in Basic Life Support and Advanced Cardiac Life Support (ACLS). These may be complemented by courses in first aid, water safety, and lifesaving offered by the American Red Cross. Basic Life Support should be a mandatory requirement for all personnel working in an exercise setting, whereas ACLS is essential in medical programs dealing with high risk populations.

In 1994, the American Nurses Association offered its first certification exam in cardiac rehabilitative nursing. Other professional organizations such as the American Heart Association, the American College of Cardiology, the American Medical Association, the American Alliance for Health, Physical Education, Recreation and Dance, the American Council on Exercise, the Aerobics and Fitness Association of America, the National Strength and Conditioning Association, the National Academy of Sports Medicine, and the National YMCAs also provide educational materials and sponsor conferences to update exercise professionals.

To keep abreast of current trends and new developments in the field of exercise science, continuing education is a must. To encourage interest and participation in continuing education, program directors should consider implementing career ladders. Each "rung" of the ladder may have specific educational and proficiency criteria. Attaining certification, continuing education credits and/or an educational degree could be rewarded with salary increases/bonuses, conference time, increased responsibility and promotions.

Staff can also identify learning needs within their facility and develop their own in-services. Presentation of new products or research findings can be shared with peers over lunchtime conferences. A staff member can be designated to be a liaison with product representatives to obtain the latest pamphlets to aid in staff/client education.

Programs can invest in professional journals related to their fields. Some journals offer continuing education credits through self tests based on specific articles. In addition, programs may want to develop their own professional newsletter which can be distributed locally or nationally. This would encourage professional writing, research, and the exchange of ideas.

Attendance at professional conferences should be strongly encouraged, and, when possible, staff should be compensated for conference fees and time off from work. Programs can also develop continuing education workshops independently or in collaboration with other exercise facilities.

To maintain life support skills, role playing and practice drills should be regularly conducted to keep staff apprised of their role in emergency situations. These drills can be used to refine and clarify individual responsibilities in the event of medical problems or cardiovascular complications that may arise.

CONCLUSION

Despite the increasing body of evidence documenting the salutary effects of regular aerobic exercise, the claim that exercise has "addictive properties," and the fact that most individuals believe that regular exercise is good for them, less than half of all Americans participate in physical activity at sufficient levels to improve cardiorespiratory fitness, or, for that matter, general health. While many persons can be motivated to initiate an exercise regimen, few sustain the interest and enthusiasm needed to maintain participation.

Exercise must be recognized as a lifetime pursuit and not a program of 10-12 weeks' duration with long-lasting residual effects. The individual must develop an attitude toward exercise that reinforces adherence. Primary care physicians, physical therapists, nurses, exercise physiologists, and other health professionals can play a critical role in favorably modifying the exercise habits of the persons they counsel. The key lies in recommending and designing programs that are safe, effective, and enjoyable. The challenge is a formidable one. ❏

BIBLIOGRAPHY •

1. American Association of Cardiovascular and Pulmonary Rehabilitation. *Guidelines for Cardiac Rehabilitation Programs*, 2nd Ed. Champaign, IL: Human Kinetics Publishers, 1995.
2. American College of Sports Medicine. *Guidelines for Exercise Testing and Prescription*, 4th Ed. Philadelphia, PA: Lea & Febiger, 1991.
3. American College of Sports Medicine. "Position stand: Exercise for patients with coronary artery disease." *Med Sci Sports Exer* 26(3):i-v, 1994.
4. American College of Sports Medicine. "Position stand: The recommended quantity and quality of exercise for developing and maintaining muscular fitness in healthy adults." *Med Sci Sports Exer* 22:265-274, 1990.
5. Blair, S.N., Kohl, H.W., Paffenbarger, R.S., et al. "Physical fitness and all-cause mortality: A prospective study of healthy men and women." *JAMA* 262:2395-2401, 1989.
6. Borg, G. "Psychophysical bases of perceived exertion." *Med Sci Sports Exer* 14:377-381, 1982.

7. Boyd, M.D., Feldman, R.H.L. "Health information seeking and reading and comprehension abilities of cardiac rehabilitation patients." *J Cardiac Rehabil* 4(8):343-347, 1984.

8. Daltroy, L.H. "Improving cardiac patient adherence to exercise regimens: A clinical trial of health education." *J Cardiac Rehabil* 5(1):40-49, 1985.

9. DeBusk, R.F. "Why is cardiac rehabilitation not widely used?" *Western J Med* 156:206-208, 1992.

10. DeBusk, R.F., Haskell, W.L., Miller, N.H., et al. "Medically directed at-home rehabilitation soon after clinically uncomplicated acute myocardial infarction: A new model for patient care." *Am J Cardiol* 55:251-257, 1985.

11. DeBusk, R.F., Stenestrand, U., Sheehan, M., et al. "Training effects of long versus short bouts of exercise in healthy subjects." *Am J Cardiol* 65:1010-1013, 1990.

12. Franklin, B.A. "Program factors that influence exercise adherence: Practical adherence skills for the clinical staff." In *Exercise Adherence*. Dishman, R.K. (Ed). Champaign, IL: Human Kinetics Publishers, 1988.

13. Franklin, B.A., Gordon, S., Timmis, G.C. "Amount of exercise necessary for the patient with coronary artery disease." *Am J Cardiol* 69:1426-1432, 1992.

14. Franklin, B.A., Gordon, S., Timmis, G.C. (Eds). *Exercise in Modern Medicine*. Baltimore, MD: Williams & Wilkins, 1989.

15. Franklin, B.A., Oldridge, N.B., Stoedefalke, K.G., et al. *On the Ball: Innovative Activities for Adult Fitness & Cardiac Rehabilitation Programs*. Carmel, IN: Benchmark Press, Inc., 1990.

16. Franklin, B.A., Reed, P.S., Gordon, S., et al. "Instantaneous electrocardiography: A simple screening technique for cardiac exercise programs." *Chest* 96:174-177, 1989.

17. Heinzelman, F., Bagley, R.W. "Response to physical activity programs and their effects on health behavior." *Public Health Rep* 85:905-911, 1970.

18. Higgins, J.C., Ades, P.A. "Cardiac rehabilitation: Clinical benefits and referral patterns." *Intern Med* 14(8):10-16, 1993.

19. Oldridge, N.B., Donner, A.P., Back, C.W., et al. "Predictors of dropout from cardiac rehabilitation. Ontario Exercise Heart Collaborative Study." *Am J Cardiol* 51:70-74, 1983.

20. Oldridge, N.B., Jones, N. "Contracting as a strategy to reduce drop out in exercise rehabilitation." *Med Sci Sports* 13:125-126, 1981.

21. Owens, P.M., Porter, K.A., Frost, C.D., et al. "Determination of the readability of educational materials for patients with cardiac disease." *J Cardiopul Rehabil* 13(1):20-24, 1993.

22. Pollock, M.L., Gettman, L., Milesis, C., et al. "Effects of frequency and duration of training on attrition and incidence of injury." *Med Sci Sports* 9:31-36, 1977.

23. Prochaska, J., Di Clemente, C. "Transtheoretical therapy, toward a more integrative model of change." *Psych Theory Res Prac* 19:276-288, 1982.

24. Rejewski, W.J., Kenney, E.A. *Fitness Motivation: Preventing Participant Dropout*. Champaign, IL: Life Enhancement Publications, 1988.

25. Statistical Abstracts of the United States. U.S. Department of Commerce. 113th ed: 255, 1993.

26. Wenger, N.K. "Home versus supervised exercise training after myocardial infarction and myocardial revascularization procedures." *Prac Cardiol* 15(5):47-53, 1989.

27. Wilmore, J.H. "Individual exercise prescription." *Am J Cardiol* 33:757-759, 1974.

EPILOGUE

•••••••••••••••••••••••••••••••••••

TEN GUIDELINES FOR SENSIBLE EXERCISE

1. *Define your exercise goals.* Identify what you expect to accomplish from your exercise program (e.g., improve aerobic fitness, lose weight, improve upper body muscular fitness, etc).

2. *Engage in a sound exercise regimen.* Base your exercise prescription on scientifically based information, for example, on the guidelines developed by the American College of Sports Medicine.

3. *Focus on safety at all times.* Be sensitive to the need for safety. For example, you should obtain appropriate clearance before initiating an exercise program; adhere to established exercise guidelines; err on the side of conservatism whenever in doubt—particularly when beginning your program; and properly use all exercise equipment (refer to Appendices B, C and D).

4. *Assess your overall fitness level.* Evaluate how fit you are before starting your exercise program and at periodic intervals (e.g., approximately every six months) thereafter.

5. *Strive for total fitness.* Include activities for all the components of health-related fitness—cardiorespiratory fitness, muscular fitness, body composition, and flexibility—in your exercise program.

6. *Eat sensibly.* Keep in mind that a sound nutrition program goes hand-in-hand with a sound exercise regimen.

7. *Do not overtrain.* Avoid doing too much, too hard, too soon (refer to Appendix E for a listing of the common signs or symptoms of overtraining)—keep in mind that exercise is not a contest; the primary goal of your exercise program should be to enable you to achieve the objectives which are important to you.

8. *Record your training progress.* Keep a detailed record of your exercise efforts. Such a record can serve several purposes, including allowing you to accurately evaluate the effectiveness of your exercise program on an on-going basis; helping to motivate you; providing you with a "status" report; etc.

9. *Make exercise a habit.* Establish a pattern of exercising on a regular basis—you'll receive the greatest benefits in your health and fitness level when you make exercise an integral part of your lifestyle.

10. *Make your exercise program enjoyable.* Select activities that you enjoy—if you like what you're doing, you will substantially increase the likelihood that you will adhere to the program.

Appendix A

GLOSSARY OF SELECTED
FITNESS TERMS

A GLOSSARY OF
SELECTED FITNESS TERMS*

(Note: This glossary includes an overview of words pertaining to exercise, health, medicine, nutrition, physiology, etc.)

Acclimation
A program undertaken to induce acclimatization to new environmental conditions such as changes in temperature or altitude.

Acclimatization
The body's gradual adaptation to a changed environment, such as higher temperatures or lower pressures (from high altitude).

Acute
Sudden, short-term, sharp or severe. Cf. chronic

Adaptation
The adjustment of the body (or mind) to achieve a greater degree of fitness to its environment. Adaptations are more persistent than an immediate response to the new stimuli of the environment. Cf. response.

Adherence
Sticking to something. Used to describe a person's continuation in an exercise program. Cf. compliance.

Adipose tissue
Fat tissue.

Aerobic
Using oxygen.

Aerobic activities
Activities using large muscle groups at moderate intensities that permit the body to use oxygen to supply energy and to maintain a steady state for more than a few minutes. Cf. steady state.

Aerobic endurance
The ability to continue aerobic activity over a period of time.

Aerobic power
See maximal oxygen uptake.

Aerobic total
A measure of the number of calories an individual expends during a Crossrobic™ training workout. The long-term impact of a Crossrobic training workout on weight control is optimal because users burn calories while building lean muscle mass—the tissue most responsible for burning calories.

Agonist
A muscle which directly engages in an action around a joint which has another muscle that can provide an opposing action (antagonist).

Amino acids
The building blocks of protein. Twenty different amino acids are required by the body. Cf. essential amino acids.

Anabolic
Pertaining to the putting together of complex substances from simpler ones, especially to the building of body proteins from amino acids.

---

* Adapted from <u>Fitness Management Products & Services Source Guide.</u> 8(3): 195-206, 1992.

Anabolic steroids
A group of synthetic, testosterone-like hormones that promote anabolism, including muscle hypertrophy. Medical uses include promotion of tissue repair in severely debilitated patients, but their use in athletics is considered unethical and carries numerous serious health risks.

Anabolism
The process of combining simple substances to build living matter by the cells. For example, combining amino acids into proteins to build muscle cells. Cf. catabolism, metabolism.

Anaerobic
Not using oxygen.

Anaerobic activities
Activities using muscle groups at high intensities that exceed the body's capacity to use oxygen to supply energy and which create an oxygen debt by using energy produced without oxygen. Cf. oxygen.

Anaerobic endurance
The ability to continue activity over a period of time (much shorter time than with aerobic activity).

Anaerobic threshold
The point where increasing energy demands of exercise cannot be met by the use of oxygen, and an oxygen debt begins to be incurred.

Anatomy
The science of the structure of the human body.

Anemia
A subnormal number or hemoglobin content of red blood cells caused when blood loss exceeds blood production. Symptoms may include fatigue, pale complexion, light headedness, palpitations, and loss of appetite.

Angina
A gripping, choking, or suffocating pain in the chest (angina pectoris), caused most often by insufficient flow of oxygen to the heart muscle during exercise or excitement. Exercise should stop, and medical attention should be obtained.

Anorexia
Lack of appetite. Anorexia nervosa is a psychological and physiological condition characterized by inability or refusal to eat, leading to severe weight loss, malnutrition, hormone imbalances, and other potentially life-threatening biological changes.

Antagonist
A muscle that can provide an opposing action to the action of another muscle (the agonist) around a joint.

Anthropometry
The science dealing with the measurement (size, weight, proportions) of the human body.

Aquatics
Exercise or sports activities in or on the water.

Arrhythmia
Any abnormal rhythm of the heart beat. Since some causes of arrythmia may have serious health consequences, exercisers experiencing irregular heart beats should be referred for medical evaluation.

Arteriosclerosis
Thickening and hardening of the artery walls by one of several diseases. Cf. atherosclerosis.

Artery
Vessel which carries blood away from the heart to the tissues of the body.

Arthritis

Inflammation of the joints which causes pain, stiffness and limitation of motion. May be symptomatic of a systemic disease, such as rheumatoid arthritis, which can affect all age groups. Cf. osteoarthritis.

Atherosclerosis

A very common form of arteriosclerosis, in which the arteries are narrowed by deposits of cholesterol and other material in the inner walls of the artery. Cf. arteriosclerosis.

Atrophy

Reduction in size, or wasting away, of a body part, organ, tissue or cell. Cf. hypertrophy.

Ballistic movement

An exercise movement in which part of the body is "thrown" against the resistance of antagonist muscles or against the limits of a joint. The latter, especially, is considered dangerous to the integrity of ligaments and tendons.

Basal metabolic rate

The minimum energy required to maintain the body's life function at rest. Usually expressed in calories per hour per square meter of body surface. Cf. met.

Biofeedback

A process which permits a person to see or hear indicators of physiological variables, such as blood pressure, skin temperature, or heart rate, which may allow the person to exert some control over those variables. Often used to teach relaxation techniques.

Blood pressure

The pressure exerted by the blood on the wall of the arteries. Maximum and minimum measures are used: The systolic pressure reaches a maximum just before the end of the pumping phase of the heart; the diastolic pressure (minimum) occurs late in the refilling phase of the heart. Measures are in the millimeters of mercury (as 120/80). Cf. hypertension.

Body composition

The proportions of fat, muscle, and bone making up the body. Usually expressed as percent of body fat and percent of lean body mass.

Body density

The specific gravity of the body, which can be tested by underwater weighing. Compares the weight of the body to the weight of the same volume of water. Result can be used to estimate the percentage of body fat.

Bradycardia

Slow heart beat. A well-conditioned heart will often deliver a pulse rate of less than 60 beats per minute at rest, which would be considered bradycrotic by standard definitions. Cf. tachycardia.

Bursa

A cushioning sac filled with a lubricating fluid that alleviates friction where there is movement between muscles, between tendon and bone, or between bone and skin.

Bursitis

The inflammation of a bursa, sometimes with calcification in underlying tendon.

Calisthenics

A system of exercise movements, without equipment, for the building of strength, flexibility and physical grace. The Greeks formed the word from "kalos" (beautiful) and "sthenos" (strength).

Calorie cost

The number of Calories burned to produce the energy for a task. Usually measured in Calories (kcal) per minute.

APPENDIX

• • •

Calorie

The Calorie used as a unit of metabolism (as in diet and energy expenditure) equals 1,000 small calories, and is often spelled with a capital C to make that distinction. It is the energy required to raise the temperature of one kilogram of water one degree Celsius. Also called a kilocalorie (kcal).

Capillary

The tiny blood vessels that receive blood flow from the arteries, interchange substances between the blood and the tissues, and return the blood to the veins.

Carbohydrate

Chemical compound of carbon, oxygen and hydrogen, usually with the hydrogen and oxygen in the right proportions to form water. Common forms are starches, sugars, cellulose, and gums. Carbohydrates are more readily used for energy production than are fats and proteins.

Carbon dioxide

A colorless, odorless gas that is formed in the tissues by the oxidation of carbon, and is eliminated by the lungs. Its presence in the lungs stimulates breathing.

Cardiac

Pertaining to the heart.

Cardiac output

The volume of blood pumped out by the heart in a given unit of time. It equals the stroke volume times the heart rate.

Cardiac rehabilitation

A program to prepare cardiac patients to return to productive lives with a reduced risk of recurring health problems.

Cardiopulmonary resuscitation (CPR)

A first-aid method to restore breathing and heart action through mouth-to-mouth breathing and rhythmic chest compressions. CPR instruction is offered by local Heart Association and Red Cross units, and is a minimum requirement for most fitness-instruction certifications.

Cardiorespiratory endurance

See aerobic endurance.

Cardiovascular

Pertaining to the heart and blood vessels.

Carotid Artery

The principal artery in both sides of the neck. A convenient place to detect a pulse.

Catabolism

The process of breaking down complex substances into simpler parts by the cells. For example, breaking down carbohydrates or fats for use in energy expenditure. Cf. anabolism, metabolism.

Cellulite

A commercially created name for lumpy fat deposits. Actually this fat behaves no differently from other fat; it is just straining against irregular bands of connective tissue.

Cholesterol

A steroid alcohol found in animal fats. This pearly, fatlike substance is implicated in the narrowing of the arteries in atherosclerosis. Plasma levels of cholesterol are considered normal between 180 and 230 milligrams per 100 milliliters. Higher levels are thought to pose risks to the arteries.

Chronic

Continuing over time.

Circuit training

A series of exercises, performed one after the other, with little rest between. Resistance training in this manner increases strength while making some contribution to cardiovascular endurance as well. (It remains controversial as to whether a significant cardiovascular benefit will be achieved in the absence of very consistent motivation or close supervision of the sessions).

Collateral circulation

Blood circulation through small side branches that can supplement (or substitute for) the main vessel's delivery of blood to certain tissues.

Compliance

Staying with a prescribed exercise program. (Often used in a medical setting.) Cf. adherence.

Concentric action

Muscle action in which the muscle is shortening under its own power. This action is commonly called "positive" work, or, redundantly, "concentric contraction." Cf. eccentric action, isometric action.

Concussion

An injury from a severe blow or jar. A brain concussion may result in temporary loss of consciousness and memory loss, if mild. Severe concussion causes prolonged loss of consciousness and may impair breathing, dilate the pupils and disrupt other regulatory functions of the brain.

Conditioning

Long-term physical training.

Connective tissue

A fibrous tissue that binds together and supports the structures of the body. Cf. fascia, joint capsules, ligament, tendon.

Contraindication

Any condition which indicates that a particular course of action (or exercise) would be inadvisable.

Cool down

A gradual reduction of the intensity of exercise to allow physiological processes to return to normal. Helps avoid blood pooling in the legs and may reduce muscular soreness.

Coronary arteries

The arteries, circling the heart like a crown, that supply blood to the heart muscle.

Coronary heart disease (CHD)

Atherosclerosis of the coronary arteries.

Cross-sectional study

A study made at one point in time. Cf. longitudinal study.

Crossrobic™ total

The combined score of the aerobic and strength totals that a user earns during a Crossrobic workout. Whichever total is higher at the completion of your workout indicates which element received the greater training emphasis. Cf. Crossrobic training, aerobic total, strength total.

Crossrobic training

A type of exercise training that enables individuals to engage in both aerobic conditioning and strength training in a single workout. Cf. Crossrobics® CardioSquat™, Crossrobics Kayak™.

Crossrobics CardioSquat

An exercise machine which enables individuals of all ages and fitness levels to simultaneously engage in aerobic conditioning and lower body strength training (refer to Appendix C-1).

APPENDIX

• • •

Crossrobics® Kayak™
An exercise machine which enables individuals of all ages and fitness levels to simultaneously engage in aerobic conditioning and upper body strength training (refer to Appendix C-2).

Defribrillator
A device used to stop weak, uncoordinated beating (fibrillation) of the heart and allow restoration of a normal heart beat. Part of the "crash cart" at cardiac rehabilitation program sites.

Dehydration
The condition resulting from the excessive loss of body water.

Detraining
The process of losing the benefits of training by returning to a sedentary life.

Diastole
Relaxation phase of the heart. Cf. systole.

Diastolic blood pressure
The minimum blood pressure that occurs during the refilling of the heart. Cf. blood pressure.

Diet
The food one eats. May or may not be a selection of foods to accomplish a particular health or fitness objective.

Diuretic
Any agent which increases the flow of urine. Used inadvisedly for quick weight loss, diuretics can cause dehydration.

Dry-bulb thermometer
An ordinary instrument for indicating temperature. Does not take into account humidity and other factors that combine to determine the heat stress experienced by the body. Cf. wet-bulb thermometer, wet-globe temperature.

Duration
The time spent in a single exercise session. Duration, along with frequency and intensity, are factors affecting the effectiveness of exercise.

Dyspnea
Difficult or labored breathing.

Eccentric action
Muscle action in which the muscle resists while it is forced to lengthen. This action is commonly called "negative" work, or "eccentric contraction," but, since the muscle is lengthening the word "contraction" is misapplied. Cf. concentric action, isometric action.

Efficiency
The ratio of energy consumed to the work accomplished. Exercisers utilizing the same amounts of oxygen may differ in their speed or amount of weight moved in a given time because of differing efficiencies.

Electrocardiogram (EKG, ECG)
A graph of the electrical activity caused by the stimulation of the heart muscle. The millivolts of electricity are detected by electrodes on the body surface and are recorded by an electrocardiograph.

Electrolyte
A substance which, in solution, is capable of conducting electricity. Certain electrolytes are essential to the electrochemical functioning of the body.

Endurance
The capacity to continue a physical performance over a period of time. Cf. aerobic endurance, anaerobic endurance.

Energy
The capacity to produce work.

Epidemiological studies

Statistical study of the relationships between various factors that determine the frequency and distribution of disease. For example, such studies have linked exercise to reduced mortality.

Epiphyseal plates

The sites of new bone growth, separated from the main bone by cartilage during the growth period. This is a potential injury site to be avoided in prescribing exercise to prepubescent individuals.

Epiphyses

The ends of long bones, usually wider than the shaft of the bone.

Ergometer

A device that can measure work consistently and reliably. Stationary exercise cycles were the first widely available devices equipped with ergometers, but a wide variety of endurance-training machines now have ergometric capacity.

Essential amino acids

Those amino acids that the body cannot make for itself. They are: isoleucine, leucine, lysine, methionine, phenylalanine, tryptophan, and valine.

Essential hypertension

Hypertension without a discoverable cause. Also called primary hypertension. Cf. hypertension.

Estrogen

The sex hormone that predominates in the female, but also has functions in the male. It is responsible for the development of female secondary sex characteristics, which have an effect on female responses to exercise. Cf. testosterone.

Exercise

Physical exertion of sufficient intensity, duration, and frequency to achieve or maintain fitness, or other health or athletic objectives.

Exercise prescription

A recommendation for a course of exercise to meet desirable individual objectives for fitness. Includes activity types, duration, intensity, and frequency of exercise.

Exercise program director

Certification as exercise program director by the American College of Sports Medicine indicates the competency to design, implement, and administer preventive and rehabilitative exercise programs, to educate staff in conducting tests and leading physical activity, and to educate the community about such programs. Must have all the competencies of the certified fitness instructor, exercise test technologist, and exercise specialist.

Exercise specialist

A person certified by the American College of Sports Medicine as having the competency and skill to supervise preventive and rehabilitative exercise programs and prescribe activities for patients. Must also pass the ACSM standards for exercise test technologist.

Exercise technologist

A person certified by the American College of Sports Medicine as competent to administer graded exercise tests, calculate the data, and implement any needed emergency procedures. Must have current CPR certification.

Expiration

Breathing air out of the lungs. Cf. inspiration, respiration.

Extension

A movement which moves the two ends of a jointed body part away from each other, as in straightening the arm. Cf. flexion.

APPENDIX

• • •

Extensor
A muscle that extends a jointed body part.

Faint
See syncope.

Fascia
Connective tissue which surrounds muscles and various organs of the body.

Fast-twitch fibers
Muscle fiber type that contracts quickly and is used most in intensive, short-duration exercises, such as weightlifting or sprints. Cf. slow-twitch fibres.

Fat
1. A white or yellowish tissue which stores reserve energy, provides padding for organs, and smooths body contours. 2. A compound of glycerol and various fatty acids. Dietary fat is not as readily converted to energy as are carbohydrates.

Fat-free weight
Lean body mass.

Fatigue
A loss of power to continue a given level of physical performance.

Fitness
The state of well-being consisting of optimum levels of strength, flexibility, weight control, cardiovascular capacity and positive physical and mental health behaviors, that prepare a person to participate fully in life, to be free from controllable health-risk factors and to achieve physical objectives consistent with his/her potential. Cf. wellness.

Fitness center
A place furnished with space and equipment, where leadership and supervision are offered to further the fitness objectives of participants.

Fitness Instructor
A person who directs classes or individuals in the performance of exercise. Certification by the American College of Sports Medicine indicates the competency to identify risk factors, conduct submaximal exercise tests, recommend exercise programs, lead classes, and counsel with exercisers. Works with persons without known disease. CPR certification is required.

Fitness testing
Measuring the indicators of the various aspects of fitness. Cf. graded exercise test, physical work capacity.

Flexibility
The range of motion around a joint.

Flexion
A movement which moves the two ends of a jointed body part closer to each other, as in bending the arm. Cf. extension.

Foot-pound
The amount of work required to lift one pound one foot.

Frequency
How often a person repeats a complete exercise session (e.g. 3 times per week). Frequency, along with duration and intensity, affect the effectiveness of exercise.

Functional capacity
See maximal oxygen uptake.

Glucose
Blood sugar. The transportable form of carbohydrate, which reaches the cells.

Glycogen
The storage form of carbohydrate. Glycogen is used in the muscles for the production of energy.

Golgi tendon organ

Organs at the junction of muscle and tendon that send inhibitory impulses to the muscle when the muscle's contraction reaches certain levels. The purpose may be to protect against separating the tendon from bone when a contraction is too great. Cf. muscle spindle, proprioceptor.

Graded exercise test (GXT)

A treadmill, or cycle-ergometer, test that delivers heart rate, ECG, and other data. Workload is gradually increased until an increase in workload is not followed by an increase in oxygen consumption; this identifies the individual's maximal oxygen uptake. Allows the prescribing of exercise to the individual's actual, rather than estimated, heart rate or aerobic capacity. Requires medical supervision. Cf. physical work capacity.

Growth hormone

Human growth hormone (HGH), somatotrophin, is produced by the pituitary to promote growth in many body cells. To treat children with growth disorders, it has been obtained from primate sources or synthesized. There are reports of abuse by athletes, although there is no clear benefit in taking the hormone and there are serious side effects, such as acromegaly, from dosages only slightly larger than those given to children.

Hamstrings

The group of muscles at the back of the thigh, and their tendons.

Health history

See medical history.

Health risk appraisal

A procedure that gathers information about a person's behaviors, family history, and other characteristics known to be associated with the incidence of serious disease, and uses that information to compare the individual's present risks with the lower risks that could be achieved by changing certain behaviors.

Heart attack

An acute episode of any kind of heart disease.

Heart rate

Number of heart beats per minute.

Heart rate reserve

The difference between the resting heart rate and the maximal heart rate.

Heat cramps

Muscle twitching or painful cramping, usually following heavy exercise with profuse sweating. The legs, arms, and abdominal muscles are the most often affected.

Heat exhaustion

Caused by dehydration (and sometimes salt loss). Symptoms include dry mouth, excessive thirst, loss of coordination, dizziness, headache, paleness, shakiness, and cool and clammy skin.

Heat stroke

A life threatening illness when the body's temperature-regulating mechanisms fail. Body temperature may rise to over 104 degrees F, skin appears red, dry, and warm to the touch. The victim has chills, sometimes nausea and dizziness, and may be confused or irrational. Seizures and coma may follow unless temperature is brought down to 102 degrees within an hour.

Heat syncope

Fainting from the heat. When a lot of blood is sent to the skin for cooling, and the person becomes inactive enough to allow blood to pool in the legs, the heart may not receive enough blood to supply the brain. Once the person is in a horizontal position, consciousness is regained quickly.

High blood pressure
See hypertension.

High-density lipoprotein (HDL)
A type of lipoprotein that seems to provide protection against the buildup of atherosclerotic fat deposits in the arteries. Exercise seems to increase the HDL fraction of total cholesterol. HDL contains high levels of protein and low levels of triglycerides and cholesterol. Cf. lipoprotein, low-density lipoprotein.

Homeostasis
The tendency of the body to maintain its internal systems in balance. Example: A buildup of carbon dioxide increases the respiration rate to eliminate it and draw in more oxygen.

Hormone
A chemical, secreted into the blood stream, that specifically regulates the function of a certain organ of the body. Usually, but not always, secreted by an endocrine gland.

Horsepower
A workrate measure equal to 746 watts, or about 550 foot-pounds per second.

Hyperglycemia
Abnormally high level of glucose in the blood (high blood sugar). The clinical hallmark of diabetes mellitus. Usually defined as a blood sugar value exceeding 140 mg/dl.

Hypertension
Persistent high blood pressure. Readings as low as 140/90 millimeters of mercury are considered a threshold for high blood pressure by some authorities. Cf. blood pressure.

Hyperthermia
Body temperatures exceeding normal. See heat cramps, exhaustion, heat stroke, heat syncope. Cf. hypothermia.

Hypertonic
Describes a solution concentrated enough to draw water out of body cells. Cf. osmolarity.

Hypertrophy
An enlargement of a body part or organ by the increase in size of the cells that make it up. Cf. atrophy.

Hypervitaminosis
Undesirable symptoms caused by an excess of certain vitamins.

Hypoglycemia
Abnormally low level of glucose in the blood (low blood sugar). May lead to shakiness, cold sweats, goose-bumps, hypothermia, hallucinations, strange behavior, and, in extreme cases, convulsions and coma.

Hypothermia
Body temperature below normal. Usually due to exposure to cold temperatures, especially after exhausting ready energy supplies. Cf. hyperthermia.

Hypotonic
Describes a solution dilute enough to allow its water to be absorbed by body cells. Cf. osmolarity.

Hypoxia
Insufficient oxygen flow to the tissues, even though blood flow is adequate. Cf. ischemia.

Iliac crest
The upper, wide portion of the hip bone.

Infarction
Death of a section of tissue from the obstruction of blood flow (ischemia) to the area. Cf. myocardial infarction.

Inflammation

Body's local response to injury. Acute inflammation is characterized by pain, with heat, redness, swelling and loss of function. Uncontrolled swelling may cause further damage to tissues at the injury site.

Informed consent

A procedure for obtaining a client's signed consent to a fitness center's prescription and leadership of his/her program. Includes a description of the objectives and procedures, with associated benefits and risks, stated in plain language, with a consent statement and signature line in a single document.

Inspiration

Breathing air into the lungs. Cf. expiration, respiration.

Intensity

The rate of performing work; power. A function of energy output per unit of time. Examples: Aerobic exercise may be measured in VO_2, METs, or heart rate; short-duration anaerobic exercise may be measured in foot-pounds per minute or other units of work measurement. Intensity, along with duration and frequency, affect the effectiveness of exercise.

Interval training

An exercise session in which the intensity and duration of exercise are consciously alternated between harder and easier work. Often used to improve aerobic capacity and/or anaerobic endurance in exercisers who already have a base of endurance training.

Ischemia

Inadequate blood flow to a body part, caused by constriction or obstruction of a blood vessel. Cf. hypoxia.

Isokinetic contraction

A muscle contraction against a resistance that moves at a constant velocity, so that the maximum force of which the muscle is capable throughout the range of motion may be applied. Cf. isotonic contraction.

Isometric action

Muscle action in which the muscle attempts to contract against a fixed limit. This is sometimes called "isometric contraction," although there is not appreciable shortening of the muscle.

Isotonic contraction

A muscle contraction against a constant resistance, as in lifting a weight. Cf. isokinetic contraction.

Joint capsules

A sac-like enclosure around a joint that holds synovial fluid to lubricate the joint.

Ketosis

An elevated level of ketone bodies in the tissues. Seen in sufferers of starvation or diabetes, and a symptom brought about in dieters on very low carbohydrate diets.

Kilocalorie (kcal)

A measure of the heat required to raise the temperature of one kilogram of water one degree Celsius. A large Calorie, used in diet and metabolism measures, that equals 1,000 small calories.

Kilogram (kg)

A unit of weight equal to 2.204623 pounds; 1,000 grams (g).

Kilogram-meters (kgm)

The amount of work required to lift one kilogram one meter.

Kilopond-meters (kpm)

Equivalent to kilogram-meters, in normal gravity.

APPENDIX

• • •

Lactate
Lactic acid.
Lactic acid
The end product of the metabolism of glucose for the anaerobic production of energy.
Lean body mass
Lean body weight.
Lean body weight
The weight of the body, less the weight of its fat.
Ligament
The fibrous, connective tissue that connects bone to bone, or bone to cartilage, to hold together and support joints. Cf. tendon.
Lipid
A number of body substances that are fat or fat-like.
Lipoprotein
Combination of a lipid and protein. Cholesterol is transported in the blood plasma by lipoproteins. Cf. high-density lipoprotein, low-density lipoprotein.
Longitudinal study
A study which observes the same subjects over a period of time. Cf. cross-sectional study.
Lordosis
The forward curving of the spine at the neck (cervical spine) and lower back (lumbar spine). Often used to refer to an abnormally increased curvature of the lumbar spine.
Low blood sugar
See hypoglycemia.
Low-density lipoprotein (LDL)
A lipoprotein carrying a high level of cholesterol, moderate levels of protein and low levels of triglycerides. Associated with the building of atherosclerotic deposits in the arteries. Cf. lipoprotein, high-density lipoprotein.
Lumbar
Pertaining to the lower back, defined by the five lumbar vertibrae, just above the sacrum.
Maintenance load
The intensity, duration and frequency of exercise required to maintain an individual's present level of fitness.
Max VO_2
See maximal oxygen uptake.
Maximal heart rate
The highest heart rate of which an individual is capable. A broad rule of thumb for estimating maximal heart rate is 220 (beats per minute) minus the person's age (in years). Cf. graded exercise test.
Maximal oxygen uptake
The highest rate of oxygen consumption of which a person is capable. Usually expressed in milliliters of oxygen per kilogram of body weight per minute. Also called maximal aerobic power, maximal oxygen consumption, maximal oxygen intake. Cf. $VO_{2\ max}$.
Maximal tests
An exercise test to exhaustion or to levels of oxygen uptake or heart rate that cannot increase further with additional work loads. Cf. graded exercise test.
Medical history
A list of a person's previous illnesses, present conditions, symptoms, medications and health risk factors. Used to prescribe appropriate exercise programs. Persons whose responses indicate they may be in a high-risk category should be referred for medical evaluation before beginning an exercise program.

Medical referral

Recommending that a person see a qualified medical professional to review their health status and determine whether medical treatment is needed or whether a particular course of exercise and/or diet change is safe.

Met

A measure of energy output equal to the resting metabolic rate of a resting subject. Assumed to be equal to an oxygen uptake of 3.5 milliliters per kilogram of body weight per minute, or a caloric expenditure of 50 Kcalories per square meter of body surface per hour. Hard exercise, for example, requires up to eight METs of energy expenditure, which equals eight times the resting energy requirement.

Metabolism

The total of all the chemical and physical processes by which the body builds and maintains itself (anabolism) and by which it breaks down its substances for the production of energy (catabolism).

Minimum daily requirement (MDR)

The minimum amounts of protein, vitamins and minerals considered necessary to maintain health. Cf. recommended daily allowance.

Monounsaturated fat

Dietary fat whose molecules have one double bond open to receive more hydrogen. Found in many nuts, olive oil, and avocados. Cf. polyunsaturated fat, saturated fat, unsaturated fat.

Motor neuron

A nerve cell which conducts impulses from the central nervous system to a group of muscle fibers to produce movement.

Motor unit

A motor neuron and the muscle fibers activated by it.

Muscle group

Specific muscles that act together at the same joint to produce a movement.

Muscle spindle

Organ in a muscle that senses changes in muscle length, especially stretches. Rapid stretching of the muscle results in messages being sent to the nervous system to contract the muscle, thereby limiting the stretch. Cf. Golgi tendon organ, proprioceptor.

Musculotendinous

Pertaining to or composed of muscle and tendon.

Myocardial infarction

A common form of heart attack, in which the blockage of a coronary artery causes the death of a part of the heart muscle. Cf. infarction.

Myositis

Inflammation of a skeletal muscle.

Myositis ossificans

The deposit of bony materials in the muscle. Bruises from contact sports may result in this condition. Severe bruises should be iced, and evaluated by a physician.

Nutrients

Food and its specific elements and compounds that can be used by the body to build and maintain itself and to produce energy.

Nutrition

The processes involved in taking in and using food substances.

Obesity

Excessive accumulation of body fat.

One repetition maximum (1 RM)

The maximum resistance with which a person can execute one repetition of an exercise movement. Cf. repetition.

Osmolarity
The concentration of a solution participating in osmosis. (E.g., a sugar-water solution of high osmolarity is concentrated enough to draw water through the membranes of the digestive tract to dilute the sugar.) Cf. hypertonic, hypotonic.

Osmosis
The movement of fluid through a membrane, tending to equalize the concentrations of the solutions on both sides. Cf. osmolarity.

Ossification
The formation of bone. The turning of cartilage into bone (as in the joints). Cf. myositis ossificans, osteoarthritis.

Osteoarthritis
A noninflammatory joint disease of older persons. The cartilage in the joint wears down, and there is bone growth at the edges of the joints. Results in pain and stiffness, especially after prolonged exercise. Cf. arthritis.

Overload
Subjecting a part of the body to efforts greater than it is accustomed to, in order to elicit a training response. Increases may be in intensity or duration.

Overuse
Excessive repeated exertion or shock which results in injuries such as stress fractures of bones or inflammation of muscles and tendons.

Oxygen (O_2)
The essential element in the respiration process to sustain life. The colorless, odorless gas makes up about 20 percent of the air, by weight at sea level.

Oxygen consumption
See oxygen uptake.

Oxygen debt
The oxygen required to restore the capacity for anaerobic work after an effort has used those reserves. Measured by the extra oxygen that is consumed during the recovery from the work.

Oxygen deficit
The energy supplied anaerobically while oxygen uptake has not yet reached the steady state which matches energy output. Becomes oxygen debt at end of exercise.

Oxygen uptake
The amount of oxygen used up at the cellular level during exercise. Can be measured by determining the amount of oxygen exhaled as compared to the amount inhaled, or estimated by indirect means.

Peak heart rate
The highest heart rate reached during a work session.

Perceived exertion
See rating of perceived exertion.

pH
A measure of acidity, relating to the hydrogen ion (H+) concentration. A pH of 7.0 is neutral; acidity increases with lower numbers, and alkalinity increases with higher numbers. Body fluids have a pH of about 7.3.

Physical conditioning
A program of regular, sustained exercise to increase or maintain levels of strength, flexibility, aerobic capacity, and body composition consistent with health, fitness or athletic objectives.

Physical fitness
The physiological contribution to wellness through exercise and nutrition behaviors that maintain high aerobic capacity, balanced body composition, and adequate strength and flexibility to minimize risk of chronic health problems and to enhance the enjoyment of life.

Physical work capacity (PWC)
An exercise test that measures the amount of work done at a given, submaximal heart rate. The work is measured in oxygen uptake, kilopond meters per minute, or other units, and can be used to estimate maximal heart rate and oxygen uptake. Less accurate, but safer and less expensive than the graded exercise test.

Plyometric
A type of exercise that suddenly preloads and forces the stretching of a muscle an instant prior to its concentric action. An example is jumping down from a bench and immediately springing back up.

PNF stretch
See proprioceptive neuromuscular facilitation stretch.

Polyunsaturated fat
Dietary fat whose molecules have more than one double bond open to receive more hydrogen. Found in safflower oil, corn oil, soybeans, sesame seeds, sunflower seeds. Cf. monounsaturated fat, saturated fat, unsaturated fat.

Power
Work performed per unit of time. Measured by the formula: work equals force times distance divided by time. A combination of strength and speed. Cf. strength.

Primary risk factor
A risk factor that is strong enough to operate independently, without the presence of other risk factors. Cf. risk factor, secondary risk factor.

Prime mover
The muscle or muscle group that is causing the movement around a joint. Cf. agonist.

Progressive resistance exercise
Exercise in which the amount of resistance is increased to further stress the muscle after it has become accustomed to handling a lesser resistance.

Pronation
Assuming a face-down position. Of the hand, turning the palm backward or downward. Of the foot, lowering the inner (medial) side of the foot so as to flatten the arch. The opposite of supination.

Proprioceptive neuromuscular facilitation (PNF) stretch
Muscle stretches that use the proprioceptors (muscle spindles) to send inhibiting (relaxing) messages to the muscle that is to be stretched. Example: The contraction of an agonist muscle sends inhibiting signals that relax the antagonist muscle so that it is easier to stretch. (Term was once applied to a very specific therapeutic technique, but now is being widely applied to stretch techniques such as slow-reversal-hold, contract-relax, and hold-relax.)

Proprioceptor
Self-sensors (nerve terminals) that give messages to the nervous system about movements and position of the body. Proprioceptors include muscle spindles and Golgi tendon organs.

Protein
Compounds of amino acids that make up most of the body's cells and perform other physiological functions. Cf. amino acids, essential amino acids.

Pulmonary
Pertaining to the lungs.

Quadriceps
A muscle group at the front of the thigh connected to a common tendon that surrounds the knee cap and attaches to the tibia (lower leg bone). The individual muscles are the rectus femoris, vastus intermedius, vastus lateralis, and vastus medialis. Acts to extend the lower leg.

Radial pulse
The pulse at the wrist.

APPENDIX

• • •

Rating of perceived exertion
A means to quantify the subjective feeling of the intensity of an exercise. Borg scales, charts which describe a range of intensity from resting to maximal energy outputs, are used as a visual aid to exercisers in keeping their efforts in the effective training zone.

Recommended dietary allowance (RDA)
The protein, vitamin, and mineral amounts considered adequate to meet the nutrition needs of 98 percent of the healthy population. Established by the National Research Council of the National Academy of Sciences. The RDA is calculated to exceed the needs of most people.

Rectus femoris
The long, straight muscle in the front of the thigh which attaches to the knee cap. Part of the quadriceps muscle group.

Rehabilitation
A program to restore physical and psychological independence to persons disabled by illness or injury in the shortest period of time.

Renal
Pertaining to the kidney.

Repetition
An individual completed exercise movement. Repetitions are usually done in multiples. Cf. one repetition maximum, set.

Residual volume
The volume of air remaining in the lungs after a maximum expiration. Must be calculated in the formula for determining body composition through underwater weighing.

Resistance
The force which a muscle is required to work against.

Respiration
Exchange of oxygen and carbon dioxide between the atmosphere and the cells of the body. Includes ventilation (breathing), exchange of gasses to and from the blood in the lungs, transportation of the gasses in the blood, the taking in and utilizing of oxygen, and the elimination of waste products by the cells. Cf. expiration, inspiration, ventilation.

Response
An immediate, short-term change in physiological functions (such as heart-rate or respiration) brought on by exercise. Cf. adaptation.

Retest
A repetition of a given test after passage of time, usually to assess the progress made in an exercise program.

Risk factor
A behavior, characteristic, symptom or sign that is associated with an increased risk of developing a health problem. Example: Smoking is a risk factor for lung cancer and coronary heart disease. Cf. primary risk factor, secondary risk factor.

Saturated fat
Dietary fats whose molecules are saturated with hydrogen. They are usually hard at room temperature and are readily converted into cholesterol in the body. Sources include animal products as well as hydrogenated vegetable oils.

Screening
Comparing individuals to set criteria for inclusion in a fitness program, or for referral to medical evaluation.

Secondary risk factor
A risk factor that acts when certain other risk factors are present. Cf. primary risk factor, risk factor.

Sedentary

Sitting a lot; not involved in any physical activity that might produce significant fitness benefits.

Set

A group of repetitions of an exercise movement done consecutively, without rest, until a given number, or momentary exhaustion, is reached. Cf. repetition.

Shin splints

Pain in the front of the lower leg from inflammation of muscle and tendon tissue caused by overuse. Cf. overuse.

Sign

An indicator of disease found in physician's examination or tests; and objective indicator of disease. Cf. symptom.

Slow-twitch fibers

Muscle fiber type that contracts slowly and is used most in moderate-intensity, endurance exercises, such as distance running. Cf. fast-twitch fibers.

Somatotrophin

See growth hormone.

Spasm

The involuntary contraction of a muscle or muscle group in a sudden, violent manner.

Specificity

The principle that the body adapts very specifically to the training stimuli it is required to deal with. The body will perform best at the specific speed, type of contraction, muscle-group usage, and energy-source usage it has become accustomed to in training.

Spot reducing

An effort to reduce fat at one location on the body by concentrating exercise, manipulation, wraps, etc. on that location. Research indicates that any fat loss is generalized over the body, however.

Sprain

A stretching or tearing of ligaments. Severity ratings of sprains are: first-degree, partial tearing; third-degree, complete tears. Cf. strains.

Static contraction

See isometric action.

Steady state

The physiological state, during submaximal exercise, where oxygen uptake and heart rate level off, energy demands and energy production are balanced, and the body can maintain the level of exertion for an extended period of time.

Strain

A stretching or tearing of a musculotendinous unit. Degrees of severity include: first-degree, stretching of the unit; second-degree, partial tearing of the unit; third-degree, complete disruption of the unit. Cf. sprain.

Strength

The amount of muscular force that can be exerted. (Speed and distance are not factors of strength.) Cf. power.

Strength total

A measure of the relative strength training emphasis of a Crossrobic™ training workout, based on the number of tons lifted, adjusted for differences in body weight and workout duration.

Stress

The general physical and psychological response of an individual to any real or perceived adverse stimulus, internal or external, that tends to disturb the individual's homeostasis. Stress that is excessive or reacted to inappropriately, may cause disorders.

APPENDIX

• • •

Stress fracture
A partial or complete fracture of a bone because of the remodeling process's inability to keep up with the effects of continual, rhythmic, nonviolent stresses on the bone. Cf. overuse.

Stress management
A group of skills for dealing with stresses imposed on an individual without suffering psychological distress and/or physical disorders.

Stress test
See graded exercise test.

Stretching
Lengthening a muscle to its maximum extension; moving a joint to the limits of its extension.

Stroke volume
The volume of blood pumped out of the heart by the ventricles in one contraction.

Submaximal
Less than maximum. Submaximal exercise requires less than one's maximum oxygen uptake, heart rate, or anaerobic power. Usually refers to intensity of the exercise, but may be used to refer to duration.

Supination
Assuming a horizontal position facing upward. In the case of the hand, it also means turning the palm to face forward. The opposite of pronation.

Symptom
Any evidence by which a person perceives that he/she may not be well; subjective evidence of illness. Cf. sign.

Syncope
Fainting. A temporary loss of consciousness from insufficient blood flow to the brain.

Syndrome
A group of related symptoms or signs of disease.

Systole
The contraction, or time of contraction, of the heart. Cf. diastole.

Systolic blood pressure
Blood pressure during the contraction of the heart muscle. Cf. blood pressure.

Tachycardia
Excessively rapid heart rate. Usually describes a pulse of more than 100 beats per minute at rest. Cf. bradycardia.

Taper down
See cool down.

Target heart rate (THR)
The heart rate at which one aims to exercise at a THR of 60 to 90 percent of maximum heart rate reserve.

Tendon
The fibrous connective tissue that connects muscle to bone. Cf. ligament.

Tendonitis
Inflammation of a tendon.

Testing protocol
A specific plan for the conducting of a testing situation; usually following an accepted standard.

Testosterone
The sex hormone that predominates in the male, is responsible for the development of male secondary sex characteristics, and is involved in the hypertrophy of muscle. Cf. estrogen.

Training
Subjecting the body to repeated stresses with interspersed recovery periods to elicit growth in its capacity to handle such stresses.

Training zone
See target heart rate.

Twitch
A brief muscle contraction caused by a single volley of motor neuron impulses. Cf. fast-twitch fibers, slow-twitch fibers.

Unsaturated fat
Dietary fat whose molecules have one or more double bonds to receive more hydrogen atoms. Replacing saturated fats with unsaturated fats in the diet can help reduce cholesterol levels. Cf. monounsaturated fat, polyunsaturated fat, saturated fat.

Valsalva maneuver
A strong exhaling effort against a closed glottis, which builds pressure in the chest cavity that interferes with the return of the blood to the heart. May deprive the brain of blood and cause fainting.

Vasoconstriction
The narrowing of a blood vessel to decrease blood flow to a body part.

Vasodilation
The enlarging of a blood vessel to increase blood flow to a body part.

Vein
A vessel which returns blood from the various parts of the body back to the heart.

Ventilation
Breathing. Cf. expiration, inspiration, respiration.

Vertigo
Sensation that the world is spinning or that the individual is revolving; a particular kind of dizziness.

Vital capacity
Maximal breathing capacity; the amount of air that can be expired after a maximum inspiration; the maximum total volume of the lungs, less the residual volume.

Vital signs
The measurable signs of essential bodily functions, such as respiration rate, heart rate, temperature, blood pressure, etc.

Vitamins
A number of unrelated organic substances that are required in trace amounts for the metabolic processes of the body, and which occur in small amounts in many foods.

$\dot{V}O_{2\,max}$
Maximum volume of oxygen consumed per unit of time. In scientific notation, a dot appears over the V to indicate "per unit of time." Cf. maximal oxygen uptake.

Warm-up
A gradual increase in the intensity of exercise to allow physiological processes to prepare for greater energy outputs. Changes include: rise in body temperature, cardiovascular and respiratory system changes, increase in muscle elasticity and contractility, etc.

Watt
A measure of power equal to 6.12 kilogram-meters per minute.

Wellness
A state of health more positive than the mere absence of disease. Wellness programs emphasize self-responsibility for a lifestyle process that realizes the individual's highest physical, mental, and spiritual well-being.

APPENDIX

• • •

Wet-bulb thermometer

A thermometer whose bulb is enclosed in a wet wick, so that evaporation from the wick will lower the temperature reading more in dry air than in humid air. The comparison of wet- and dry-bulb readings can be used to calculate relative humidity. Cf. dry-bulb thermometer, wet-globe temperature.

Wet-globe temperature

A temperature reading that approximates the heat stress which the environment will impose on the human body. Takes into account not only temperature and humidity, but radiant heat from the sun and cooling breezes that would speed evaporation and convection of heat away from the body. Reading is provided by an instrument that encloses a thermometer in a wetted, black copper sphere. Cf. dry-bulb thermometer, wet-bulb thermometer.

Work

Force times distance. Measured in foot-pounds and similar units. Example: Lifting a 200-pound barbell 8 feet and lifting a 400-pound barbell 4 feet each require 1,600 foot-pounds of work.

Work measures

See foot-pounds, kilogram-meters.

Workout

A complete exercise session, ideally consisting of warm-up, intense aerobic and/or strength exercises, and cool-down.

Workrate

Power. The amount of work done per unit of time. Can be measured in foot-pounds per second, watts, horsepower, etc.

Appendix B

• •

GUIDELINES FOR EXERCISING ON THE STAIRMASTER® VERTICAL CLIMBING SYSTEMS

• •

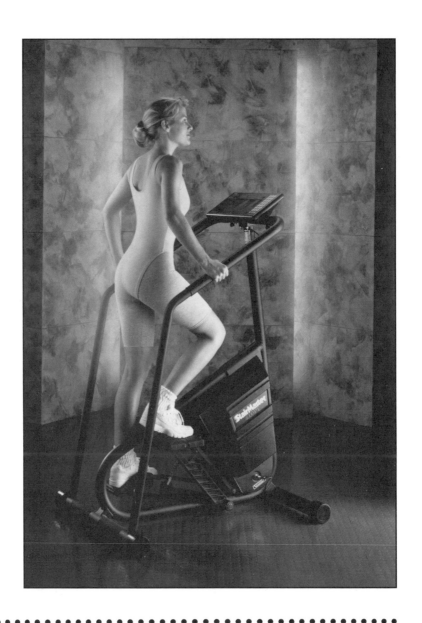

APPENDIX B-1

• •

HOW TO PROPERLY USE
THE STAIRMASTER® 4000PT®
AND THE STAIRMASTER® 4000CT®

The 4000 PT* exercise system is an independent step-action, vertical climbing machine which provides a safe, effective, and functional exercise training and testing modality for individuals of all ages and fitness levels. It features a unique, patented geometry that provides a pedal rate of descent which closely replicates the metabolic demands of actual stair climbing while ensuring that the impact loads are reduced to an orthopaedically safe level. In fact, the impact loads while exercising on a 4000 PT are no greater than walking on level terrain and considerably less than climbing either actual stairs or other stair climbing machines. The specific geometry of the 4000 PT is responsible for the "feel" which made it the exercise machine that revolutionized the fitness industry in the 1980s. You can derive the most benefits from your stair climbing efforts by adhering to the following guidelines:

- Warm up with light calisthenics and easy stretching exercises for at least five minutes before beginning your exercise program.
- Step up (do not push down) with one foot at a time. Try to keep the pedals in the middle of the range of motion; do not let the pedals touch the floor or contact the upper stop.
- Relax as much as possible while exercising and maintain an erect posture. Use the handrails for balance. Don't lock your elbows or lean on the console. Supporting your weight will reduce the exercise intensity and overestimate the number of calories you've burned. Leaning forward will place your back in a compromised position.
- Select a stepping rate (or intensity level) that allows you to stay in the middle of the range of motion for the pedals. Faster is not always better. Exercise at a level that is consistent with your fitness level.
- Continue to cool down after you complete your workout by walking and stretching for at least five minutes.

---

* These guidelines also apply to the StairMaster® 4000CT®

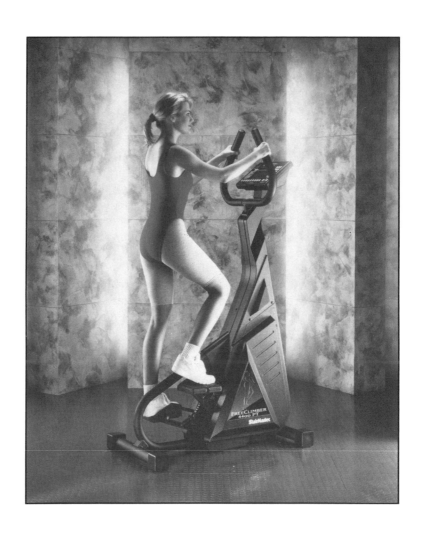

APPENDIX B-2

• •

HOW TO PROPERLY USE THE STAIRMASTER® FREECLIMBER® 4400PT™ EXERCISE SYSTEM

The StairMaster FreeClimber 4400 PT exercise system is the next generation stair climbing machine. The FreeClimber offers better conditioning results than any other climber on the market, yet provides users with the same unique "feel" as the 4000 PT. Featuring the same patented geometry as the 4000 PT, the FreeClimber tightly controls the rate of descent of the pedals to allow an extremely wide range of users to exercise within their comfort zone. Furthermore, the FreeClimber provides a more balanced involvement of the quadriceps, hamstrings, and gluteals and encourages a more upright exercise posture than the 4000 PT. Because it elicits a greater degree of involvement of the muscles of the lower body (particularly the gluteals), you can get a better workout. This enhanced level of muscle mass involvement allows users to achieve higher levels of exercise intensities (burn more calories) at correspondingly lower levels of perceived exertion. You can derive the most benefits from your efforts on the 4400 PT by adhering to the following guidelines:

- Warm up with light calisthenics and easy stretching exercises for at least five minutes before beginning your exercise program.
- Step up (do not push down) with one foot at a time. Try to keep the pedals in the middle of the range of motion; do not let the pedals touch the floor or contact the upper stop.
- Relax as much as possible while exercising and maintain an erect posture. Use the handrails for balance. Don't lock your elbows or lean on the console. Supporting your weight will reduce the exercise intensity and overestimate the number of calories you've burned. Leaning forward will place your back in a compromised position.
- Select a stepping rate (or intensity level) that allows you to stay in the middle of the range of motion for the pedals. Faster is not always better. Exercise at a level that is consistent with your fitness level.
- Continue to cool down after you complete your workout by walking and stretching for a least five minutes.

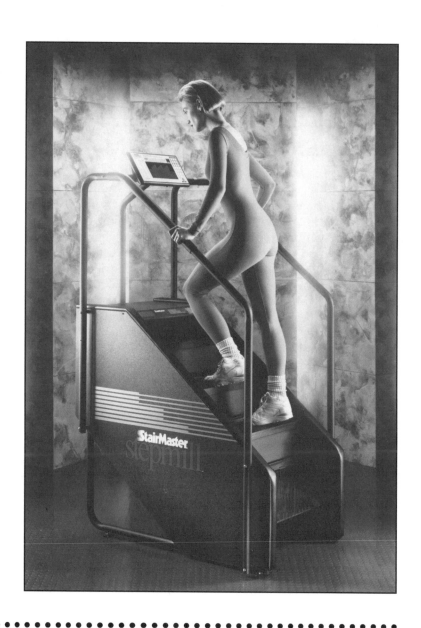

APPENDIX B-3

HOW TO PROPERLY USE THE STAIRMASTER® STEPMILL® 7000 PT™ EXERCISE SYSTEM

The Stepmill 7000 PT exercise system is a fixed-height, vertical treadmill which has a patented revolving staircase which conditions and strengthens the heart and the major muscle groups of the lower body without the orthopaedic trauma associated with other forms of weight-bearing exercise. The joint impact forces produced on the Stepmill 7000 PT have been observed, for example, to be up to five times less than those that occur on a treadmill at comparable exercise intensities. Featuring a diverse array of motivational and challenging conditioning programs, the Stepmill 7000 PT can accommodate individuals of a wide range of ages and fitness levels. It also offers a user-friendly, submaximal aerobic fitness test that is based on the proven physiological relationship between heart rate, oxygen uptake, and work rate. The Stepmill 7000 PT is a highly reliable, cost-efficient exercise training and testing alternative to a treadmill. To gain the most from exercising on the Stepmill, you should adhere to the following guidelines:

- Warm up with light calisthenics and easy stretching exercises for at least five minutes before beginning your exercise program.
- Hold onto the handrails with both hands. Step onto the bottom step while pulling yourself up with your arms. The stairs will move at a very slow rate while you enter data into the console.
- Step up (do not push down) with one foot at a time; try to stay near the top of the staircase while climbing.
- Relax as much as possible while exercising and maintain an erect posture. Use the handrails for balance. Do not lock your elbows or lean on the console. Supporting your weight will reduce the exercise intensity and overestimate the number of calories you've burned. Leaning forward will place you in an inappropriate body posture.
- Select a stepping rate (or intensity level) that allows you to stay near the top of the staircase. Faster is not always better. Exercise at a level that is consistent with your fitness level.
- Continue to cool down after you complete your workout by walking and stretching for at least five minutes.

Appendix C

GUIDELINES FOR EXERCISING ON THE STAIRMASTER® CROSSROBICS® CONDITIONING SYSTEMS

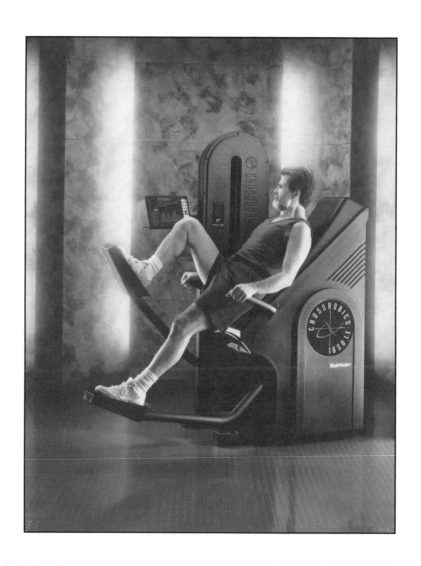

APPENDIX C-1

• •

HOW TO PROPERLY USE THE STAIRMASTER® CROSSROBICS® 1650 LE™ CARDIOSQUAT™ CONDITIONING SYSTEM

The StairMaster Crossrobics 1650 LE CardioSquat conditioning system is an exercise machine which enables individuals of all ages and fitness levels to engage in both aerobic conditioning and strength training in a single workout. Employing the patented Crossrobic™ loading mechanism, the CardioSquat machine provides you with the capability to separately select and control the amount of weight (resistance) used and the speed at which you perform the exercise. This capability, in concert with the wide range of resistance and exercise movement speed levels offered by the machine, allows you to simultaneously achieve the aerobic conditioning benefits of exercising on any conventional aerobic tool and the superior strength gains inherent from performing the squat exercise. Research has shown that exercising on the CardioSquat produces aerobic conditioning benefits that are equivalent to exercising on a treadmill, while simultaneously developing the major muscle groups of the lower body (gluteals, quadriceps, and hamstrings).

- Straddle the pedal arms, place your buttocks against the seat pad, and keep your feet on the floor.
- Select an exercise program option and enter the requested data.
- The suggested starting weight for "first time" users is three plates for women or five plates for men; adjust the resistance level (number of plates) as desired for subsequent workouts.
- Mount the machine by grasping the handrails and then moving your feet up and onto the pedals.
- Start exercising by taking long, deep alternating strides—push through the pedals with your heels.
- Keep the gray arrow on the weight stack suspended in the gray zone on the decal located on the weight stack cover.
- Keep in mind that the deeper the stride you take (i.e., the farther you bring your leg back), the greater the exercise range of motion you will achieve and the more muscle mass you will use on the down stroke; the greater the level of muscle mass involved, the easier the exercise.
- If the weight stack touches the bottom, either step faster or press the speed decrease button (the down arrow) on the console.
- If the weight stack clicks at the top, either decrease your rate of stepping by taking a slight pause between steps or press the speed increase button (the up arrow) on the console.
- Dismount the machine by first allowing both pedals to return to the fully upright position; then restraddle the pedal arms and step over them while moving away from the machine.

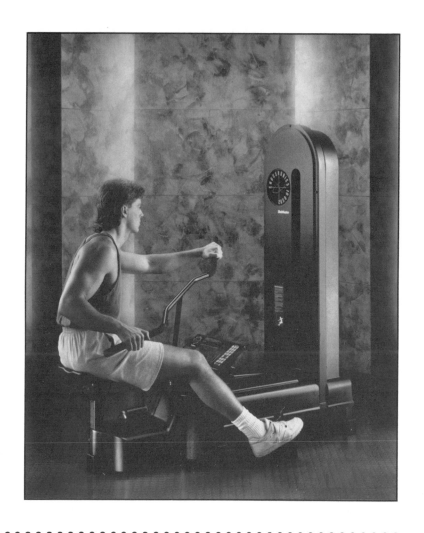

APPENDIX C-2

HOW TO PROPERLY USE THE STAIRMASTER® CROSSROBICS® 2650 UE™ KAYAK™ CONDITIONING SYSTEM

The StairMaster Crossrobics 2650 UE Kayak conditioning system is an exercise machine which involves having users perform a continuous series of modified kayak paddling movements. The Kayak is an extraordinarily safe and effective exercise tool which allows individuals of all ages and fitness levels to engage in both aerobic conditioning and strength training in a single workout. By enabling you to condition and strengthen the heart and the major muscle groups of the torso and upper extremities in a time-efficient manner, the Kayak provides you with the means to achieve meaningful results (e.g., stronger back and torso, stronger shoulder girdle region, greater energy and stamina, etc.) in the shortest amount of time possible. In fact, the movement pattern on the Kayak elicits 30% more muscle mass involvement than traditional arm ergometers. In general, you should adhere to the following basic guidelines and techniques when using the Kayak:

- Sit down close to the handlebar pivot, then place your feet in a comfortable position.
- Select an exercise program and enter the requested data.
- The suggested starting weight for "first-time" users is three plates for women and five plates for men; adjust the resistance level (number of plates) desired for subsequent workouts.
- Grasp the handlebar comfortably with your hands evenly spaced approximately shoulder-width apart, and bring the handlebar to an upright position.
- Alternate pulling down and back with one arm while pushing up and forward with the other arm (visualize paddling a kayak). A complete stroke will bring your forward hand across the center line of your body.
- Keep the gray arrow on the weight stack suspended in the gray zone on the decal located on the weight stack cover.
- If the weight stack touches the bottom, either paddle faster or press the speed decrease button (the down arrow) on the console.
- If the weight stack clicks at the top, either decrease your rate of paddling by taking a slight pause between strokes or press the speed increase button (the up arrow) on the console.
- Maintain a relatively erect posture while you exercise.

Note: The movement pattern of the Kayak allows for relatively large differences in exercise style between individuals without an appreciable reduction in workout safety or effectiveness.

APPENDIX D

• •

GUIDELINES FOR EXERCISING ON THE STAIRMASTER® GENERAL EXERCISE SYSTEMS

• •

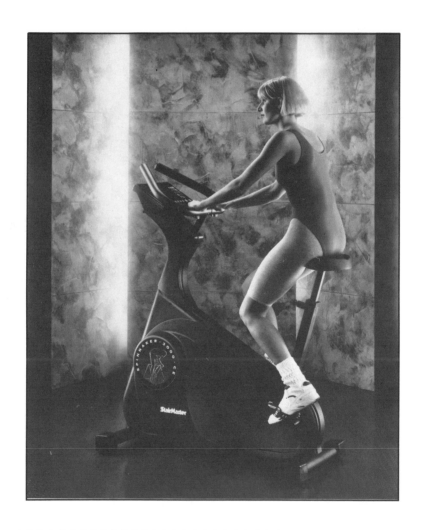

APPENDIX D-1

• •

HOW TO PROPERLY USE THE STAIRMASTER® SPINNAKER™ 3000 CE™ CYCLE ERGOMETER

The StairMaster Spinnaker 3000 CE cycle ergometer is a stationary cycle that duplicates the "feel" and conditioning effects of outdoor bicycle riding. It features a drive train mechanism that converts air pressure into resistance to provide a smooth, comfortable exercise experience. The drive train mechanism on the Spinnaker cycle ergometer reduces the pedal force required to maintain the pedal rate at critical points during the cycle stroke, thereby reducing the stress placed on the user's knees. The Spinnaker cycle ergometer with its unique programming options is designed to be a safe, challenging, and enjoyable exercise modality for individuals of all ages and fitness levels. The Spinnaker cycle ergometer also features two testing program options—a modified YMCA submaximal testing protocol for predicting maximal aerobic capacity and a modified Wingate test for assessing anaerobic fitness. When you exercise on the Spinnaker 3000 CE, you should adhere to the following basic guidelines to ensure that your efforts are safe, effective, and enjoyable:

- Position the seat so that at the bottom of the pedal stroke your knee is slightly bent when the ball of your foot is on the pedal.
- Release the seat adjustment knob to lower or raise the seat as needed. Note: Make sure the seat post retaining pin is fully engaged before sitting on the seat.
- Adjust the pedal footstraps so that they fit snugly around your feet.
- Pedal the bike. After five seconds, the word "accept?" will appear on the console with an arrow pointing to the enter button. Press the enter button to accept the exercise program (basic exercise). Two dots, representing your bike, will appear at the bottom of the screen. You are pedaling around a quarter-mile loop. The elapsed time in minutes and seconds is shown in the middle of the screen. Stop pedaling to the end of the program.
- Pedal in a circular motion, pulling up with one foot while pushing down with the other one. This technique is more efficient than simply pushing only on the downstroke.

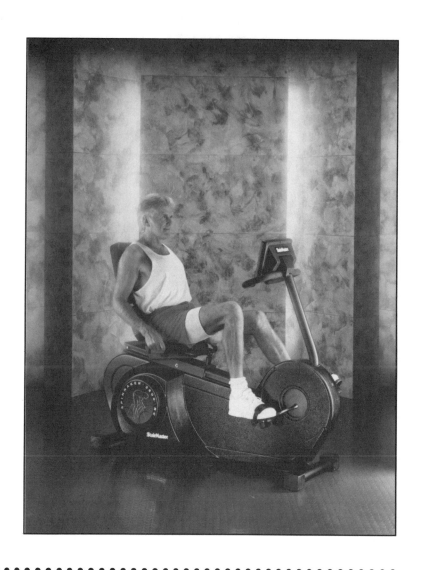

APPENDIX D-2

• •

HOW TO PROPERLY USE
THE STAIRMASTER®
SPINNAKER™ 3600 RC™
RECUMBENT CYCLE

Unlike traditional recumbent cycles which focus exclusively on comfort, the StairMaster Spinnaker 3600 RC exercise system was designed for both comfort and safety—particularly for the knees. A major disadvantage of traditional recumbent cycles is that they place a considerable load on the quadriceps (resulting in localized muscular fatigue and knee strain) and limit exercise performance before the heart and lungs are stressed to a level sufficient to produce an aerobic training effect. Because the Spinnaker 3600 RC (due to its unique resistance mechanism) does not place high loads at low speeds on the quadriceps, it tends to be more easily tolerated by deconditioned individuals. The Spinnaker 3600 RC features the same unique and challenging training and testing program options as the Spinnaker 3000 CE cycle ergometer. You can receive the most benefits from your exercise efforts performed on the Spinnaker 3600 RC by adhering to the following basic guidelines:

- Sit on the seat and place both feet onto the pedals and into the footstraps. Pedal slowly and stop when one leg is fully extended. The knee on your extended leg should be slightly bent.
- To adjust your seat, lift up on the lever in front of the seat. Slide the seat forward or backward as needed. Release the lever to lock the seat in position.
- Adjust the pedal footstraps so that they fit snugly around your feet.
- Pedal the bike. After five seconds, the word "accept?" will appear on the console with an arrow pointing to the enter button. Press the enter button to accept the exercise program (basic exercise). Two dots, representing your bike, will appear at the bottom of the screen. You are pedaling around a quarter-mile loop. The elapsed time in minutes and seconds is shown in the middle of the screen. Stop pedaling to the end of the program.
- Pedal in a circular motion, pulling up with one foot while pushing down with the other one. This technique is more efficient than simply pushing only on the downstroke.

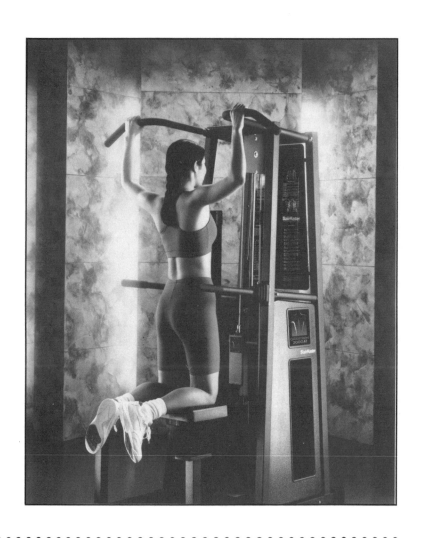

APPENDIX D-3

HOW TO PROPERLY USE THE STAIRMASTER® GRAVITRON® 2000 AT™ UPPER BODY EXERCISE SYSTEM

The Gravitron 2000 AT upper body exercise system is a compact upper body conditioning machine which features a weight stack that can provide users with lift assistance so that they can reduce the total amount of their body weight that they actually lift—by up to 180 pounds—while performing chin-ups, pull-ups, and dips. It features a linear tracking mechanism that facilitates the application of constant user-assistance force throughout the exercise movement. The Gravitron 2000 AT provides a functional basis for development of upper body muscular fitness. Dips and pull-ups/chip-ups are considered to be among the most functional exercises for the upper body through a full range of movement when performed correctly. They require individuals to lift their body weight against the force of gravity—a concept that has great application to sports and activities of daily living. With a minimum ceiling height requirement of less than eight feet, the Gravitron 2000 AT is the perfect addition to any exercise facility or home. The following guidelines provide the basic information and instruction that you need to safely and effectively use the Gravitron 2000 AT:

- Place the weight stack pin in the appropriate plate. For the first workout, women should lift 20-25% of their body weight; men should lift 50-55%.
- Hold onto the dip bars with both hands. Step up onto the assistance steps. Kneel on the knee pad, one leg at a time. Keep your arms in an elbows-locked position, with your back straight (this represents the starting exercise position).
- Perform bar dips by bending your elbows until your upper arms are parallel with the floor. Return to the starting position by straightening your elbows. Repeat nine more times for a total of 10 repetitions (reps). The 10 reps are one set. Reach up, one hand at a time, and grasp the chin-up bar. Pull-ups are performed with your palms facing away from you. Chin-ups are performed with your palms facing you. Both exercises work the same muscles, but at slightly different angles. Perform a 10-rep set and return to the starting position.
- Perform three sets of both dips and pull-ups (chin-ups). Each set should consist of a minimum of 10 reps of each exercise. Alternate one set of dips with one set of pull-ups (chin-ups).
- Dismount the Gravitron 2000 AT by stepping onto the assistance steps and carefully allowing the weight stack to lower to its resting position.
- Perform all the exercises in a controlled manner and through a full range of motion. Go all the way down and all the way up, but don't let the weights touch.
- Exercise at a level of assistance which challenges you. The tenth rep of each set should be the last one you could perform with the proper form. Decrease the level of assistance when you can comfortably do 10 reps in each set.

STAIRMASTER® SPORTS/MEDICAL PRODUCTS, INC.

OFFICES IN THE UNITED STATES

CORPORATE HEADQUARTERS
12421 Willows Road NE, Suite 100
Kirkland, WA 98034
(800) 635-2936 or (206) 823-1825
FAX (206) 823-9490

CUSTOMER SERVICE
12421 Willows Road NE, Suite 100
Kirkland, WA 98034
(800) 331-3578 or (206) 823-1825
FAX (206) 814-0601

EAST REGION
(800) 772-0089
(914) 564-6011
FAX (914) 564-8157
Serving: Connecticut, Maine,
Massachusetts, New Hampshire,
New Jersey, New York,
Pennsylvania, Rhode Island,
Vermont

SOUTHEAST REGION
(800) 448-5040
(813) 531-5040
FAX (813) 539-1342
Serving: Alabama, Delaware, Florida,
Georgia, Maryland, Mississippi,
No. & So. Carolina, Tennessee,
Virginia, Washington DC

MIDWEST REGION
(800) 950-2814
(216) 425-4833
FAX (216) 425-4829
Serving: Illinois, Indiana, Iowa,
Kentucky, Michigan, Minnesota,
Ohio, West Virginia, Wisconsin

WEST REGION
(800) 829-9993
(805) 495-6414
FAX (805) 498-2314
Serving: Arizona, Alaska, Arkansas,
California, Colorado, Hawaii, Idaho,
Kansas, Louisiana, Missouri, Montana,
Nebraska, Nevada, New Mexico,
No. & So. Dakota, Oklahoma, Oregon,
Texas, Utah, Washington, Wyoming